Lippincott's Nursing Guide to

EXPERT ELDER CARE

Lippincott's Nursing Guide to

EXPERT ELDER CARE

Wolters Kluwer | Lippincott Williams & Wilkins
Health

Philadelphia • Baltimore • New York • London
Buenos Aires • Hong Kong • Sydney • Tokyo

Staff

Publisher
Chris Burghardt

Clinical Director
Joan M. Robinson, RN, MSN

Creative Director
Doug Smock

Product Manager
Diane Labus

Clinical Project Manager
Beverly Ann Tscheschlog, RN, MS

Editor
Margaret Eckman

Clinical Editors
MaryAnn Foley, RN, BSN
Collette Bishop Hendler, RN, MS, CIC

Copy Editor
Heather Ditch

Design Assistant
Kate Zulak

Associate Manufacturing Manager
Beth J. Welsh

Editorial Assistants
Karen J. Kirk, Jeri O'Shea, Linda K. Ruhf

Printed in China.

LNGEEC01-070110

ISBN-13: 978-1-60547-627-8
ISBN 10: 1-60547-627-7

Library of Congress CIP information
Lippincott's nursing guide to expert elder care.
    p. ; cm.
  Other title: Nursing guide to expert elder care
  Includes bibliographical references and index.
  ISBN 978-1-60547-627-8
 1. Geriatric nursing. I. Lippincott Williams & Wilkins. II. Title: Nursing guide to expert elder care.
  [DNLM: 1. Geriatric Nursing—methods. 2. Aged—physiology. 3. Aged—psychology. 4. Nursing Care—methods.
WY 152 L765 2011]
  RC954.L57 2011
  618.97'0231—dc22

                                                        2010008990

Contents

Contributors and consultants

Wanda Bonnel, RN, PhD
Associate Professor
University of Kansas School of Nursing
Kansas City, Kans.

Julie A. Calvery-Carman, RN, MS
Instructor
University of Arkansas-Fort Smith
Fort Smith, Ariz.

Anne W. Davis, RN, PhD
Professor of Nursing
East Central University
Ada, Okla.

Margaret "Marge" Dean, RN, CS-BC,
   GNP-BC, MSN
Geriatric Nurse Practitioner
Faculty Associate, Geriatrics Division
Texas Tech University Health Sciences Center
Amarillo, Tex.

Laurie S. DeGroot, RN, MSN, GCNS-BC
Program Leader and Nursing Instructor
North Iowa Area Community College
Mason City, Iowa

Mara Ferris, RN, MS, CS, CPHQ, EMT
President (Geriatric Nurse Specialist,
   Consultant, and Educator)
AGE: Association for Gerontologic Education
Exeter, N.H.

Rhonda Gall, MSN, GNP-C
Faculty Nursing
Bowie State University
Bowie, Md.

Ann S. McQueen, RNC, MSN, CRNP
Family Nurse Practitioner
Health Link Medical Center
Southampton, Pa.

Roseanne Hanlon Rafter, RN, MSN,
   GCNS, BC
Director of Nursing Professional Practice
Chestnut Hill Hospital
Philadelphia

Peggy Thweatt, RN, MSN
Nursing Faculty
Medical Careers Institute, LPN Program
Newport News, Va.

Karen Zulkowski, RN, DNS, CWS
Associate Professor
Montana State University
Billings, Mont.

Foreword

Look around any health care waiting room or hospital corridor in the United States, and it's easy to see the "graying" of America as Baby Boomers—now official members of the elder population—have quickly become an all-too familiar sight. Although many Boomers are relatively healthy and approach health care from a more preventive perspective, many seek care for aging-related problems—often the same problems faced by their more senior elderly counterparts, patients of the GI Generation and Silent Generation.

Many Baby Boomers also have current health issues complicated by lifestyle choices made in their younger adult years, which can pose special challenges to the nurses caring for them. This massive group of computer-literate, tech-savvy patients is well informed, outspoken, and not afraid to ask questions or seek medical care. And they seem to be entering the health care arena in droves, making care of the aging Boomer the latest challenge faced by nurses and other clinicians.

Experienced nurses and nursing students need up-to-date information and expert advice on how to meet the unique challenges of older adults, and *Lippincott's Nursing Guide to Expert Elder Care* delivers that and so much more. With its engaging, easy-to-read style, this book offers a comprehensive view of today's elders (from young Boomers to the very old) and provides practical information, guidelines, helpful tools, and good sage advice on how to care for every segment of this fast-growing population in all clinical settings—hospital, long-term care, hospice, and home care.

One quick glance at the table of contents for this text reveals the scope of important topics covered. Chapter 1, "the Graying of America," offers an overview of the current trends and issues affecting older adults (including financial concerns, dealing with technology, and retirement) as well as theories on the aging process and societal attitudes toward aging. Chapter 2, "Promoting a Healthy Life," covers healthy lifestyle choices, preventive care, immunizations, safety issues, living arrangements, and insurance options as ways to help older adults maintain their health and independence for as long as possible. In Chapter 3, "Assessing the Older Adult," you'll find general principles and guidelines for conducting a thorough head-to-toe physical and mental health assessment and a variety of useful tools to document the older patient's findings and responses. Chapter 6, "Common Disorders: A Systematic Approach," provides a detailed account, by body system, of the most common disorders affecting elderly patients (includes information on causes and incidence, pathophysiology, assessment findings, complications, treatments, and nursing considerations). Other chapters offer timely information, assessment tips, care guidelines, and evaluative tools on such topics as nutrition, medication use, sexuality (yes, older adults still have sex), caregiving, elder abuse, and end-of-life issues.

Throughout *Lippincott's Nursing Guide to Expert Elder Care,* you'll find numerous anatomic illustrations, charts, lists, case studies, documentation forms, and other handy visual tools. Each chapter includes a Timeline featuring personalities, historical events, and interesting tidbits pertinent to the topic of discussion, which you can use as a starting point for conversations with your elderly patients. Graphic logos in the text and sidebars help identify need-to-know information at a glance: Cultural considerations, Healthy living, Medication alert, and Nutrition tips. And, finally, in the appendices, you'll find a handy list of resources and helpful teaching aids that can be given to patients and their caregivers.

The Baby Boomers are a very different generation from the quiet, peaceful ones that preceded them. This group protested overseas conflicts, openly smoked marijuana, experimented with LSD, and surfed the internet. They also advocated women's lib and enjoyed the freedom of sex with the advent of birth control pills. In many ways, they have different health care issues and require a whole new set of nursing tools to keep them as healthy as possible. This group most likely won't go quietly (or gentle) into that long-term-care setting of a good night regardless of their compromised health or living conditions. They are generally well informed and well armed with a multitude of pointed questions about their health care. They will confront you with the latest information on whatever medication they are taking or the particular ailment they have. And they are eager to learn, which means nurses must diligently maintain their knowledge base to anticipate questions, respond intelligently, and provide quality care. I'm sure you'll turn to *Lippincott's Nursing Guide to Expert Elder Care* as a handy reference time and time again.

Margaret "Marge" Dean, RN, CS-BC,
GNP-BC, MSN
Geriatric Nurse Practitioner
Faculty Associate, Geriatrics Division
Texas Tech University Health Sciences Center
Amarillo, Tex.

The Graying of America

I f someone asked you to picture a "typical" patient, who would come to mind? Would you imagine a young man or woman coming in for a routine physical? Would you envision a middle-aged man, maybe in his 40s, hospitalized for coronary bypass surgery? A pediatrician's office full of children? Or perhaps a nursery full of newborns?

Now picture graying hair on that man or woman getting a physical. The bypass surgery patient is as likely to be in his 60s as in his 40s. And as for the nursery? Try imagining a long-term care facility instead. Nowadays, the number of people entering the ranks of old age far surpasses the number of babies being born. In fact, since the 1900s, the percentage of people in the United States age 65 and older has quadrupled.

The report *The State of Aging and Health in America 2007*, issued by the Centers for Disease Control and Prevention (CDC), indicates that this population will continue to grow. By 2030, the report estimates that the number of Americans age 65 and older will more than double, reaching 71 million, about 20% of the total U.S. population. In some states, it's likely that a quarter of the population will be 65 or older.

What does this mean for you as a nurse? It means that, over time, you're more likely to be caring for elderly patients. It means that you'll need to understand the specific health issues that older patients face in order to offer these patients the care they need. And it means you'll have a chance to help these patients improve their health and quality of life.

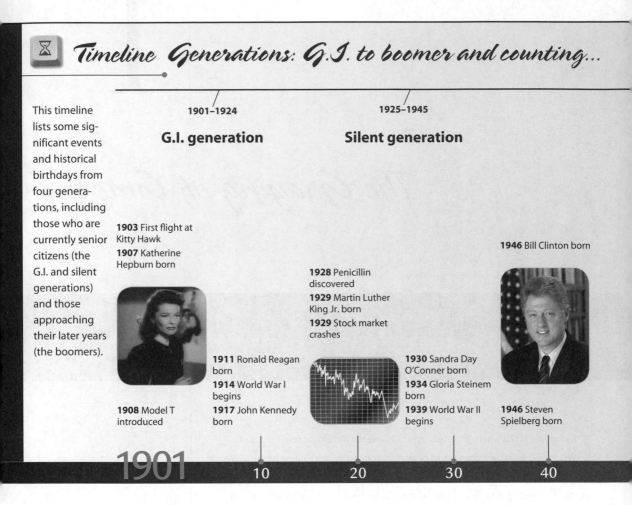

Timeline Generations: G.I. to boomer and counting...

This timeline lists some significant events and historical birthdays from four generations, including those who are currently senior citizens (the G.I. and silent generations) and those approaching their later years (the boomers).

1901–1924

G.I. generation

1925–1945

Silent generation

1903 First flight at Kitty Hawk

1907 Katherine Hepburn born

1908 Model T introduced

1911 Ronald Reagan born

1914 World War I begins

1917 John Kennedy born

1928 Penicillin discovered

1929 Martin Luther King Jr. born

1929 Stock market crashes

1930 Sandra Day O'Conner born

1934 Gloria Steinem born

1939 World War II begins

1946 Bill Clinton born

1946 Steven Spielberg born

1901   10   20   30   40

A Healthy Objective

The U.S. Department of Health and Human Services looks closely at the health needs and trends of our population, developing a set of health objectives for the United States every 10 years. *Healthy People 2010*, the current set of health objectives, seeks to assess the major preventable threats to health and wellness and to develop ways to reduce these threats, with the goals of increasing the quality and length of life and eliminating health disparities. The upcoming *Healthy People 2020* will continue to pursue these goals in the next decade, goals that are essential for an aging population.

The State of Aging and Health in America 2007 report uses the goals from *Healthy People 2010* in its assessment of the overall health of older Americans. It looks at 15 health indicators—including health status, health behaviors, preventive care and screening, and injuries—to determine the overall health of older adults in the United States. (See *Assessing the health of older adults in the United States*, page 4.) These indicators provide nurses with specific areas where they can make a difference in helping older patients improve their health.

1946–1954

Older boomers

1950 Korean War
begins
1950 Era of
McCarthyism
1952 Polio vaccine
created

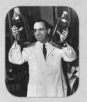

1955 Bill Gates born
1957 *Sputnik* invented

1955–1964

Younger boomers

1960 Lasers
invented
1961 Barak Obama
born
1962 Cuban missile
crisis

1963 Martin Luther
King makes "I have
a dream" speech in
Washington, D.C.
1963 President
Kennedy assassinated
1964 The Beatles
come to New York

50   60   1964

The Cost Factor

In the United States, the cost of providing health care for an older patient is three to five times the cost for a patient younger than age 65. By 2030, the nation's health care spending is projected to increase by 25%, largely because of our growing aging population.

A big part of the reason for that projected rise in cost is the continuing increase in life expectancy. In 2005, the average life expectancy for all races was 80.4 years for women and 75.2 years for men, with an average of 77.8 years for both sexes. Compare that with the average life expectancy in 1900: only 47.3 years. That's an average increase of 30 years overall, 35 for women.

Fortunately, the elderly today typically enjoy greater health than their counterparts did a few generations ago. However, the process of aging still presents challenges, calling for us to help patients maintain healthy lifestyles at a cost that's affordable to both individuals and society. To help control those costs while also improving and preserving the health of older adults, we must find ways to shift the emphasis from expensive acute care to preventative health care. To understand the different kinds of care the elderly

ASSESSING THE HEALTH OF OLDER ADULTS IN THE UNITED STATES

The report *The State of Aging and Health in America 2007* uses 15 key indicators to assess the overall health of older Americans. Nurses are encouraged to help improve and preserve the health of older patients by striving to lower the incidence of unhealthy practices, behaviors, and events in these areas.

Health Status
- Physical health
- Mental distress
- Oral health
- Disability

Health Behaviors
- Leisure time
- Intake of fruits and vegetables
- Obesity
- Smoking

Preventive Care and Screening
- Flu vaccine
- Pneumonia vaccine
- Mammogram
- Colorectal cancer screening
- Keeping up-to-date on selective preventive screenings
- Cholesterol screening

Injuries
- Hip fracture

Centers for Disease Control and Prevention and The Merck Company Foundation. *The State of Aging and Health in America 2007.* Whitehouse Station, N.J.: The Merck Company Foundation, 2007.

need, it helps to understand the different groups that make up the older population.

From One Generation to the Next

Geriatrics (from *geras*, the Greek word for "old age") is the branch of medicine that focuses on health promotion and the prevention and treatment of disease in older adults. Currently, the older adult segment consists of several groups, ranging from the very old, often very frail, G.I. generation, to the silent generation, to the relatively young boomers, who are just beginning to join the ranks of senior citizens. Each group has distinct characteristics formed by the unique challenges of their time, each requires a different approach to health care delivery, and each presents its own challenges to nurses and other health care providers striving to promote healthy, successful aging. And the oldest of these groups—and the one that typically requires the most care—is a fast-growing one, according to the U.S. Census Bureau, and projected to grow even faster in

years to come. (See *Current and projected growth rates for people age 65 and over.*)

G.I. Joes (and Janes)

The G.I. generation, typically defined as those born between 1901 and 1924, consists of those age 85 and older who compose most of the frail elderly. This group came of age during World War I and the Great Depression, and as a result, they learned self-sufficiency and understood the need for public unity in the face of adversity. They achieved a higher education level than those born earlier, with an increasing number of teenagers completing high school. The G.I. generation trusted their government, respected authority, and believed in community support. As adults, they wore suits and had a sense of formality. They were the creative force behind such national groups as the American Association of Retired Persons (AARP) and the National Council of Senior Citizens. In the health care arena, they saw the start of Medicare and Medicaid and the expansion of Social Security.

CURRENT AND PROJECTED GROWTH RATES FOR PEOPLE AGE 65 AND OVER

The chart below shows the increasing growth rate of people age 65 and older since the beginning of the last century. As the 21st century continues, the growth rate is projected to jump, with more than 85 million Americans reaching or passing age 65 by the year 2050.

Number of people age 65 and over, by age-group, selected years 1900–2006 and projected 2010–2050

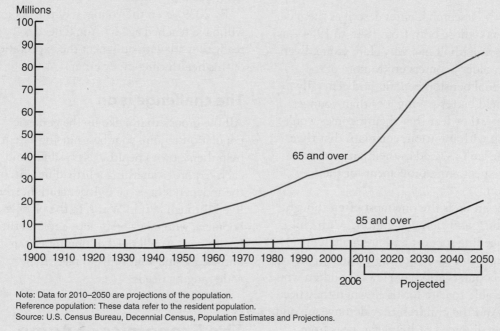

Note: Data for 2010–2050 are projections of the population.
Reference population: These data refer to the resident population.
Source: U.S. Census Bureau, Decennial Census, Population Estimates and Projections.

Talkin' 'bout my generation

The so-called silent generation, generally considered to be born between 1925 and the mid 1940s, faced different challenges. Arriving on the scene shortly before the Great Depression and during World War II, they experienced a changing nation, with more women entering the workforce and, eventually, more people working overall. They used many of the technologies developed in World War II to help the nation progress.

As these technologies continued to develop, new ideas and changing morals challenged this generation. Women's roles were changing too, with Margaret Sanger championing birth control during the 1930s, eventually underwriting the research needed to develop a birth control pill. The silent generation produced fewer children than previous ones.

Some great—and certainly not very silent—leaders came from this generation, including Martin Luther King Jr. and Gloria Steinem. The men and women of the silent generation lived through Cold War, and they watched the Civil Rights movement unfold on their televisions and in their communities.

On the health care front, they experienced the advent of antibiotics to control infection and the development of a hospital system that delivered better care. When surveyed, older adults from the silent generation make it clear that they're on a mission to stay healthy, with 81% stating that they're in good to excellent health.

The boomers—Part I

The Pew Research Center describes the older boomers—those born from 1946 to 1954—as the gloomier half of a very glum group. Even though older boomers enjoy more of the traditional pension benefits and generally have held better-paying jobs than younger boomers, they fear that their incomes won't keep up with inflation, complain that their lifestyle isn't as good as their parents', and don't expect an improvement for their children.

This group is the one most often thought of as the "sandwich generation," with children needing support and financial help at the same time as one or more elderly parents. Older boomers also have fewer children who will be able to care for them when they need help. And the children they do have are quite possibly divorced or living far away from them.

For older boomers, the challenge seems to be keeping healthy so that they can stay independent as long as possible. Making good health choices early on will make all the difference in maintaining their health as they age. Helping them to reach this goal are a variety of medical advances—including a huge drop in the rate of cardiovascular disease, which has decreased by two-thirds since 1950.

The boomers—Part II

The younger boomers, born between 1955 and 1964, are the most recent group to approach the ranks of older adults. Still middle-aged,

they demonstrate yet another perspective on life and health. They bring with them a more holistic notion of health care and are more open to exploring alternative medicine. Younger boomers are often empowered patients, willing to take an active part in their health care and ready to collaborate with their health care providers.

By 2029, even the youngest of the boomers will have reached age 65. You'll need to be ready to work with and meet the expectations of this health care–savvy group.

The challenge is on

All the groups that make up the geriatric population require your best nursing care to help them stay as healthy as possible. And each requires something a little different, from the independent, stoic G.I. generation, who lived through World War I, to the prosperous boomers, who take a very active role in their health care. You'll need to fine-tune your knowledge and your skills to meet their wide-ranging needs.

The Economics of Aging

An older patient's economic situation significantly impacts his health. Not surprisingly, the CDC confirms that those with incomes near or below the federal poverty level experience poorer health than those with higher incomes. Poor or inadequate nutrition, substandard housing, exposure to environmental hazards, and decreased access to and use of health care services can all lead to unhealthy lifestyles and poorer health. From 2004 to 2005, those age 65 and older were the only age-group to see their poverty rate actually rise.

Not only does poverty lead to poor health, but illness can lead to poverty. Many who experience long-term or significant acute illness lose income because they can't work or care for themselves.

Creating a safety net

Before the advent of such social support programs as Social Security, those age 65 and older were more likely than any other age-group to live in poverty. After the introduction of social support programs, the poverty rate declined rapidly for older adults until it leveled off in 1974 and remained level into the start of this century. However, despite the safety net, the poverty rate for those 65 and older increased slightly to 10.1%, or 3.6 million people, with 9.5 million older adults (26.7%) considered to be near-poor.

THE DOCTOR IS IN

Other government social support programs that help prevent the elderly from falling below the poverty line include Supplemental Security Income, housing programs, and energy assistance. One program—Medicare—focuses specifically on improving access to health care.

Started in 1965, Medicare is a U.S. government health insurance program that provides hospital, medical, and surgical benefits for adults age 65 and older and for those with certain disabilities or chronic renal failure. Medicare Part A provides basic hospital insurance, Part B (which carries a monthly fee) covers physician services, and Part D (which also costs extra) offers a prescription drug plan.

Medicare Part C, the Medicare Advantage Plan, is a little different. Approved by Medicare and run by private companies, Part C combines the benefits of Parts A and Part B but also provides funds for managed care organizations and prescription drugs. It also carries a monthly fee. You can read more about Medicare in the next chapter.

BRIDGING THE GAP

But Medicare doesn't cover everything. Although it pays for general health care and some prescription drugs, it still doesn't cover dental or vision care, some routine and preventive medicine, and unskilled long-term care. However, that is changing, with Medicare beginning to cover several preventive care services, such as mammograms and glaucoma screenings.

Medicare also covers only about 70% of medical costs, leaving the patient responsible for the remaining 30%. Some older adults can afford supplemental, or Medigap, insurance policies to cover the shortfall. State Medicaid programs can help some poorer adults, covering medical visits and pharmacy needs for those who qualify. Coverage and financial and other qualifications for Medicaid vary from state to state. More information about Medicare and Medicaid appears in the next chapter.

GIVE ME A (TAX) BREAK

Certain tax breaks also help older adults, including an end to paying Social Security taxes. Also, government and Social Security pensions are usually tax exempt, and those over age 65 can take advantage of extra tax deductions as well as a one-time capital gains tax exclusion when they sell their home.

Other financial options geared toward older adults include reverse mortgages, in which a bank provides monthly payments to the homeowner in exchange for the proceeds from the eventual sale of the house, although such plans have restrictions and limitations. Some poorer adults may qualify for assistance programs that can help with housing costs. The food stamp program can help with food costs and, in more severe cases, food pantries offer some support.

When the safety net fails

Unfortunately, many older adults are wary about receiving anything from the government, and others don't want to disclose personal financial information. As a result, many who qualify for these programs don't take advantage of them.

In some of these cases, adult protective services (APS) may step in when family members or others suspect that an older adult needs help. But the APS can't do much for an older adult unless he accepts help or is legally proven to be no longer mentally competent to make health and legal decisions for himself. This leaves many older adults who may really need help to care for themselves as best they can.

LOOKING AT THE LONG TERM

Many older adults—particularly boomers—are creating their own safety nets with long-term care insurance policies. Some businesses offer these increasingly popular policies as an option in benefits packages. These policies cover the growing costs of long-term care, including assisted-living and private home care.

But those who don't have such coverage, including most of the frail elderly, have more limited access to good care and often face overwhelming costs. Such patients typically have to "spend down" their assets, including their home, to get to the point where state assistance from Medicaid will step in. This can place a burden not only on the older patient but also on family members and others helping to care for and support him.

Promoting Successful Aging

How can you help older adults in this complex situation? One way is to promote the idea of healthy, successful aging. Teach older adults how to reach their optimal health status. Help them understand that, even though their bodies are aging, they can still maintain or improve their health. Show your older patients how to face health challenges instead of letting those challenges overwhelm them, and help them move toward a healthier life.

Tap into technology

For some of your older patients, technology can help. Many older adults aren't really comfortable using computers, cell phones, and other electronic devices, but many—particularly older boomers just now approaching retirement—are happy to take advantage of the latest technology.

For these patients, technology offers several advantages. E-mail, for instance, allows many clinics to stay in closer touch with older patients. It also gives patients a chance to ask health care questions without waiting for a return phone call from a health care practitioner or for their next physician's appointment. You can maintain contact with patients by e-mail or text messaging, monitoring a patient's compliance with a drug and treatment regimen, passing on health education tips, or using text message alerts such as "medication" or "time to exercise" to help keep patients on track.

You can also guide patients to reputable Web sites, forums, and chat rooms that can offer resources and help with medical concerns; of course, make sure you steer patients toward sites that provide accurate information, and caution them about misinformation on the Web. When suggesting technology as a resource, keep in mind that a patient with arthritis may have trouble with a keyboard, particularly the smaller keyboards on some phones.

INTERNET USE ACROSS THE GENERATIONS

How do people of different ages use the Internet? What age-group uses text messaging the most? Who shops online? Do older adults check out health care Web sites more often than younger people?

The Pew Research Center answers these questions in *Generations Online in 2009*, a report that examines how older Americans use technology. The report finds that, although Internet use is higher among younger Americans, a surprising number of older adults—including those from the oldest generations—do use the Internet and other technologies for everything from research to online banking and shopping. The full report is available online at http://www.pewinternet.org/Reports/2009/Generations-Online-in-2009.aspx

Technology can improve an older adult's quality of life in other ways, too. For instance, some seniors may appreciate banking or making travel arrangements online, and keeping in touch with family and friends by e-mail can combat loneliness. (See *Internet use across the generations*.)

Speak out

You can also pass on your knowledge in other ways. Offer to speak at church groups or senior citizen centers to teach older adults how to advocate and care for themselves. Write education pieces for independent living center newsletters and town newspapers. With a little exploration, you'll find many ways to promote successful aging.

Taking on New Roles

Older adults have had to play many parts as they've moved through life. Right now, older adults are being called on to take on some surprising new roles as they move toward and into retirement. Some older adults will become primary caregivers for aging parents, many will experience their adult children take on the role of parent for them—and some will need to become parents for their own grandchildren. All of these new roles have an impact on health.

Parenting, take two

Many older adults are finding themselves pressured into assuming the role of primary caretaker for their grandchildren. Currently, 6 million grandparents live in households with grandchildren ages 18 and younger, and about 2.4 million grandparents act as primary caregivers for their grandchildren. Causes for these "skipped-generation" households range from economic issues to parental abuse of drugs or alcohol. And, because a third of parents are single parents, many older adults have to provide a home not just for grandchildren, but for their adult children.

Taking on this responsibility can significantly affect an older adult's struggles to remain healthy and financially solvent. Besides limiting personal freedom, the economic burden of caring for grandchildren (and sometimes adult children) forces many grandparents to postpone or even cancel retirement plans. And, because establishing legal guardianship can be an emotional and expensive process, many grandparents omit this step. If the grandparent then falls ill, their grandchildren may be left in a sort of legal limbo, with no clear guardian.

Where can a grandparent turn for help? The Area Agency on Aging offers excellent support and problem-solving resources and sponsors support groups for older adults raising their grandchildren. These groups allow older adults facing similar situations to share their experiences and support one another, which can help reduce the impact of stress on their overall health.

When the child becomes the parent

As life spans increase, more and more households consist of four, even five generations, with older adults caring for their even older parents. More commonly, middle-aged family members may find themselves "sandwiched" between raising their own children and providing care for their parents, leaving the older adults who need their care and support to feel like a burden on their adult children. If such a household isn't carefully arranged so that the burden doesn't fall too heavily on one generation, the situation can compromise everyone's health.

TAXI SERVICE

Caring for an older parent may start simply enough, with the older parent still living on his own but needing a ride to medical appointments and the pharmacy or grocery store. Even this situation can be stressful for both parties, with the older parent feeling reluctant to ask for help, sometimes doing without needed groceries or medications rather than burden his child. And when the older parent does ask, he must accommodate his needs to fit into his adult child's schedule. As for the caregiver (typically a daughter), she must take extra time to accommodate her parent's needs, often time she doesn't have. Both parties need to openly discuss the situation and arrive at a mutually acceptable plan, which may include alternative methods of transportation, such as senior service vans.

MOVING IN...

Some older parents find their finances stretched thin trying to cover household expenses and any extra care they may need.

Adult children, who may have their own money worries, may try to help pay for living expenses but find that the best financial solution is for the older parent to move in with them. If not carefully thought out, the new living situation can easily lead to increased stress for everyone sharing the home. Even after the parent moves in, the living situation requires open, ongoing discussion and planning to solve evolving problems.

Honestly addressing some basic questions can help a family decide if having an older parent and adult child share a household will work:

- Does the the parent require physical care? What kind of care?
- How much and what type of living space is available?
- Does someone need to care for the older adult while other family members are at work?
- Will the new living situation place excessive stress on the older adult, the adult child, or other members of the household?

...AND MOVING OUT

When the parent needs more help than the adult child can provide, the family faces some difficult decisions. Discussing the situation before it becomes a crisis—including emotional repercussions, such as guilt on the part of the adult caregiver—can help the family make better decisions.

The Area Agency on Aging and state health and long-term care regulatory offices can help. They offer handouts and support services to help the family select an appropriate assisted living situation or long-term care setting.

Aging Milestones

We pass countless milestones as we journey through life—graduations, first jobs, moving, marriage, the birth of a child. For older adults, two of the most significant milestones are retirement and the death of a spouse.

The process of retirement

Many boomers fear that they may never reach retirement, what with disappearing pension funds, the Social Security system's predicted shortfall, and the potential failure of the Medicare system. Nevertheless, most of us hope for and try to plan for eventual retirement. The process of retirement has several phases.

REMOTE PHASE

The time when a person starts thinking about retirement is called the *remote phase*. For some, this phase starts early on, with a longing for the time and freedom to pursue personal interests.

The remote phase typically begins when a person starts to grapple with the financial aspects of retirement and begins to plan accordingly. The person may meet with a financial advisor or with someone from his company's human resources department to begin planning.

NEAR PHASE

In the *near phase*, the older adult sets the date for retirement and makes specific plans to leave his job. During this phase, the adult may work through feelings of grief over leaving a role that provided a sense of responsibility and possibly a social outlet. A person typically alternates between excitement and fear as the actual day approaches.

HONEYMOON PHASE

Upon first entering retirement, the new retiree may feel euphoric, as if beginning an indefinite vacation. During this phase, he begins to complete tasks and enjoy hobbies and pastimes that he didn't have time for while employed.

DISENCHANTMENT PHASE

The honeymoon phase eventually ends, and the retiree may become disenchanted with retirement, especially if his expectations for retirement haven't been fulfilled. Those with the greatest expectations for retirement risk feeling the greatest disappointment. Some may even slip into depression.

REORIENTATION PHASE

After a period of disenchantment, the retiree may review his situation and make changes to make his lifestyle more enjoyable. He may, for instance, pursue new pastimes, take part in community service, or take steps to improve his health or financial situation.

STABILITY PHASE

In the *stability phase*, the retiree has developed a fulfilling and comfortable retirement routine. Some enter this phase immediately after the honeymoon phase; others may take years before discovering a fulfilling routine. Some people never achieve this phase.

TERMINATION PHASE

The *termination phase* marks the end of retirement. It may end because the retiree returns to work, perhaps because of a need for extra income. Or the retiree may become too ill or disabled to enjoy an independent, productive lifestyle.

HELPING TO EASE THE TRANSITION

By taking a few simple steps, you can help make the transition to retirement for the older, healthy adult a success. For instance, you can counsel a new retiree about ways to make his retirement more meaningful, such as referrals to community agencies that could benefit from his expertise, yet still give him the freedom to choose when and how he wants to volunteer. Such volunteering promotes a sense of belonging and feelings of self-worth.

Helping a patient forced into retirement because of a health issue can be more challenging. Such a patient typically needs monitoring for depression at each health care visit. If a Geriatric Depression Scale score or clinical observation points to possible depression, he'll need further evaluation and may be prescribed an antidepressant. Despite health issues, the patient may be able to take part in some type of volunteer activity.

For all new retirees, you'll need to keep an eye out for depression, which can lead to unhealthy lifestyle choices. It can be hard to spot signs of depression in a brief interview at the hospital or clinic; you may want to use the *Try This* assessment tools developed by the Hartford Institute of Geriatric Nursing to help identify depression and alcohol abuse. Identifying such behaviors early on allows for interventions to help improve the situation and prevent further damage to the patient's health.

Death of a spouse

The death of a spouse is devastating at any age, and can be even more overwhelming when a couple has been together for decades. The person left behind can feel lost in grief and completely alone after sharing a lifetime with a spouse. Such grief takes time and the support of family and friends to gradually lessen.

THE WOMAN LEFT BEHIND

Typically, the wife is the one who survives. Women generally outlive men by about 7 years, with most married women becoming widows before they reach age 80. Because elderly widows greatly outnumber single elderly men, the chances they'll remarry are slim.

Older widows, who are less likely to have worked outside the home and may not have a strong support group, face particular challenges. Many from the G.I. generation never learned how to manage household finances or keep a house in good repair. An older widow may need family or friends to intervene and help with health care and other decisions. A widow from the boomer generation typically fares better in making such decisions because she's more likely to have held a job and managed the financial and physical upkeep of her home.

THE WIDOWER'S TALE

Currently, older widowers are greatly outnumbered by older widows. Many widowers remarry within a year of their spouse's death; those who don't tend to be more vulnerable and subject to depression, which can lead to unhealthy lifestyle choices. White men in particular are at risk for suicide after the death of a spouse and require close observation.

As boomers age, this situation may change. Male boomers typically enjoy better health than men from previous generations and should live longer. As a result, the ratio of widows to widowers will likely decrease, perhaps leading to more remarriages.

OFFERING SKILLED HELP

Whether it's the husband or the wife who's left behind, you'll need to call on many skills to help your patient through this difficult transition. Offer support where you can, and determine if the patient has family or friends who can help with the adjustment to living alone. Watch for signs of depression and difficulty coping, and provide referrals or intervene where necessary.

Theories of Aging

We can all see the effects of aging on our minds and bodies. But what causes our bodies to age, how does the aging adult function in society as he ages, and how does a person develop psychologically as he ages? Several biological theories attempt to explain what causes physical aging. Various psychosocial theories examine the interactive relationship between society and the older adult, and two major psychological theories focus on how a person adapts to and copes with the different stages of life.

Biological theories

A complex process, aging results in cellular and molecular changes that affect the body's ability to function and resist disease. Biological theories of aging include genetic, cross-link, wear-and-tear, free-radical, and immunity theories.

GENETIC THEORY

The genetic theory hypothesizes that the body's genetic codes contain programmed instructions that regulate the reproduction and death of cells and help determine a person's overall lifespan. The genes in the human body switch on and off, determining what happens to a person's ability to function as they age. The continuing study of the human genome may reveal more answers about the genetic theory.

CROSS-LINK THEORY

According to the cross-link theory, proteins, deoxyribonucleic acid (DNA), and other structural molecules develop inappropriate attachments, or *cross-links*, to one another as a person ages. These unnecessary links decrease the elasticity of proteins and other molecules. Normally, enzymes called *proteases* break down proteins that are damaged or no longer needed, but the presence of cross-links inhibits this protease activity. As a result, these damaged and unneeded proteins remain, causing such age-related changes as cataracts and wrinkling.

Some nutritionists believe that changing from a high-sugar, high-carbohydrate diet to one lower in sugars and other carbohydrates may slow the development of cross-links.

WEAR-AND-TEAR THEORY

Wear-and-tear theory focuses on the process of metabolic waste product accumulation or nutrient deprivation that damages DNA synthesis, which, in turn, results in molecular and organ malfunction. Stress factors, such as smoking, alcohol abuse, poor diet, and muscle strain, can exacerbate the wearing-out process. Osteoarthritis, a degenerative joint disease, is an age-related process explained by the wear-and-tear theory.

According to this theory, cells and organs have vital parts that wear out with years of use. It states that each person's body has a "master clock" that controls these cells and organs, which slows down with time. This process reduces the body's ability to repair damage from environmental assaults and such lifestyle choices as smoking and alcohol abuse. Such damaging lifestyle choices not only cause premature aging, but place a person at risk for early development of disease such as osteoarthritis.

FREE-RADICAL THEORY

In free-radical theory, oxygen-free radicals—highly reactive molecules that contain an extra charge—cause an accumulation of damage to the body that results in aging. These oxygen-free radicals can result from the normal metabolism of oxygen or from other causes, such as oxidation of pesticides, pollutants, or the ozone; free radicals can also generate more free radicals.

The body naturally produces antioxidants that help protect against free-radical damage. Some nutritionists propose taking extra antioxidants, such as beta-carotene and vitamins C and E, to boost this protection.

IMMUNITY THEORY

Normally, the immune system prevents atypical cells from forming and protects against the invasion of microorganisms. Immunity theory suggests that aging results from a programmed decline in the immune system, particularly the thymus and the immunocompetent cells in the bone marrow. This decreased effectiveness of the aging immune system results in increased susceptibility to developing infections, cancer, and autoimmune diseases, such as rheumatoid arthritis and lupus erythematosus.

Older adults can combat some of the effects of a declining immune system by receiving an annual flu vaccine and periodic tetanus boosters and by maintaining a healthy diet, exercising regularly, and limiting exposure to environmental assaults, such as smoke or dust.

Psychosocial theories

Psychosocial theories describe how society and older adults influence each other. They include the disengagement, activity, subculture, person-environment fit, and age-stratification and age-integration theories.

DISENGAGEMENT THEORY

Disengagement theory maintains that an elderly adult withdraws, or disengages, from society at the same time as society disengages from him. The theory suggests that this mutual withdrawal occurs because the older adult and society don't see any benefit in continuing to engage with one another.

The theory assumes that older adults accept—even embrace—this separation from society. However, although the transfer of power from older to younger adults is a necessary rite of passage, many question the assumption that this mutual separation must take place. An older person's health and culture play a key role in how much he can continue participating in

society, and many suggest that disengagement wouldn't need to occur if older adults had adequate health care and financial resources, and if society accepted and respected older adults.

ACTIVITY THEORY

In contrast to disengagement theory, activity theory maintains that, to age successfully, an adult must remain active. Activity promotes mental, social, and physical well-being—and, perhaps most importantly, the sense of well-being that results when a person feels his life matters and is making a difference.

Unfortunately, sometimes an older adult can't actively take part in society because of a physical or mental disability. When this happens, the adult is more likely to lapse into depression or develop an unhealthy lifestyle. Such an adult may need extra support to remain as active and involved as possible.

SUBCULTURE THEORY

Older adults often create a subculture with others of a similar age who share similar beliefs, habits, and expectations. The subculture theory maintains that an older adult will interact more with other older adults in his subculture than he will with people from other age-groups. Within these subcultures, status tends to hinge on one's mobility and health rather than on education, occupation, or economic success. One example of a successful subculture is the AARP, which has a membership of over 34 million people.

PERSON-ENVIRONMENT FIT THEORY

This theory evaluates a person's competence (including his ego strength, health, motor skills, cognitive ability, and sensory-perceptual capacity) in relationship to his environment. An older person who has a higher level of competence can usually tolerate greater demands or stimulus from his environment. Activity directors and therapists may use this theory to plan appropriate activities for elderly adults with disabilities.

AGE-STRATIFICATION AND AGE-INTEGRATION THEORY

This theory looks at the ways those born in a particular generation tend to stratify into groups of the same age, or *cohorts*—the way, for instance, most of those who grew up in the silent generation and experienced the Great Depression as children share a strong sense of what it's like to do without, a sense they carry with them even as they grow old, and a sense that most of those who were young in the more affluent 1950s don't share. The theory also looks at the flip side: how people of different ages integrate, learning from and teaching each other by interacting in families, in public, at work, and in some social situations. How much people of different ages stratify into cohort groups and how well they integrate with other age-groups changes over time and varies within and between societies, but the theory suggests that age shouldn't dictate a person's role in society.

Psychological theories

The two major psychological theories of aging—Erik Erikson's developmental theory and Carl Jung's theory of individualism—look at the different stages people pass through as they age. To age successfully, they suggest, a person must use adaptation and coping skills. A person must find ways to deal with the normal changes that occur as one grows old, including retirement, the deaths of one's partner and friends, and one's own health issues.

ERIKSON'S DEVELOPMENTAL STAGES OF AGING

Erikson describes eight stages of psychological development that extend from birth to death. To age successfully, a person must complete each stage satisfactorily. (See *Erikson's stages of development.*)

ERIKSON'S STAGES OF DEVELOPMENT

Erik Erikson theorized that, to fully develop, a person must pass through eight stages of development, from infancy through old age. The chart below describes these eight stages.

AGE	STATE OF DEVELOPMENT	DEVELOPMENTAL WORK AT THAT STAGE
Infant	Trust vs. mistrust	Needs maximum comfort with minimal uncertainty to trust himself, others, and the environment
Toddler	Autonomy vs. shame and doubt	Works to master physical environment while maintaining self-esteem
Preschooler	Initiative vs. guilt	Begins to initiate, not imitate, activities; develops conscience and sexual identity
School-age child	Industry vs. inferiority	Tries to develop a sense of self-worth by refining skills
Adolescent	Identity vs. role confusion	Tries integrating many roles (child, sibling, student, athlete, worker) into a self-image under pressure from role models and peers
Young adult	Intimacy vs. isolation	Learns to make personal commitment to another, such as spouse, friends, or partner
Middle-age adult	Generativity vs. stagnation	Seeks satisfaction through productivity in career, family, and civic interests
Older adult	Integrity vs. despair	Reviews life accomplishments, deals with loss, and prepares for death

By the time a person reaches the developmental tasks of old age, he should have mastered the earlier tasks. If he hasn't, he may face problems with the final tasks of aging. For instance, if he hasn't had a fulfilling marriage or career, he'll need to resolve his issues with these life tasks before he can move on to the tasks of old age—reviewing his life's accomplishments and preparing for death. A failure to have resolved earlier tasks of aging becomes more obvious as a person approaches the later stages of life. A frustrated older adult still struggling with finding intimacy or achieving generativity is more likely to fall into depression, develop anger issues, and make poor lifestyle choices that result in poor health.

JUNG'S THEORY OF INDIVIDUALISM

Jung looks at aging as a life span of personality development rather than simply meeting basic needs. He suggests that, in old age, a person turns inward to review his life's accomplishments and examine his beliefs. The older adult who ages successfully develops the ability to accept the past and adjust to his declining physical functioning. He's able to accept the loss of friends and relatives and recognize that he, too, is moving toward death. He expects nurses and other health care professionals to deal with him realistically about his health, help him maintain that health as long as possible, and help him adjust as his health declines.

Attitudes Toward Aging

The views on the worth of an older adult vary from country to country. In some places, older adults are revered for their knowledge; in others, they've become nearly invisible, ignored by the general population. In the United States, attitudes have evolved over the centuries and vary among subcultures.

A shift toward youth

During the early 1600s, older people in the United States were respected, even venerated. However, the median age at that time was only 16 years, and average life expectancy was only until the ripe old age of 35.

In the late 1700s, however, attitudes began to shift, with people beginning to fear aging (*gerontophobia*) and idealize youth. According to the then-popular form of evangelical Protestantism, young people could mend their ways and repent their sins, but older people were seen as long past the age of redemption, and their wisdom wasn't valued.

The working world was also shifting from an agrarian society, where older people owned and ran farms, to an industrial society that depended on younger, stronger laborers. Physicians considered aging to be an "incurable disease," even into the early 1900s. Being old was considered both a medical and a social problem until around 1930. At that time, physicians began to realize that aging is a process and not a disease, and a trend toward viewing longer life with some enthusiasm started. And as living conditions improved, people could begin to live longer, healthier lives.

Living longer

In the mid 1940s, attention turned to the populations' increasing life expectancy. For the first 30 years after World War II, the United States benefited from an economy that brought about a tremendous increase in national wealth and living standards, with workers more likely to have health insurance. Medical strides included further development of antibiotics and progress in curing some diseases that caused disability or early death. People began to realize that living longer meant they would have to take steps to live healthier lives.

It also meant that both individuals and society would have to be able to meet the economic needs of the growing elderly population. Professional groups began to form to address issues of aging. By the 1950s, researchers and physicians were studying the social, economic, and medical implications of aging and looking for ways to improve the health and living conditions of the elderly.

Research studies began to focus on the problems of aging. Starting in the 1980s and continuing into the current century, the focus has shifted to helping the growing older population to remain as healthy and independent as possible. This not only decreases older people's dependence on costly medical support for chronic illnesses but also helps them enjoy healthy, successful lives in their later years.

Ageism

Despite such progress, many people still hold prejudices toward and misconceptions about the elderly. An extreme form of gerontophobia, *ageism* is discrimination against and prejudice toward someone based solely upon age. Someone exhibiting agism typically views older people as unattractive, unproductive, and unintelligent. Ageism can lead to destructive, irrational behavior toward older people and a devaluing of their contributions to society.

Like other forms of discrimination, ageism stems from stereotypes and misconceptions. Such stereotypes include beliefs that all older people are:

- uncreative
- asexual
- socially isolated
- in a state of mental and physical decline
- a familial and economic burden
- biologically inferior
- senile
- hard of hearing
- sick
- disabled
- either cranky or very tranquil.

Age discrimination takes place in the workforce, with many employers refusing to hire older workers. It also happens in the marketplace; for instance, some banks won't grant loans or mortgages to older borrowers. (See *Identifying ageism*, page 18.)

Even some health care professionals are guilty of ageism. Researchers have found that health care providers typically offer older patients less health care information than younger patients. Whether because of a lack of interest or an education shortfall, some health care practitioners seem to feel that older patients don't need the same level of evaluation and treatment as younger patients. National efforts are underway to correct this situation and improve health care of older adults. (See *Could I be ageist?*, page 19.)

Aging anxiety

Aging anxiety refers to fears of and concerns about growing old. Although not everyone experiences it, it can affect middle-aged and even young adults.

Concerns about financial well-being, changes in physical appearance, social losses, and declines in cognitive ability, health, and physical functioning can all trigger aging anxiety. It's often fueled by perceived stereotypes of older individuals.

Our culture's interest in antiwrinkle creams, facelifts, and hair transplants reflects aging anxiety. Likewise, an increased focus on health, including exercise and diet, may also result from anxiety over aging.

Cultural attitudes

Every culture has different beliefs and behaviors that influence their health. Different cultures also have different attitudes toward aging.

IDENTIFYING AGEISM

The survey below helps identify victims of ageism. To administer the survey, tell the patient to place a number in each blank to signify how frequently he has experienced each situation, using the following scale: 0 = never, 1 = once, and 2 = more than once. (Note: The term *age* refers to advanced age.)

_____ 1. I was told a joke that pokes fun at old people.

_____ 2. I was sent a birthday card that pokes fun at old people.

_____ 3. I was ignored or not taken seriously because of my age.

_____ 4. I was called an insulting name related to my age.

_____ 5. I was patronized or "talked down to" because of my age.

_____ 6. I was refused rental housing because of my age.

_____ 7. I had difficulty getting a loan because of my age.

_____ 8. I was denied a position of leadership because of my age.

_____ 9. I was rejected as unattractive because of my age.

_____ 10. I was treated with less dignity and respect because of my age.

_____ 11. A waiter or waitress ignored me because of my age.

_____ 12. A doctor or nurse assumed my ailments were caused by my age.

_____ 13. I was denied medical treatment because of my age.

_____ 14. I was denied employment because of my age.

_____ 15. I was denied a promotion because of my age.

_____ 16. Someone assumed I could not hear well because of my age.

_____ 17. Someone assumed I could not understand because of my age.

_____ 18. Someone told me, "You're too old for that."

_____ 19. My house was vandalized because of my age.

_____ 20. I was victimized by a criminal because of my age.

Age: _____

Sex: Male_____ Female_____

Highest educational level completed: _____

Survey © Copyright 2000 by Erdman Palmore

Adapted from Palmore, E. *The Ageism Survey*. Durham, N.C.: Duke Center for the Study of Aging, 2000. (From Miller, C.A. *Nursing for Wellness in Older Adults 5th ed.*, Philadelphia: Lippincott Williams & Wilkins, 2009, Chapter 1, page 6, Figure 1-1. Used with permission.)

AFRICAN-AMERICANS

In many African-American families, the older adult plays a critical role in the extended family, often caring for grandchildren. Older adults are valued and treated with respect. To survive old age is considered a personal triumph and accomplishment that demonstrates a person's strength, faith, and resourcefulness.

ASIAN-AMERICANS

Asian-Americans include those of Japanese, Chinese, Korean, and Vietnamese descent. Most Asian-Americans believe that the elderly should be respected. They also believe that children are obligated to care for older parents, with the oldest son shouldering the responsibility. Adult children usually consult their parents before making important decisions. Older women usually make health care decisions for the family.

Most Chinese-Americans view the family as more important than the individual; personal independence isn't highly valued. Older adults are respected for their longevity and wisdom, and it's expected that the family will care for its older members.

Culture Among older adult Korean-Americans, smiling a lot shows a lack of respect or intelligence.

GERMAN-AMERICANS

In the German-American culture, children are expected to help their parents remain in their own homes as long as possible. Eventually, elderly parents typically live with their children, perhaps moving from the home of one child to the home of another.

HISPANICS

Hispanics include those of Mexican, Cuban, and Puerto Rican descent. Family is important in this culture, and blended communal families are common. When older adults can no longer care for themselves, they usually move in with their children. Old age is seen as a time for the older person to enjoy what he's accomplished during life.

In Puerto Rican families, elders are honored, respected, and admired and viewed as figures of wisdom.

Culture Many older Hispanics avoid eye contact, fearing the "evil eye."

NATIVE AMERICANS

When older Native Americans can no longer care for themselves, they're typically cared for by younger adults. In this culture, the term "elder" refers not just to age, but to physical and social status. Elders are shown respect and valued as leaders, teachers, and advisors to the young.

| 🏳 *Culture* | Native Americans avoid direct eye contact because it's viewed as confrontational.

Making a Difference

Now that you've seen the many aspects involved in caring for older adults, you can turn to the chapters that follow to find a wealth of information that you can use in your everyday practice. You'll find theories on aging along with practical information to help you provide the best care possible to your older patients.

But you already have one of the most important skills: the ability to listen, with patience and caring. Taking the time to really hear your older patients' concerns will help you partner with them to find the most appropriate health care options. Couple the information you'll find in this book with your nursing skills and the ability to listen, and you'll provide your older patients with care that will really make a difference.

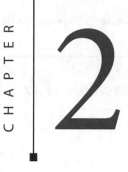

Promoting a Healthy Life

The World Health Organization defines health as not merely the absence of disease or infirmity, but the state of complete physical, mental, and social well-being—a definition that applies to people of all ages. For you as a nurse, that means doing more than treating the ailments of aging; it means finding ways to help your older patients live truly healthy lives.

In your practice, you'll find many opportunities to promote health. For instance, when caring for an elderly patient in a clinic or performing discharge teaching, make it a point to teach about issues pertinent to his age, health, and culture. Look for chances to teach the older patient how proper nutrition and exercise can help him maintain his independence. Instruct a male patient how to perform a testicular self-exam, and a female patient, a breast self-exam. Provide information on smoking cessation, if indicated. Teach the patient on how to cope with the effects of aging, such as decreased mobility and hearing loss. Several organizations that promote healthy aging can help both you and the older patient. (See *A resource guide to healthy aging*, page 24.)

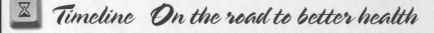

Timeline *On the road to better health*

Review this timeline for health promotion milestones and other interesting health-related facts.

1933 Schwinn introduces the balloon tire, which becomes the bicycle industry standard in 1935

1921-1927 First vaccines introduced for diphtheria, pertussis (whooping cough), and tuberculosis

1927 Babe Ruth hits 60 home runs in one season

1944 First widely used sunscreen (Red Vet Pet) developed and later acquired by Coppertone (marketed as Bain de Soleil)

1904 National Tuberculosis Association (later renamed the American Lung Association) founded to encourage the prevention and cure of TB

1913 American Society for the Control of Cancer (renamed the American Cancer Society) founded

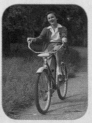

1936 Jesse Owens wins 4 gold medals at Berlin summer Olympics

1900   10   20   30   40

An Ounce of Prevention

One of the most important steps in maintaining health is prevention. Many organizations—such as the American Cancer Society (ACS), the Agency for Healthcare Research and Quality, and The United States Prevention Services Task Force (USPSTF)—provide guidelines for assessing and preventing disease. Make sure your older patients know what steps they can take to help prevent disease, including undergoing routine screening and testing, receiving immunizations for certain diseases, and identifying and reducing health risks.

A test in time...

Keeping current with routine tests and screenings can help the older patient detect problems early on, when they're more manageable. Commonly recommended routine screenings include vision and hearing tests; breast, cervical, colorectal, and prostate cancer screening; and depression and dementia screening.

BREAST CANCER

Almost half of all breast cancers occur in women age 65 and older. The ACS recommends mammography screening every 2 years for women ages 40 to 49 and annually for women age 50 and older.

The USPSTF recommends that women older than age 70 continue to be screened annually. However, some women in this group who have other disease processes that limit their life expectancy may not benefit from this additional screening, so some agencies recommend

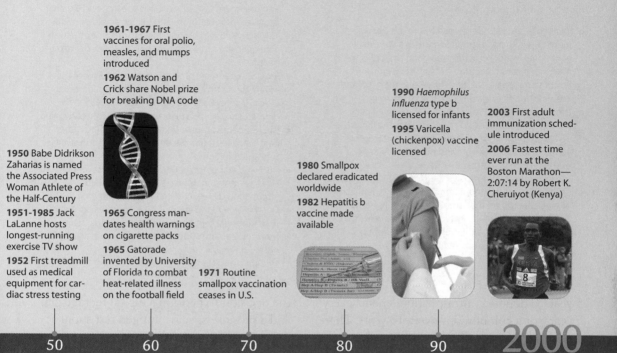

1961-1967 First vaccines for oral polio, measles, and mumps introduced

1962 Watson and Crick share Nobel prize for breaking DNA code

1950 Babe Didrikson Zaharias is named the Associated Press Woman Athlete of the Half-Century

1951-1985 Jack LaLanne hosts longest-running exercise TV show

1952 First treadmill used as medical equipment for cardiac stress testing

1965 Congress mandates health warnings on cigarette packs

1965 Gatorade invented by University of Florida to combat heat-related illness on the football field

1971 Routine smallpox vaccination ceases in U.S.

1980 Smallpox declared eradicated worldwide

1982 Hepatitis b vaccine made available

1990 *Haemophilus influenza* type b licensed for infants

1995 Varicella (chickenpox) vaccine licensed

2003 First adult immunization schedule introduced

2006 Fastest time ever run at the Boston Marathon— 2:07:14 by Robert K. Cheruiyot (Kenya)

50   60   70   80   90   2000

screening only those over age 70 who have a life expectancy of more than 10 years.

The American Geriatrics Society recommends that mammography be offered to women with at least 5 years of life expectancy up to age 85. Beyond age 85, they recommend screening only those in excellent health.

CERVICAL CANCER

The ACS recommends that women older than age 70 who have had three or more negative cervical cytology tests over the previous 10 years no longer receive cervical cancer screening. The USPSTF recommends screening for women who have never been screened or whose screening history is unavailable. For women who have been adequately screened, they suggest stopping screening after age 65.

Every patient's sexual history needs review before deciding to stop cervical cancer screening. For instance, women who have multiple sexual partners or a new partner should continue cervical cancer screening. Regardless of whether a woman receives cervical cancer screening, she should still receive a bimanual and vulvar exam. Unfortunately, many women don't receive this once they stop the cervical cancer screening.

COLORECTAL CANCER

Starting at age 50 for both men and women, the ACS recommends yearly fecal occult blood tests or a fecal immunochemical test. They also recommend one of the following: a flexible sigmoidoscopy or a computed tomography colonography (virtual colonoscopy) every

A RESOURCE GUIDE TO HEALTHY AGING

Several groups have developed programs and resources that promote healthy aging. Here are a few of these programs and resources:

- *Healthy People 2010,* developed by the U.S. Department of Health and Human Services, is a statement of national health objectives designed to identify the most significant preventable threats to health and to establish national goals to reduce these threats. *Healthy People 2020* will focus on goals for the following decade.
- The Healthy Aging Project, part of the Centers for Medicare and Medicaid Service, reviews the literature on health promotion and disease prevention interventions for older people and publishes evidence-based health care recommendations.
- The Program of All-Inclusive Care for the Elderly (PACE) provides an integrated, community-based, multidisciplinary care model that emphasizes health promotion for older adults. It centers around the belief that, whenever possible, older people benefit from being cared for in their own communities.

- *The Pocket Guide to Staying Healthy at 50+,* put out by the U.S. Department of Health and Human Services and the Agency for Healthcare Research and Quality, provides information, health tips, and guidelines for staying healthy for people age 50 and older. It's available online at http://www.pueblo.gsa.gov/cic_text/health/50plus/50plus.pdf.
- The U.S. Department of Health and Human Services has a Web site at http://healthfinder.gov/prevention called *Quick Guide to Healthy Living.* The site has a section for older adults that offers several guidelines for healthy living.
- The National Resource Center for Safe Aging offers best practices that have been identified to showcase safe aging initiatives.
- The National Center for Chronic Disease Prevention and Health Promotion provides a variety of health-related information to help older adults maintain their health.
- The National Association of Area Agencies on Aging is an umbrella organization that advocates the need for resources and support services to be available for older Americans.

5 years, a double contrast barium enema every 5 years, or a colonoscopy every 10 years. These guidelines may be adjusted based on the patient's personal history of polyps and family history of colon cancer.

PROSTATE CANCER

About 75% of all diagnosed cases of prostate cancer occur in men over age 65. The ACS recommends that every man over age 40 have a digital rectal examination as part of a regular annual checkup. For men over age 50, the ACS recommends an annual prostate-specific antigen blood test. If either of these tests are abnormal, the patient needs a complete evaluation.

 Culture African-American men have a 66% higher prostate cancer rate than white men and are more than twice as likely to die from prostate cancer.

Because prostate cancer grows slowly when it occurs in elderly men—taking about 10 years before causing noticeable problems—some feel

the decision to perform a digital rectal exam and a prostate-specific antigen test should depend on the patient's life expectancy. The patient should be consulted about whether or not to undergo these tests.

ALCOHOL USE AND MISUSE

Older adults should be screened for excessive alcohol use. Besides increasing the risk for falls and accidents, excessive drinking complicates medical conditions commonly found in older adults, such as diabetes, gastroesophageal reflux disease, and hypertension. The National Institute on Alcohol Abuse and Alcoholism recommends that men and women age 65 and older consume no more than seven alcoholic drinks per week.

You can use screening tests, such as the Short Michigan Alcoholism Screening Test—Geriatric version, to screen patients for alcohol abuse. It's often used in outpatient settings. (See *The Short Michigan Alcoholism Screening Test—Geriatric version.*)

THE SHORT MICHIGAN ALCOHOLISM SCREENING TEST—GERIATRIC VERSION

You can use the Short Michigan Alcoholism Screening Test—Geriatric Version (SMAST-G) to screen older patients' alcohol abuse. Have the patient check off either "yes" or "no" next to each question. A score of 2 or more "yes" answers indicates alcohol misuse.

Question	Response	
	YES	NO
Do you ever underestimate how much you drink when you talk with others?		
After you have had a few drinks, do you sometimes skip a meal because you don't feel hungry?		
Is your shakiness or tremors relieved by a few drinks?		
Is it hard for you to remember parts of the day or night after drinking alcohol?		
Do you usually take a drink to relax or calm your nerves?		
Do you drink to take your mind off your problems?		
After experiencing a loss in your life, have you ever increased your drinking?		
Has a doctor or nurse ever said they were worried or concerned about your drinking?		
Have you ever made rules to manage your drinking?		
Does having a drink help when you feel lonely?		
TOTAL SMAST-G SCORE (0–10)		

Adapted from Blow, F.C. "Short Michigan Screening Test—Geriatric Version," Ann Arbor: University of Michigan (1991). © The Regents of the University of Michigan, 1991. University of Michigan Alcohol Research Center. Reprinted with permission.

VISION AND HEARING

One of the goals of *Healthy People 2010*, a set of national health objectives put out by the U.S. Department of Health and Human Services, is to reduce the incidence of visual impairment from diabetic retinopathy, glaucoma, and cataracts. Everyone between ages 18 and 50 should be screened every 2 years (yearly for a patient at risk) for visual impairment and disability. After age 50, everyone should receive yearly testing for glaucoma or other eye problems.

Unless a person has a suspected problem, he shouldn't need an annual hearing test. But if he has signs of diminishing hearing, he should undergo audiometric testing.

DEMENTIA

Although a patient doesn't typically undergo dementia screening as part of a routine exam, a noncompliant patient or one who has difficulty following directions should be screened. Concern about a patient expressed by family members or other caregivers should also trigger dementia screening.

Although the Montreal Cognitive Assessment is a useful assessment tool for dementia, the Mini-Cog test can serve as a quick

USING THE MINI-COG WITH AN OLDER ADULT

The Mini-Cog is a simple, 3-minute preliminary screening tool that helps indicate whether a patient may have mild cognitive impairment, dementia, or early-stage Alzheimer's. If you suspect any type of dementia, refer the patient for further testing. The test consists of three parts.

First Part

Ask the patient to name three items and then repeat them back to you (e.g., an apple, a watch, and a penny). If the patient can't repeat the three items after two tries, immediately refer him for further evaluation. If he can complete this task, move on to next part.

Second Part

Ask the patient to draw a clock. The clock should consist of a normal, round shape with the numbers arrayed correctly around the inside, as on a typical analogue clock. This section of the test evaluates executive thinking, or the ability to perform multiple steps in a procedure.

Third Part

After the patient finishes drawing the clock, ask him to repeat the items from the first part of the test.

Scoring

Give the patient 1 point for each item recalled after drawing the clock, and then take a look at the clock drawing (see first and second figures). For the clock test, give the patient 1 point each for:

- drawing a closed circle
- including all the correct numbers
- placing the numbers correctly
- including the hands in the correct position.

The patient needs to include all items on the clock test for it to be considered completely correct; if he's incorrect on one or two items, refer him for further evaluation.

Interpreting the Results

Follow these guidelines for interpreting the test results.

- If the patient can't recall any words after drawing the clock, he has a score of 0 and has a positive result for cognitive impairment. He should be referred for further evaluation.
- If the patient scores 1 to 2 points and has drawn an abnormal clock, he's positive for cognitive impairment and needs further evaluation.
- If the patient scores 1 to 2 points and has drawn a normal clock, he's negative for cognitive impairment.

The low score on recalling items indicates possible dementia, and he should be retested.

- If the patient scores 3 points on the recall of items and has drawn a normal clock, he most likely doesn't have dementia.

What to do Next

Whenever you administer this screening test, keep in mind that it only indicates whether or not to refer the patient on for further testing: It doesn't confirm dementia. It may instead indicate that the patient is suffering from another type of illness, such as depression, hypothyroidism, or any number of illnesses that present as Alzheimer's.

Normal-looking Clock: Indicative of Executive Thinking

Abnormal-looking Clocks: Indicates Need for Further Testing

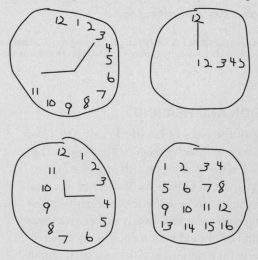

Borson, S., et al. "The Mini-Cog: A Cognitive 'Vital Signs' Measure for Dementia Screening in Multi-lingual Elderly," *International Journal of Geriatric Psychiatry*, 15(11): 1021-1027, 2000.

screening tool when time is an issue. This easily administered test combines components of the recognition of familiar objects and recall with a clock-drawing test. It indicates whether the patient needs further evaluation for Alzheimer's disease or dementia. (See *Using the Mini-Cog with an older adult*.)

BONE DENSITY

The risk for osteoporosis increases with age, with women at greatest risk after menopause and men after age 70. Let your older patients know that bone density testing, a simple, noninvasive, painless procedure, is covered by Medicare. You can also encourage them to take calcium and vitamin D supplements to lessen the risk for osteoporosis.

Immunizations: Keeping current

Both the Advisory Committee on Immunization Practices and the American Academy of Family Physicians recommend annual influenza immunizations for adults age 50 and over. Adults age 65 and over should also receive a one-time dose of the pneumococcal vaccine. And an older patient at higher risk—such as a patient with multiple myeloma or leukemia—can have the vaccine repeated every 6 years.

An older patient at risk for hepatitis, such as someone with end-stage renal disease, should receive the hepatitis B vaccine. And all adults over age 60 should receive a single dose of zoster vaccine, even if they don't have a history of herpes zoster infection.

Unless contraindicated, even patients with chronic medical conditions can be vaccinated. Also, remind your older patients that they should receive the tetanus-diphtheria immunization, which is frequently overlooked in older patients. Let them know that they'll need a booster dose of this vaccine every 10 years.

Reducing the risk

A key aspect of promoting health and wellness is recognizing and reducing the risks that can threaten health. The first step is identifying and assessing the environmental risks and lifestyle choices that can contribute to injury or the development of disease in older patients. Risk assessment tools include general tools you can use with older adults as well as tools tailored to fit the older patient's health or degree of frailty.

Specific risk assessment tools include those for assessing the risk of falls (the biggest safety risk for older adults), incontinence, heart disease, pressure ulcers, and abuse and neglect. One excellent tool provided by the American Heart Association, for instance, assesses the risk of heart disease and heart attack. It poses questions about medical history, blood pressure, weight, blood sugar, and family history of heart disease and then calculates the risk based on the respondent's answers.

Once you've identified the risks, you can take steps to reduce them and help your older patients stay healthy. The most important steps include keeping patients physically safe, particularly from falling; helping them find the appropriate level of physical activity and exercise; and teaching them how they can stay safe and continue on their own to learn about ways they can maintain—even improve—their health.

STEPPING UP TO SAFETY

It's a given that you want to promote safety for all your patients. However, older patients can face particular risks, including the risk of drug interactions or adverse effects and the possibility of abuse in the very frail elderly. Among the greatest risk to the elderly are falls and fires.

Healthy living — Identifying Risk Factors for Falling

Below you'll find a list of key risk factors for falling in older adults. Use it to evaluate whether your older patients are at risk.

- History of previous falls
- Absence of railings or grab bars
- Ataxia
- Being female and age 75 or older
- Diabetes mellitus
- Dizziness
- Edema
- Fatigue
- Foot problems
- Gait disturbance
- Highly polished floors
- Impaired vision
- Inadequate environmental lighting
- Incontinence
- Medications (antihypertensives, antidepressants, antipsychotics, diuretics, sedatives, tranquilizers, or multiple medications)

- Mood disturbance
- Multiple diagnoses
- Neurologic disease
- Newly admitted to a facility
- Nocturia
- Orthopedic disease
- Paralysis
- Parkinsonism
- Peripheral vascular disease
- Physical disability
- Poor environmental design
- Postural hypotension
- Presence of an I.V. line or indwelling urinary catheter
- Stroke
- Transient ischemic attacks
- Unfamiliar environment
- Unstable cardiac condition
- Use of a mobility aid
- Use of a restraint

The fallout from falls

The single most common safety issue older adults face is falling. In fact, it's such a problem that the Federal government passed the Elder Fall Prevention Act of 2002 to provide funds for research on—and public education and services to prevent—falls in the elderly. In older adults, falling is the leading cause of injury, hospital admissions for injury, and death from trauma. According to the Centers for Disease Control and Prevention (CDC), over 250,000 adults over age 65 suffer a hip fracture each year.

Of those who fall and escape injury, most develop a fear of falling called *post-fall syndrome.* This fear can make it more difficult for an older adult to perform his usual activities of daily living (ADLs), leading to unnecessary dependency, social isolation, loss of function, and poor quality of life. It can also make the older adult less willing to ambulate, which can reduce muscle tone and actually increase the risk of further falls.

Many factors contribute to the high incidence of falls in older adults, including changes related to aging, risks from mobility aids, adverse effects from medications, environmental hazards, unsafe caregiving, clothing that can trip the patient, and the effects of disease. (See *Identifying risk factors for falling.*) Taking some simple steps to modify the environment—such as installing grab bars in the bathroom, improving lighting, and removing throw rugs that can cause tripping—can reduce the risk and improve the older adult's level of functioning.

Changes from aging

As adults age, several changes that typically occur can increase the risk of falling.

For instance, difficulty differentiating shades of the same color (such as blues, greens, and violets), cataracts, poor night vision, and reduced visual capacity make it more likely that an older adult simply won't see something that might trip him. Reduced toe and foot lift during stepping, an altered center of gravity (which can lead to impaired balance), and slowed reaction time all make falling more likely. Urinary frequency that makes nighttime trips to the bathroom necessary also increases the risk of falling.

The risk from mobility aids

Using canes or walkers incorrectly can contribute to falls. Wheelchair use can also increase the risk if the patient or caregiver hasn't been taught how to use the wheelchair properly—including how to work the brakes—or if wheelchair hasn't been prescribed or properly fitted. A physical therapist can help to make sure the equipment is properly fitted and used.

Medications

Medications, particularly those that can cause dizziness, vertigo, drowsiness, orthostatic hypotension, and incontinence (such as antihypertensives, antipsychotics, sedatives, and diuretics), can increase the risk for falls.

Make sure you review the patient's medications (see chapter 5, Medication: The Right Prescription), and encourage him or his caregiver to bring all the patient's prescribed medications, over-the-counter drugs, and herbal supplements to his health care appointments.

Environmental hazards

Wet or recently waxed floors, poor lighting, throw rugs, and objects on the floor or in the person's path can all contribute to falls. Emphasize the importance of keeping all pathways for the older adult safe and clear of obstacles.

The caregiver's role

A caregiver who doesn't fully understand potential risks—including the risk of falling—won't be able to give an older adult the safest care. You can help the caregiver understand the particular risks and appropriate care, including how to anticipate problems and how to remain calm and keep the patient calm. This can help keep problem behaviors from developing, behaviors that can put both the patient and caregiver at risk.

Clothing

Long robes, long pant legs, and shoes and socks that don't fit well can all contribute to falls. Help the older adult understand the importance of wearing clothing that fits well and isn't too long.

Disease

Several diseases cause symptom that interfere with an older adult's ability to move or perceive his surroundings, increasing the risk of falling. Depression, orthostatic hypotension, mood disturbances, confusion, weakness, incontinence, reduced cerebral blood flow, edema, ataxia, dizziness, brittle bones, and paralysis can all contribute to falls and injury. Teach the patient and his caregiver about these effects, and offer suggestions for coping with these symptoms.

Fire

Fire also poses a particular risk to older adults, with adults age 65 and older twice as likely to die in a house fire as other adults. Just like other adults and children, older adults should be taught how to prevent fires and plan an escape route in case of a fire.

The National Fire Protection Association, with assistance from the CDC, has developed

Healthy living — Preventing and Escaping From Fires

Adults age 65 and older have an increased risk of dying in a house fire. Help them minimize their risk by teaching them these rules:

- Make sure your home has working smoke detectors. Replace the batteries at least twice a year, and never disable the monitor when cooking.
- Use caution around open flames or cigarettes, and never leave either unattended. Empty all smoking materials into a metal container, making sure the materials can't smolder or combust.
- Never smoke in bed.
- Check extension cords for frayed or loose plugs. Never remove a plug from an outlet by pulling on the cord. Be careful not to overload an outlet.

- Never wear long or loose sleeves when cooking. Keep baking soda and a pot lid handy, and use them to extinguish a cooking fire if one develops. Never use water to extinguish a cooking fire, especially if oil or grease is involved.
- If there is a fire, don't use the elevator.
- Have an escape plan ready before a fire occurs. Plan more than one exit route if possible. Have a flashlight, a whistle, and a pair of glasses (if you're vision-impaired) at the bedside.
- If you have a physical disability that limits your ability to ambulate, make sure you have a backup plan for escaping from your home.
- Don't try to fight the fire yourself. Escape first, and then call the fire department.

a fire and fall injury prevention program directed at older adults. Called *Remembering When*, the program uses games, trivia, and humor to teach older adults how to safeguard themselves and their homes from fire and how to escape a fire safely. (See *Preventing and escaping from fires*.)

GETTING PHYSICAL

Staying safe is crucial for older adults, but it's also essential for them to maintain physical health. Regular physical activity can extend an older adult's years of independence, improve his quality of life, and reduce disability. Regular exercise increases strength, promotes and helps maintain muscle mass, and improves balance, coordination, and joint flexibility. It can also help an older adult regulate blood glucose levels, maintain or lose weight, lower blood pressure, improve sleep quality, and reduce stress.

Regular, moderate exercise performed for as little as 30 minutes a day provides a greater benefit than infrequent, strenuous

exercise. The particular benefits depend on the type of exercise: aerobic, stretching, or strengthening.

Workout time

Aerobic exercise promotes cardiovascular health and respiratory function by enhancing the ability of the heart, lungs, and blood vessels to deliver oxygen to all the cells of the body. Such exercises include swimming, jogging, cycling, walking, rowing, tennis, and aerobic dancing. For best results, the older adult should exercise at least three times a week for 20 minutes or more, as possible. (See *Physical activities for older adults*.)

And... stretch!

Gentle stretching exercises can improve muscle and joint flexibility. Stretching for 5 to 10 minutes before and after other exercises can also reduce muscle stiffness and soreness and prevent injury from strained muscles.

Healthy living · Physical Activities for Older Adults

The following activities can help improve aerobic capacity and strengthen muscles. The intensity of activity can be adjusted—from moderate to vigorous—to match a person's level of fitness.

Aerobic Exercises
- Walking
- Dancing
- Swimming
- Water aerobics
- Jogging
- Aerobic exercise classes
- Bicycle riding (stationary or on a bike path)
- Some gardening activities, such as raking and pushing a lawn mower
- Tennis
- Golf (without a cart)

Muscle-strengthening Exercises
- Exercises using exercise bands, weight machines, or hand-held weights
- Calisthenic exercises (in which one's body weight provides resistance to movement)
- Digging, lifting, and carrying as a part of gardening
- Carrying groceries
- Some yoga exercises
- Some tai chi exercises

U.S. Department of Health and Human Services (2008). "Physical Activity Guidelines for Americans" [Online]. Available: http://www.health.gov/paguidelines/pdf/paguide.pdf

Pump it up

Strengthening exercises can help improve stamina, balance, and flexibility, which can also reduce the risk of falling. Proper strength training requires resistance (from lifting the weight) and progression (gradually increasing the amount of weight lifted). Isometric exercises or using one's own body weight (through push-ups and pull-ups) also increase strength. As possible, the older adult should perform strengthening exercises in sets of 8 to 12 repetitions for each muscle group, at least twice a week. (See *Learning simple exercises*, pages 32 and 33.)

Before beginning any exercise program, the older adult should consult his health care provider, who can assess his health and recommend an exercise program appropriate for him. (See *Key physical activity guidelines for older adults*, page 34.)

THE SELF-TAUGHT MAN AND WOMAN

Today's older adults are, for the most part, healthier than older adults of previous generations. They're typically well informed on health issues and actively participate in their health care. Many are computer literate, readily finding health information on the Web. These healthy, physically active older adults are ready to take the lead in learning about maintaining their own health.

You can help by guiding older patients to trustworthy Web sites and other resources, such as health and fitness magazines, that offer health care and treatment information. As always, make sure to offer clear guidelines on when they should call their health care provider with questions and concerns beyond the scope of a Web site.

You can also encourage them to participate in and learn more about preventive health care practices. Teach them about such topics as proper nutrition, exercise, dental care, and smoking cessation and avoiding secondhand smoke—and then show them how they can take control and continue to learn more on their own.

(*Text continues on page 34.*)

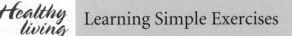

Healthy living · Learning Simple Exercises

Use these illustrations to learn—and then teach—your older patients some simple exercises. They can be performed while standing, lying, or sitting.

Standing

Hold your arms out straight and make big circles.

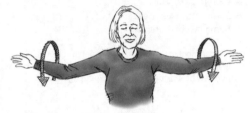

Keep your hands at your sides and bend at the waist as far as you can to the left side and then to the right.

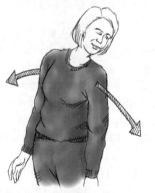

With your arms at your sides, twist your upper body at the waist toward your right while swinging your arms; repeat the movement toward your left.

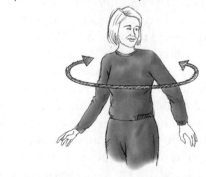

While holding onto the back of a chair, bend your knees slightly and then straighten them.

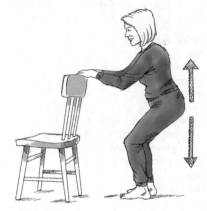

Lying Down

Lie on your back. With your arms at your sides, bend both your arms at the elbow and curl both your arms up as if making a muscle.

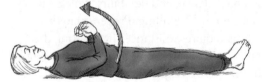

While lying on your back, raise both arms in front of your head and clap your hands together.

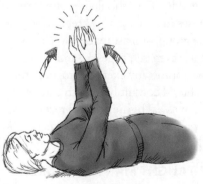

Healthy living Learning Simple Exercises (continued)

Grab one leg with both hands and pull it toward your chest slowly. Repeat with the other leg.

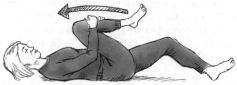

Lie on your back and stretch your arms and legs as you take a deep breath.

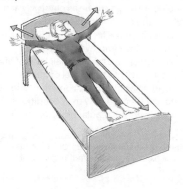

Sitting

Sit on the edge of the bed or a firm chair and bend over slowly, letting your arms dangle. Try to touch your toes. Remember to sit back slowly.

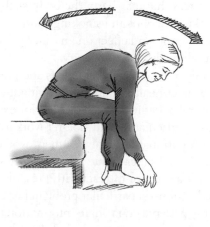

Place your hands on your hips and twist your upper body from side to side.

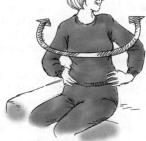

Touch your elbows together in front of you.

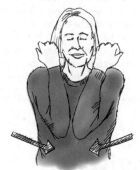

While sitting, move each of your knees up and down as if walking. Hold onto the bed or the back of the chair for balance.

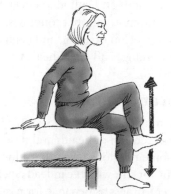

Healthy living — Key Physical Activity Guidelines for Older Adults

Exercise is crucial to maintaining health. Following are some guidelines about physical activity; the first set of guidelines applies to all adults, including older adults; the second set applies just to older adults.

All Adults
- All adults should avoid inactivity. Some physical activity is better than none, and older adults participating in any amount of physical activity gain some health benefits.
- For substantial health benefits, older adults should perform at least 150 minutes (2 hours and 30 minutes) of moderate-intensity or 75 minutes (1 hour and 15 minutes) of vigorous-intensity aerobic physical activity each week. They may also perform an equivalent combination of moderate- and vigorous-intensity aerobic activity. They should perform aerobic activity in episodes of at least 10 minutes, preferably spread throughout the week.
- For more extensive health benefits, older adults should increase their aerobic physical activity to 300 minutes (5 hours) a week of moderate-intensity or 150 minutes a week of vigorous-intensity aerobic physical activity. Or they can perform an equivalent

combination of moderate- and vigorous-intensity activity. They'll gain even more health benefits by engaging in physical activity beyond this amount.
- Older adults should also do moderate- or high-intensity muscle-strengthening activities that involve all major muscle groups 2 or more days a week. Such activities offer further health benefits.

Older Adults
- Older adults who can't do 150 minutes of moderate-intensity aerobic activity a week because of chronic conditions should still be as physically active as their abilities and conditions allow.
- Older adults at risk for falling should do exercises that maintain or improve balance.
- Older adults should match their level of effort for physical activity to their level of fitness.
- Older adults with chronic conditions should understand whether and how their conditions affect their ability to perform regular physical activity safely.

U.S. Department of Health and Human Services (2008). "Physical Activity Guidelines for Americans" [Online]. Available: http://www.health.gov/paguidelines/pdf/paguide.pdf

Outside Influences: Factoring it All in

Factors not specifically related to health can have a significant impact on health and wellness. Religious and cultural beliefs, knowledge and motivation, economics, mobility, perception of aging, and cognitive and sensory changes all affect health promotion.

Religion and culture

A person's religious beliefs can significantly affect his perception of health and illness. For instance, some religions teach that illness is a punishment for sin, which can lead a person to simply accept illness as penance for past

misdoings. Other religions teach that the body is a temple and that a believer must avoid practices that may harm the body, such as drinking alcohol and smoking. Both beliefs can have a profound effect on an older person's overall health and longevity.

Like religion, cultural beliefs and practices also affect health. If an older adult adheres to a cultural belief in home remedies, for example, and a particular remedy doesn't work as well as a traditional medical treatment would, his health may suffer. Some home remedies can even interfere or interact with prescribed medication—a particular problem because many patients don't share information about their home remedies with their health care providers.

Culture Understanding How Culture Affects Disease

Cultural beliefs and dietary practices greatly influence a person's health, including the risk for developing certain diseases. The following list shows the diseases most prevalent in certain cultures.

African-American
- Obesity (especially in women)
- Hypertension (leading to acute renal failure)

American-Indian
- Diabetes (the highest incidence among Americans)

Hispanic
- Obesity (especially in women)
- Cervical cancer
- Stomach cancer
- Diabetes

Filipino
- Hypertension

Pacific Islanders
- Hypertension
- Obesity
- Hypercholesteremia
- Cardiovascular disease

The strong cultural influence on diet affects health in a different, but no less important, way. A culture with a diet high in fat and salt will have a very different effect on a person's health over a lifetime than a culture with a diet that centers on fruits, vegetables, and grains. (See *Understanding how culture affects disease.*)

Knowledge and motivation

How much a person understands health promotion and healthy living strongly affects how well he'll be able to maintain a healthy life. If he's been taught healthy living practices from childhood—such as proper nutrition and dental care—and has had those teachings reinforced as he grows older, he has a better chance to enjoy a healthy older adulthood.

Unfortunately, cognitive disabilities that develop in some older adults can rob them of the knowledge they've learned over a lifetime. Adults with such cognitive impairments need frequent reinforcement about health promotion practices.

WHAT'S MY INCENTIVE?

Motivation also plays a key role in maintaining a healthy lifestyle. Older adults suffering from loss or grief, those with low self-esteem, and those who feel hopeless or depressed may not have the necessary incentive to maintain good health practices. Physical challenges, such as difficulty ambulating or joint pain and stiffness, can also interfere with motivation.

You can get creative to help motivate such patients. For instance, to motivate an older patient with joint stiffness, you might recommend chair exercises first, and then a short walk in a nearby garden, emphasizing how enjoyable it would be to look at the variety of flowers and birds. Or arrange a short walking trip with other older adults where they can share their knowledge and company. Such interesting activities can give older patients the motivation they need to take part in the physical activity of walking. As a bonus, they enjoy the mental stimulation of observing what's around them and of conversation with peers.

Economics

Maintaining a healthy lifestyle can be difficult for those on fixed incomes. Fresh fruits and vegetables tend to be more expensive than many processed foods, which are often high in fat and salt and low in nutritive value. Also, because many older adults can't afford private health insurance, they may neglect regular immunizations and routine health care evaluations. Medicaid and Social Security offset some, but not all, health care costs, leading some older adults to extend the time between checkups.

PINCHING PENNIES

Those with limited incomes may also attempt to perform home repairs and maintenance projects themselves instead of hiring help. Performing these types of activities places them at risk for injury, such as falls from a ladder or chair, or a wrenched back or, more dangerous still, coronary event from shoveling snow.

Suggest to these patients that they look for affordable help with these tasks as needed. They might turn to neighborhood or local senior service agencies that offer free or low-cost help for such tasks, or take recommendations for low-cost help from family, friends, or neighbors. But caution them to use only trustworthy people with good references; many see older people as easy targets they can cheat or overcharge.

Mobility

Older adults with limited mobility often can't obtain the goods or services they need to lead healthy lives. Limited transportation can also make going to the grocery store to buy healthy food, keeping health care appointments, and getting to the pharmacy difficult, even impossible.

Talk to these patients about available community and senior service resources that offer door-to-door transportation for shopping and health care appointments. Some grocery stores also offer free delivery.

Perception of aging

The perception of what to expect as a normal part of aging varies widely. Some people accept declining health as something to be expected and make no attempt to slow its progression. Others—typically those who have led healthy lifestyles—perceive aging as something they have some control over and take significant steps to stay healthy.

Those who feel more in control are typically more willing to make the lifestyle choices necessary to maintain the best health, including exercising, eating a proper diet, getting enough rest, and seeking medical attention as needed. Older adults who feel helpless or not in control, such as the recently widowed and those who lack family support, may be more fatalistic about aging and do less to maintain their health.

Cognitive and sensory changes

A decrease in sensory perception can increase an older person's risk for injury, especially in the home. For instance, an older adult with impaired vision may misread a medication label and take the wrong drug or the wrong dose, or he may not see an object on the floor and trip over it. A poor sense of smell may impair an older person's ability to smell smoke, and changes in skin sensation can lead to burns when bathing or cooking. And a person with a diminished sense of taste may eat food that's spoiled, placing him at risk for food poisoning.

An older person with cognitive impairment may forget to bathe or take medications, or he may leave a pot unattended on the stove or forget to turn off the stove when he's finished cooking. A patient with cognitive impairment may need help with ADLs to keep him from endangering himself or others. Suggest to the family of such a patient that they look into caregiving options.

Living Arrangements

An older person's living situation greatly affects his health and wellness and, in turn, an older person's health may dictate his living situation. Most older adults prefer to live in their own homes and, although some can perform their ADLs alone or with the help of a spouse, others need more assistance.

When home is best

The National Association for Home Care estimates that more than 7.6 million people in the United States need some type of home care services; of those, almost 70% are over age 65. Some older adults can care for themselves but find housework and home maintenance too much; others need help with self-care. Caregivers fall into two categories: primary caregivers, who take care of a patient's daily needs, and secondary caregivers, who help with shopping, home maintenance, and transportation.

HELP FOR FREE...

Unpaid caregivers—most often a spouse, adult child, or other family member—typically provide help for an older adult and have to take care of their own responsibilities. As mentioned in the previous chapter, most unpaid caregivers are women. When the responsibility becomes more than a caregiver can handle, the family may have to hire a paid caregiver.

...AND FOR A FEE

Several agencies provide services to the elderly. Friends, places of worship, and hospitals can provide referrals, but it's up to the family to make sure the agency is reputable. Many reputable agencies have their caregivers bonded to protect the patient against theft or loss from damage, and family members should make sure all caregivers have had background checks for criminal activity. Caregivers should also provide certification stating they're free from communicable diseases, such as tuberculosis. (See *Finding a home health agency*, and *Understanding the rights of home health patients*, page 38.)

FINDING A HOME HEALTH AGENCY

Finding a reputable and affordable home health agency can be a daunting task. The questions below can help families focus their search.

- Does the agency offer the specific health care services needed, such as nursing or therapy?
- Are staff members available to provide care at the times and for the duration needed?
- Can the agency satisfy any special needs, such as language or cultural preferences?
- Does the agency offer the personal care services needed, such as help with bathing and dressing?
- Will they help with laundry, cooking, or shopping?
- Will they help arrange additional services, such as Meals On Wheels?
- Do they have staff members available at night and on weekends for emergencies?
- Are they Medicare-certified?
- Can they clearly explain what services insurance covers, and what must be paid for out-of-pocket?
- Have staff members had background checks performed?
- Does the agency have letters from satisfied patients, family members, and physicians?

Adapted from the U.S. Department of Health and Human Services Administration on Aging, "Home Health Compare" [Online]. Available: http://www.nlm.nih.gov/medlineplus/homecareservices.html [June 3, 2009].

UNDERSTANDING THE RIGHTS OF HOME HEALTH PATIENTS

Patients of a Medicare-approved home health agency have several rights. These agencies must give the patient a copy of their rights in writing. Patients have the right to:

- choose their home health agency; however, for members of managed care plans, the choices will be limited to those with whom their insurance has contracted.
- have their property treated with respect.
- have their family or guardian act for them if they can't do it themselves.
- complain to the agency or the State Survey Agency if their treatment isn't being provided or if the staff fails to respect them or their property.
- receive a copy of their plan of care and to ask questions about the type and frequency of services they'll receive and about the staff who will administer it.

Adapted from Centers for Medicare & Medicaid Services, U.S. Department of Health and Human Services [Online]. Available: http://www.medicare.gov/HHCompare/Home.asp?dest=Nav|Home|About|WhatIs#TabTop [June 19, 2009].

AWAY FOR THE DAY

Adult day-care centers offer another alternative. These centers provide older adults with meals and structured social and recreational activities in a group setting for 8 hours during the day. Some centers also provide health-related services and therapies, and many even offer transportation to and from the facility. These centers not only help older adults maintain or increase their ability to function, but also provide a respite for home caregivers. They may also delay or even prevent the need for institutional care.

A BREAK FOR CAREGIVERS

Family members who must care for an older adult at home and still cope with their own daily responsibilities can feel stressed, isolated, and depressed. Respite care centers can offer them temporary, occasional relief. The care center provides a caregiver to stay short term or overnight with the older adult. Alternatively, the older adult can stay for a short time at a nursing home designated for respite care. Either way, the family member who usually cares for the older adult can get a much-needed break.

Home away from home: Alternative housing

Many older adults can still live independently but are happy to give up the pressures of home-ownership; they also want to know that help is available when they need it. Many of these adults opt for continuing care retirement and life-care communities. Within these communities, residents can live in single-family homes or apartments and then, as their needs change, move into assisted-living or skilled-nursing areas.

A LITTLE EXTRA HELP

Assisted-living facilities usually assist patients with three or more daily activities. Facilities vary, but most provide at least one daily meal and have 24-hour assistance available. A resident typically has one or two rooms and a bathroom; residents share common areas for meals and social activities. Other services include transportation, laundry assistance, housekeeping, personal care, and medication administration, as needed.

MORE EXTRA HELP

An older patient who needs help with several ADLs may need a nursing home or nursing facility. These institutions provide skilled nursing care on a short-time basis for people recovering from acute conditions, and intermediate and long-term care for those with chronic conditions.

Paying for it All

Most of us think of retirement as starting at age 65, but that's not always the case. Many people choose to work longer; some choose to retire earlier, at age 62 or even 55. Regardless of how old people are when they retire, they'll need to have enough income to pay for general living expenses—and enough money to cover health care costs and maintain their health.

Most adults over age 65 count on Social Security as their primary income. This Federal government program pays benefits to retired people and their survivors as well as to the disabled. Some older adults receive extra financial help from other government programs, such as Supplemental Security Income. This program pays monthly benefits to disabled, visually impaired, and elderly people who have little or no income.

Medicare

Established by the government in 1965, Medicare is a health insurance program for people age 65 or older and for those with certain disabilities or chronic renal failure. Medicare covers primarily physician and hospital care, but it also provides limited coverage for skilled nursing care at home as well as for nursing homes. Some plans also include routine immunizations and medical clinic visits. And beginning on January 1, 2006, Medicare began providing access to prescription drug coverage for all people on Medicare.

THE MEDICARE ALPHABET

Medicare has four basic parts: Part A through Part D. Each provides different coverage and benefits.

Medicare Part A covers psychiatric and medical inpatient care in a hospital or skilled nursing facility. It also covers some of the cost of durable medical equipment, such as walkers, hospital beds, or wheelchairs. Medicare Part A is free for most people, and anyone age 65 or older is eligible, as long as they've paid taxes to Medicare through payroll deductions for at least 10 years. If they haven't been employed and paid taxes for 10 years, they can get coverage by paying a monthly premium based on the number of years they did pay taxes. For instance, if a person paid taxes for fewer than 7½ years, his monthly premium would be $423. If he paid taxes for fewer than 10 years but at least 7½ years, his monthly premium would be $233.

Participants must meet a deductible each benefit period before any benefits can be paid. Once this deductible has been met, Medicare fully covers the first 60 days of a hospital stay or the first 20 days in a skilled nursing facility. After that, the participant must pay a certain amount for each additional day he's hospitalized or in the skilled nursing facility. Because of these costs, many people also buy private insurance, called Medigap insurance, to cover what Medicare doesn't.

Medicare Part B—available for a fee based on income—covers all or part of approved physician services and outpatient services, such as laboratory testing or diagnostic imaging. It also covers medically necessary ambulance services, the cost of durable medical equipment used at home, and some specialty services, such as physical or occupational therapy.

Historically, even with Medicare and Social Security benefits, many older people still couldn't afford preventive medicine or immunizations. With the current focus on wellness and health promotion, Medicare recently began to cover such preventive services as bone density measurements, mammograms, breast exams, diabetes education, glaucoma screening, Papanicolaou smears, colorectal cancer screening, prostate-specific antigen tests, digital rectal exams, pelvic exams, and influenza, hepatitis B, and pneumonia vaccinations.

Medicare Part C—known as the Medicare Advantage Plan—is a plan that's approved by Medicare and run by a variety of private companies. It combines the benefits of Parts A and B but also provides funds for managed care organizations, such as preferred provider organizations and provider-sponsored programs. The monthly fee eliminates the need for out-of-pocket expenses, such as co-payments. This plan typically includes coverage for prescription drugs.

Medicare Part D allows for drug coverage through the private market. Medicare doesn't run the plan but insists that the private insurance company providing the coverage meet certain minimum standards. As a result, the specifics of each plan vary considerably, with different co-payments, premiums, and coverage. Medicare recommends that patients review their plans with their health care provider during the open enrollment period each year (November 15 to December 31) because plans can change regularly.

Medicaid

A state-run program receiving partial federal government funding, Medicaid provides health insurance coverage for people with low incomes and limited resources. Each state determines its own eligibility requirements based on income and assets, but the federal government mandates that the Medicaid program pay for certain services, including skilled and intermediate levels of nursing home care for all eligible adults.

Private insurance

Around three-fourths of older adults buy extra medical coverage from private insurance companies. As mentioned earlier, these policies cover the co-payments and premiums for services by Medicare Parts A and B. Despite having both private and Medicare insurance coverage, most older adults currently spend about 22% of their incomes on health care.

CRITICAL THINKING QUESTIONS: HEALTH PROMOTION

Understanding the kinds of situations your older patients face, and having ideas about how to handle those situations, helps prepare you to offer your patients the best guidance you can.

Take a look at the following questions and consider your responses to these situations. As you continue to provide care to older patients, you're sure to come up with different scenarios to challenge your skills and thinking.

- What immunizations would you recommend for a 70-year-old woman in good health?
- An older boomer has recently decided to retire and care for her aging mother. What types of services would you recommend she should look into to help her give her mother the best care and still meet her own needs?
- The older boomer caring for her mother tells you she's decided to hire a home health aide. What guidelines should she follow in choosing an aid?
- Your grandmother, who has mild arthritis but is otherwise in good health, has decided she wants to take up an exercise program to improve her health. What type of exercises would you suggest to keep your grandmother active and healthy?
- An older relative asks you about the types of Medicare coverage available. What would you tell her?

A Last Word on Health Promotion

Promoting health and wellness in your older patients can be a daunting task. So many factors play into each patient's well being, and each patient and his family face many choices about health care coverage, living situations, and the details of day-to-day life. But understanding the factors that can affect an older person's health, having a firm grasp on choices available to patients and their families, and thinking beforehand about how you would handle different health care situations that an older patient might face will help you to be a powerful advocate for all your older patients. (See *Critical thinking questions: Health promotion.*)

Assessing the Older Adult

> *"The great secret that all old people share is that you really haven't changed in seventy or eighty years. Your body changes, but you don't change at all. And that, of course, causes great confusion."*
>
> —DORIS LESSING

Careful assessment lays the foundation for all patient care, no matter what age a patient is. But with older patients, assessment becomes particularly important because they have such complex needs. To identify the problems and needs of older adults, you'll need to integrate a sound theoretical knowledge of the older population with your best assessment skills.

⧗ *Timeline* *Assesment: The tools of the trade*

Nurses rely on numerous scales, indexes, and equipment to perform physical assessments on elderly patients. This timeline traces some of the advances in medical diagnostic equipment still in use today.

1901 Blood compatibility and rejection first described, leading to development of ABO blood typing

1903 First electrocardiograph machine developed

1905 Korotkoff publishes paper on use of stethoscope to auscultate systolic and diastolic blood pressures

1914-1918 World War I

1918 Lenah Higbee awarded the Navy Cross for distinguished service as superintendent of the U.S. Navy Corps

1925 Wood's lamp first used in dermatology to detect fungal infection

1928 First Pap test performed by George Papanicolaou using a vaginal speculum

1931 First electron microscope prototype built; first commercial model, the Transmission Electron Microscope, was built in 1939

1933 Albert Einstein takes position at The Institute for Advanced Study at Princeton University; he remains there until his death in 1955

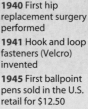

1935 Social Security enacted

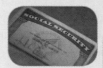

1937 National Cancer Institute founded

1940 First hip replacement surgery performed

1941 Hook and loop fasteners (Velcro) invented

1945 First ballpoint pens sold in the U.S. retail for $12.50

1900   10   20   30   40

Adapting Your Assessment: Age Makes the Difference

When assessing older patients, you'll find that they differ greatly from patients of other age-groups. Older patients also differ from each other. Age-related changes affect individuals at different times and rates, and to different degrees. To assess older patients effectively, make sure you adapt your assessment to take into account common age-related changes, role transitions, psychological adjustments, and long-term lifestyle choices that may be affecting these patients.

Many people assume that all older adults suffer from disease or disability, which, of course, isn't true. However, aging does typically bring with it an increased incidence

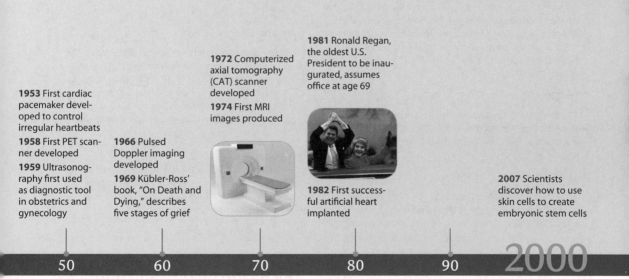

1953 First cardiac pacemaker developed to control irregular heartbeats

1958 First PET scanner developed

1959 Ultrasonography first used as diagnostic tool in obstetrics and gynecology

1966 Pulsed Doppler imaging developed

1969 Kübler-Ross' book, "On Death and Dying," describes five stages of grief

1972 Computerized axial tomography (CAT) scanner developed

1974 First MRI images produced

1981 Ronald Regan, the oldest U.S. President to be inaugurated, assumes office at age 69

1982 First successful artificial heart implanted

2007 Scientists discover how to use skin cells to create embryonic stem cells

50   60   70   80   90   2000

of chronic disease, and it may be hard to distinguish disease from normal age-related changes. What's more, patients typically have vague symptoms that aren't clearly characteristic of a particular disorder. A careful physical and psychosocial function assessment can help narrow down the cause of symptoms and provide key information about a patient's status.

Assessments can take place in various settings: hospitals, physician's offices, acute care facilities, patient homes, senior centers, adult day-care centers, and long-term care facilities. Although the setting and the patient's age don't affect the specific methods you'll use to collect data, other factors can alter your assessment. (See *Variables affecting assessment*, page 46.)

VARIABLES AFFECTING ASSESSMENT

The factors listed here affect the overall atmosphere of trust, caring, and confidentiality when assessing elderly patients.

Your Attitude

Communicating with older adults may challenge you to confront your attitudes about aging and older people. Examine your feelings and decide in advance how you'll handle them. Any prejudices you reveal will probably interfere with your efforts to communicate because older people are especially sensitive to others' reactions and can easily detect negative attitudes and impatience.

The Patient's Attitude

As you assess the patient, try to determine his attitude toward his body and health. An older person may have a distorted perception of his health problems, dwelling on them needlessly or dismissing them as normal signs of aging. He may ignore a serious problem because he doesn't want his fears confirmed. If the patient is seriously ill, the subjects of dying and death may come up during the assessment.

Language

The language you use when you assess an older patient should be tailored to that individual. Consider his educational level, culture, and other languages he may speak.

Deficits

Sensory deficits, such as hearing and vision loss, are common in older people. Other impairments, such as musculoskeletal or neurologic deficits, also appear in many cases. All of these can significantly interfere with accurate data collection. With sensory or neurologic deficits, older people may misinterpret a question or not hear it at all. With musculoskeletal deficits, discomfort or pain may keep them from focusing on your questions or instructions. As a result, they may respond incorrectly or inappropriately. If you don't take these deficits into consideration, they can cause inaccuracies in your assessment and subsequent conclusions.

Consent

Informed consent, an essential element for all patients, is especially crucial for seniors. Older patients have the right to know why you're doing the assessment, what procedures it involves, and what kinds of information you need. They have the right to refuse to answer questions or to participate in any aspect of the assessment.

Time and Energy Level

Be sure to allow enough time for your assessment. The older adult possesses a wealth of information, but generally processes these data more slowly than a younger adult would. The patient may need extra time, or even several shorter sessions, if such problems as fatigue or discomfort limit the amount of time he can meaningfully participate in the assessment.

Environment

You may need to modify the environment to suit an older patient, taking into consideration sensory or musculoskeletal changes. Take particular care to ensure that the room is quiet, well-lit, and comfortable.

Performing the Assessment: The Essential Elements

A comprehensive assessment of an older person involves two key steps: taking a thorough health history and performing a complete physical examination. This comprehensive assessment establishes the person's baseline health status, allowing you to evaluate changes in his condition over time and determine the need for support services.

The health history and interview

The first part of your assessment, the health history and interview, provide a subjective account of the older adult's present and past health status. They also initiate your relationship and establish the patient's well-being as your primary concern. The information you gather from the health history alerts you to key areas of focus for the physical examination and point to what laboratory tests the patient may need.

Talking with an older person about health concerns increases his health awareness, helps you identify knowledge deficits, and provides an opportunity for patient teaching. Because the patient may overlook important health information, make sure you interview methodically and, if possible, gather information from the patient's family members or friends. Also, make sure you include a thorough medication review—prescribed and over-the-counter (OTC) drugs as well as herbal remedies—and a history of lifestyle choices that may have had a long-term effect on the patient's health.

For those living in long-term care facilities without family support, facility staff members and past health records can provide a wealth of information about the patient.

SETTING THE STAGE

Approaching an older patient for a health history shouldn't be difficult if you anticipate his special needs. Keep the following in mind.

Timing

If possible, plan to talk with an older patient early in the day, when he's likely to be most alert. An older patient may experience "sundown syndrome," in which his capacity for clear thinking diminishes by late afternoon or early evening. Some patients even become disoriented or confused later in the day.

During the assessment, watch for signs of possible fatigue, such as sighing, grimacing, head and shoulder drooping, irritability, slouching, or leaning against something for support. If one long session is too taxing for the patient, schedule additional times and take advantage of other interactions (such as during bathing, grooming, and meals) to gather further data and confirm information you've already collected. You can clarify inconsistencies and possible inaccuracies by assessing the patient more than once and at different times of the day.

Environment

Choose a quiet area that's private, comfortable, warm enough (75° F [23.9° C] is usually comfortable for an older person), and draft-free. Make sure the area provides ample space, especially if the person uses assistive devices. Avoid bright fluorescent lighting and direct sunlight. Instead, use diffused lighting.

Keep water or other fluids for drinking on hand, and make sure the patient is close to a bathroom. Have a comfortable chair available for the patient (if he isn't on bed rest), especially if the interview may be lengthy. Because arthritis and other orthopedic disabilities may make sitting in one position for a long time uncomfortable, encourage an older person to change his position in the chair (or bed) and to move around as much as he wants to during the interview.

Deficits

If the patient wears glasses, make sure he has them before the interview begins. Pull shades and block bright light from the patient's view. Reduced visual acuity or environmentally induced blindness from bright lights, shiny floors, or direct sunlight can cause squinting or poor eye contact in an older person. During the interview, face the patient closely at eye level.

To help compensate for a hearing impairment, close the door to the room. This minimizes background noise, such as passing foot traffic, paging systems, televisions, radios, ringing telephones, and outside conversation. An older person with a hearing impairment may have difficulty understanding fast-paced speech. You may notice that he seems distracted, fails to follow the conversation, answers inappropriately, or seems puzzled by your questions—all signs that he's having trouble following you. Make sure the room is well lit so that the patient can read your lips if necessary. Determine which ear he hears better with, and speak toward that ear. If the patient wears a hearing aid, make sure it's in place and working properly.

Speak clearly and distinctly in a normal tone of voice. Don't shout, because shouting raises the pitch of your voice and may make understanding you harder, not easier. Because hearing loss from aging, called *presbycusis*, affects perception of high-pitched tones first, speaking in a low voice will help reduce its effects. Repeat facts periodically during the interview.

Communication

Always address older patients as Miss, Mrs., or Mr. followed by their surname, unless requested otherwise. Experts also recommend the use of touch. For example, shake the patient's hand when you say hello, then hold it briefly to convey concern. Use body language, touch, and eye contact to encourage participation. Be patient, relaxed, and unhurried.

Talk to the person, not at him. Tell him how long the process will take. If language poses a problem, enlist the aid of an interpreter, family member, or friend, as appropriate.

Early in the interview, try to evaluate the patient's ability to communicate and his reliability as a historian. If you have doubts, before the interview continues, ask the patient if a family member or a friend can be present. Don't be surprised if an older patient requests that someone help him; he, too, may have concerns about getting through the interview on his own. Having another person present gives you a chance to observe the patient's interaction with this person and provides more data for the history. However, it may prevent the patient from speaking freely, so plan to talk with him privately sometime during your assessment.

Provide carefully structured, open-ended questions to elicit significant information. Keep your questions concise, rephrase any question the patient doesn't understand,

and use nonverbal techniques, such as facial expressions, pointing, or touching, to enhance your meaning.

Use terms appropriate to the patient's level of understanding; don't use jargon or complex medical terms. Offer explanations in lay terms, and then use the related medical terms, if appropriate, so the patient can become familiar with them.

To foster your older patient's cooperation, take a little extra time to help him see the relevance of your questions. You may need to repeat an explanation several times during the interview, but don't repeat unnecessarily. Give the patient plenty of time to respond to your questions and directions. Remain silent to allow him time to collect his thoughts and ideas before responding.

Patience is the key to communicating with an older adult who responds slowly to your questions. But don't confuse patience with patronizing. The patient will easily perceive patronizing behavior and may interpret it as a lack of genuine concern.

Consent

Initial contact should focus on ensuring that the patient knows the assessment's purpose and how he can help during the history taking—an important step in establishing a trusting relationship.

Review all parts of the assessment with the patient, including the kinds of information you need. Explain how the information will be used and who you'll be sharing it with. Ask only for information that's relevant to the patient's condition. For example, you wouldn't obtain a detailed obstetric history from a 75-year-old woman who doesn't have a gynecologic problem. If the patient refuses to answer questions or participate, document the refusal appropriately.

After you've obtained an older adult's cooperation, you may have trouble getting him to keep his story brief. He has a lot of history to relate and may reminisce during the interview. Try to find time to let him talk; you may gather valuable clues about his current physical, mental, and spiritual health. If you must keep the history brief, remind him how much time you have available for the interview, and offer to come back another time to chat with him informally.

CURRENT HEALTH STATUS: THE HERE AND NOW

The first part of the interview explores the person's chief complaint and his current health status. Keep in mind that some older patients fail to report symptoms, and some believe symptoms that may signal a larger problem are just part of aging. And some are reluctant to report any problems because they fear a loss of independence.

- Begin your interview by asking the patient his full name, address, age, date of birth, birthplace, and contact people in case of an emergency. Record the information on an appropriate patient history form. This information can also help you gain insight into the patient's mental status, although you'll typically more fully assess mental status toward the end of the physical examination. For instance, the patient's ability to tell you his name, date of birth, and current age reflect the accuracy of his remote, recent, and immediate memory and test his ability to calculate his age.
- Record the reason for admission or the chief complaint in the person's own words. Evaluate each complaint in terms of onset, location, duration, timing, intensity, aggravating or alleviating factors, treatment measures, and lifestyle impact.
- Ask the patient about current prescription and nonprescription medications, including the name, dosage, frequency, and reason for the medication. Eliciting this information

can sometimes be a challenge because older people typically use multiple medications, placing them at risk for adverse drug reactions. Even the most oriented older adult may have difficulty remembering his medications. If he has brought any of his medications with him, ask to see them. Encourage him to bring all his medications, including OTC drugs and herbal remedies, to future appointments.

- Next, ask about treatments he's receiving, such as pulmonary treatments, wound care, or pain control.
- Finally, list devices that the person uses, such as a cane, walker, corrective lenses, or hearing aid. Ask if he has any home safety devices, such as grab rails in the shower or tub, smoke alarms, nonskid floor surfaces, and strong lighting.

MEDICAL HISTORY: WHEN PAST BECOMES PRESENT

The medical history includes an overview of the patient's general health status, a history of his adult illnesses, a record of past hospitalizations and their purpose, the frequency of visits to the physician, and previous use of medications and treatments and their purpose. Pay special attention to the patient's medication history because he probably routinely takes medication. Find out what OTC and prescription medications he has taken in the past, with dosages, if possible.

- Before asking specific questions about the medical history, ask an open-ended question such as, "How would you describe your overall health?" This can provide specific information about the patient's history and reveal how he perceives his health status.
- Try to determine the patient's reaction to previous hospitalizations. Someone who has had a bad experience may fear readmission and thus withhold important information.

- Ask about a history of cancer, surgery, trauma, falls, fractures, and cardiac, respiratory, renal, or neurologic disorders. You'll need the patient's detailed recall of major illnesses, surgical procedures, and injuries to complete the history. For example, fractures from early in his life may figure significantly now in osteoporosis. As you record his past history, try to get an idea of the amount of stress he has had recently and the way he has handled previous health problems. Don't be concerned if he can't relate this medical history chronologically; just make sure you record his age at the time each medical condition occurred. Try to develop a chronological report, including the event, date, treatment received, and physician involved. Because an older patient has typically received treatment from more than one physician, asking for physicians' names, conditions treated, and dates of treatment can yield important clues.

REVIEW OF SYSTEMS: A TOP-DOWN APPROACH

The review of systems for an older person involves asking questions that take into account the physiologic changes considered a normal part of aging. Remember that an older adult's disease presentation is typically different from that of a younger adult. For instance, an older patient's only signs and symptoms may be subtle changes in appetite and mental status.

Review all body areas and systems, using either a head-to-toe approach or the major body systems method. Either provides a systematic and organized framework, so choose the method that works best for you. The example below, using the body system approach, covers the information you need to find out.

Skin, hair, and nails

- Ask the patient about any unhealed sores, irregular moles or lesions, and any other changes.

- Ask whether his skin is dry, oily, or normal.
- Does he experience itching, easy bruising, rashes, or calluses? Rashes may be adverse effects of certain medications. Contact allergies and calluses can interfere with ambulation and other activities of daily living (ADLs).
- The patient may report typical age-related changes. For instance, his skin may seem thinner and looser (less elastic) than before, he may perspires less, and his scalp may feel dry. Also, his fingernails and toenails may have thickened and changed color slightly. Find out if he can take care of his own nails, especially his toenails.
- Ask about hair changes and loss, which may indicate chronic disease or nutritional deficiency.

Eyes

- Has the patient noticed diminished near vision (called *presbyopia*) or increased tearing?
- Ask about vision changes, especially night vision or double or blurred vision. Does he need more light than usual when reading? Does he have difficulty driving?
- Ask about corrective lenses, glaucoma, and the date of his most recent eye examination.
- Find out if has trouble taking part in enjoyable activities because of visual changes.

Ears

- Ask the patient if he has any ear pain; ideally, he should be pain-free.
- Ask about tinnitus, which can occur in older people without any hearing impairment. Tinnitus without any other clinical symptoms is considered benign.
- Ask about earwax, ear discharge, and hearing problems. Older people commonly have a harder time hearing such high-pitched sounds as smoke alarms or a small child's

voice and, in general, older people have diminished hearing. Conductive hearing loss typically results from cerumen plugs, but unilateral hearing loss calls for further investigation to rule out acoustic neuroma. Note whether the patient favors one ear, and target your speech toward his good ear; plan for a hearing aid if appropriate.

- If the patient already has a hearing aid, assess the ear canal that the hearing aid is in. Artificial devices such as hearing aids usually increase the amount of cerumen that collects, requiring regular cleaning of that ear canal. Increased hair growth in the canal, which can occur in male patients, can also increase cerumen production.

Respiratory system

- Ask about lung or breathing problems. Remember that hypoventilation and hypoperfusion from respiratory disease can produce confusion or slowed mental function in an older person.
- Ask the patient if he currently smokes or has ever smoked. If he currently smokes or used to smoke, ask for how long and how many packs he smokes or smoked each day. If he no longer smokes, ask when he quit.
- Find out if he ever feels shortness of breath on exertion or when lying down. Older people commonly experience dyspnea on exertion, but dyspnea can also result from lung infections, such as bronchitis or pneumonia.
- Does the patient have a history of respiratory diseases, such as asthma, emphysema, pneumonia, or tuberculosis? If so, ask whether he has received recurring treatment.
- If he reports trouble breathing, explore the precipitating circumstances. To assess his tolerance level, note the distances he says he can walk and the type of exertion that

usually produces dyspnea. Many patients won't mention trouble breathing unless you give them examples of when they might have trouble, such as walking up a flight of stairs.

- Does the patient cough excessively? Does the cough produce a lot of sputum? If so, what color is it? When does it occur?
- Ask if he has had bleeding from any mucous membranes. Has his sense of smell decreased?
- Record possible exposure to harmful substances by asking about his former occupation and hobbies.
- Does the patient get an annual influenza immunization? When was his last one? Did he receive a pneumococcal immunization?

Cardiovascular system

- Ask the patient whether he's gained weight recently. Do his belts, shoes, or rings feel tight, or has he noticed his ankles swelling? Also find out if he tires more easily now than before, if he has trouble breathing, and if he feels dizzy when he gets up from a chair or bed. All these symptoms indicate heart failure, which more than half of all older people suffer from to some degree.
- Check the patient's level of consciousness (LOC), noting confusion or slowed mental status. Occasionally, these are early signs of inadequate cardiac output.
- Ask about chest pain. Any pain could be angina pectoris, but remember that the patient's chief complaint may be dyspnea, chest pressure, palpitations, or even GI issues instead of the more definitive chest pain. Aging contributes to coronary artery plaque development but also promotes collateral circulation to areas deprived of perfusion. Also bear in mind that any of these signs and symptoms in an older person may indicate a disorder in another

system, such as the urinary, endocrine, musculoskeletal, or respiratory system, rather than a cardiovascular disorder. Because an older person is less sensitive to deep pain, keep in mind, too, that he may describe chest pain as heavy or dull, whereas a younger person would describe the same pain as sharp. Even if an older person is having a myocardial infarction, he may experience only confusion, vomiting, faintness, and dizziness.

- Ask the patient about any previous cardiac disease and treatment. Some older adults need prompting to remember health conditions they have had.

- Ask the patient about ADLs and signs and symptoms triggered by these activities, as well as his response to physical and emotional exertion. Reduced cardiac reserve limits an older person's ability to respond to such conditions as infection, blood loss, hypoxia-induced arrhythmias, and electrolyte imbalances. Try to correlate your assessment of the patient's ADLs and his mental status with eating or sleeping difficulties.

- Ask about adverse reactions to prescribed cardiac medications, and pay attention to symptoms that might actually be reactions to these drugs. For instance, a dry cough may result from an antiarrhythmic medication such as an angiotensin-converting enzyme inhibitor (lisinopril [Prinivil]).

- Ask about weakness, bradycardia, hypotension, and confusion, which may indicate high potassium levels; weakness, fatigue, muscle cramps, and palpitations may stem from low potassium levels.

- Question the patient about anorexia, nausea, vomiting, diarrhea, headache, rash, vision disturbances, and mental confusion, which may signal digoxin (Lanoxin) overdose.

- Complaints of lower extremity edema accompanied by fatigue may result from a calcium channel blocker; this can escalate into a serious condition if not corrected.

GI system

- Ask about changes in the patient's sense of taste. An older person may complain about a foul taste and soreness in his mouth, which can stem from a number of causes, including decreased saliva production, periodontal disease, bleeding gums, mouth lesions, dentures, smoking, vitamin deficiencies, or other more serious conditions.

- Ask the patient if his mouth is dry. Dry mouth, or *xerostomia*, may result from medications or from systemic disease, such as rheumatoid arthritis, scleroderma polymyositis, or Sjögren's syndrome.

- If the patient wears dentures, find out how comfortable they are and how well they work. An improper fit may explain a report of declining appetite.

- Ask about voice hoarseness or changes in his voice, which may indicate cancer.

- If the patient reports difficulty in swallowing, ask if he has the same degree of trouble swallowing solid foods and liquids. Does food lodge in his throat? Does he feel pain after eating or while lying flat?

- Question him about heartburn, a sour stomach or early satiety, changes in eating habits, and changes in food tolerance.

- Question him about weight loss, rectal bleeding, and elimination habits. Many medications can cause changes in elimination, and about half of older adults develop diverticulosis.

- Ask if he has had any cramplike abdominal pain in the left lower quadrant, keeping in mind that abdominal disorders commonly present atypically in older adults.

For example, diffuse abdominal pain may indicate fecal impaction. Also, although fecal incontinence is abnormal at any age, it's commonly seen in older people who abuse laxatives or who have advanced dementia or cerebrovascular disease.

- Note the presence of such devices as a feeding tube or an ostomy.

Genitourinary system

- Investigate any report of incontinence. When incontinence occurs, does the patient feel the loss of control or urge to urinate? Ask if he uses pads or experiences enuresis. If he urinates in the middle of the night, find out how often and whether the urge awakens him. Most older adults think that urinary incontinence is a result of aging, but common causes of urinary incontinence can typically be treated. They include fecal impaction, prostatic obstruction, atrophic vaginitis, infection, loss of sphincter control, and certain medications.
- Ask an older male patient about frequent urinary infections, urinary incontinence, dribbling after urination, and decrease in the size and force of the urine stream; all are common signs of prostatic obstruction. Also ask about erectile dysfunction, which may indicate underlying vascular disease or may be a result of medications.
- If the patient is an older woman, ask if she experiences vaginal itching, discharge, or pain. Ask if she performs monthly breast self-examinations and, if so, whether she has detected abnormalities. Find out when she had her last mammogram and how frequently she has them. Postmenopausal bleeding and any changes in the breast tissue or presence of breast masses are abnormal and require prompt evaluation.

Neurologic system

- Ask about any changes in coordination, strength, or sensory perception.
- Has the patient had difficulty controlling his bowels or bladder?
- Does he have headaches or has he had any seizures?
- Has he experienced temporary losses of consciousness? Loss of consciousness (*syncope*) may stem from a cardiac, neurologic, or metabolic disorder. Common complaints include a feeling of "blacking out" or complete amnesia of events during a specific time period. Ask about events that preceded the syncopal episode as well as the initial events he remembered after regaining consciousness.
- Find out if he has felt dizzy (a sensation of unsteadiness and movement within the head or of light-headedness) or experienced vertigo (a sensation that the room is rotating around the person or that the person himself is rotating). Vertigo in older adults may result from inner ear disorders, such as labyrinthitis, Ménière's disease, or benign positional vertigo, or from posterior circulatory diseases, such as vertebrobasilar insufficiency or stroke. It can even stem from medications.
- Ask about memory loss or forgetfulness.
- Find out if the patient has noticed vision or coordination changes that may make him more susceptible to falling.

Musculoskeletal system

- If the patient's chief complaint is pain associated with a fall, determine if the pain preceded the fall. Pain present before a fall may indicate a pathologic fracture.
- Does the patient have a fear of falling? If so, why? Unsteady gait may explain an older adult's fear of falling. Many older patients who have had a fall not only have

an increased risk of falling again, but fear that they may fall again, which ends up restricting their movements.

- Has the patient's gait changed?
- Does he have a deformity or wear a prosthesis?
- Ask if he has joint or lower back pain, or weakness or stiffness in an extremity. Osteoarthritis commonly accounts for an older adult's complaints of pain, stiffness, or limitation in weight-bearing joints. Focal pain may occur in a person who has another rheumatoid disease, such as rheumatoid or gouty arthritis or carpal tunnel syndrome.
- When recording the patient's history of illnesses, determine if he has a chronic disease (such as asthma or arthritis that requires treatment with steroids, which affect calcium absorption) that led to osteoporosis. If he has arthritis, he's also more likely to have an unstable gait. A patient with pernicious anemia is more likely to also have rheumatoid arthritis; he's also less able to absorb vitamin B_{12}, which leads to the loss of vibratory sensation and proprioception and can result in falls. If the patient has cancer of the breast, prostate, thyroid, kidney, or bladder, metastases to bone can lead to loss of bone strength and an increased risk of pathological fracture.

Endocrine system

- Find out if the patient has ever received a diagnosis of hyperparathyroidism or hormone imbalance. Hyperparathyroidism leads to bone decalcification and osteoporosis, and hormone imbalance can result in postmenopausal osteoporosis.
- Ask about changes in sensation, such as tingling, numbness, a sensation of pins and needles, or involuntary movements.
- Ask about cold intolerance, diabetes symptoms, a history of diabetes, and thyroid or other hormone treatments.

Hematologic and immune systems

- Find out if the patient experiences joint pain, weakness, or fatigue. Does he take walks? If so, for how long? Does he have difficulty using his hands? Do his knees bother him? Does he bruise easily? Does he have a history of deep vein thrombosis?
- Ask about current medications, and note which ones produce adverse effects similar to signs and symptoms of hematologic and immune disorders. For instance, digoxin may cause anorexia, nausea, and vomiting; aspirin can produce mucosal irritation and GI bleeding; and excessive laxative use can prevent absorption of dietary nutrients.
- Determine the patient's typical daily diet. Does he live alone and cook for himself? Because of limited income, limited resources, and decreased mobility, older people may have diets deficient in protein, calcium, and iron—nutrients essential to hematopoiesis. Even with an adequate diet, nutrients may not be metabolized because of reduced enzymes. (About 40% of people over age 60 have iron deficiency anemia.)

PSYCHOSOCIAL ASSESSMENT: GETTING AT LIFE'S DETAILS

- Begin the psychosocial assessment by asking about alcohol and tobacco use. Note the quantity and type of alcoholic beverages the patient consumes. Document tobacco use in "pack years," the number of packs smoked per day multiplied by the number of years the patient has smoked.
- Ask the patient if he has difficulty sleeping, unresolved problems, sadness, depression, or loss of interest in usual activities. A person with a major depressive disorder commonly has difficulty sleeping and changes in appetite.

- Ask an older person about his sleeping habits. When does he go to bed and when does he wake up? Does he use sleeping aids, such as medications or alcohol, to help him get to sleep? Does he take naps during the day?
- Is the patient employed? If he is, ask about his job and whether his health problems will interfere with his returning to work. Talk with him about his retirement plans, if he has any, and his attitude toward this phase of his life.
- If the patient expresses financial concerns, explore them further in a financial history. Ask if his income meets his monthly expenses for food, rent, household items, clothing, and other bills. Refer a person whose income falls below his monthly expenses to social services for assistance. Remember to ask the patient if he receives pensions or Social Security payments.
- How does the patient spend his time? What are his hobbies? How often does he see people socially? Has his activity level decreased lately?
- Does he live alone or with a spouse, family member, or friend? Does he own a home, rent, or live in a retirement, boarding, or nursing home?
- Make a point of talking with your older patient about his family and friends. Find out what significant relationships he has because these play a central role in his overall health and well-being. This part of the assessment can yield vital information about his support network. Families provide substantial help to their older members, so assessing family involvement is crucial. If the patient is hospitalized and seriously ill, or must transfer to another type of facility (such as a nursing home), he'll need the emotional support of family and friends.

If he's returning home after an illness, he may need their help.
- Does the patient rely on assistance from family or friends to perform his usual daily activities?
- What person is primarily responsible for his care? Is this person overwhelmed or stressed?
- If the patient doesn't have a family or friends he can depend on for support, record this for referral to a social services agency as appropriate. Without your intervention, loneliness may discourage an older patient from getting well. Record the names of his next of kin.
- Note the use of community resources, such as meal service, reduced-fare or free transportation for seniors, adult day care, and home health services.
- Inquire about problems or concerns regarding sexual activity. Don't ignore the subject because of the patient's age. Approach this aspect of the psychosocial assessment with the same sensitivity and respect for privacy that you would show with a younger person. Be particularly sensitive to the patient's cultural background and moral values. This is especially true for a person who may be a generation or two older than you. If the patient is reluctant to discuss his sexual activity, don't press him for information. By inquiring, you've indicated your openness to discuss sexual issues. Although a patient may not disclose information immediately, he may bring it up at a later time.

FUNCTIONAL ASSESSMENT: KEEPING THINGS IN WORKING ORDER

- Ask for a description of the patient's typical day at home, including activities, eating habits, and sleep patterns. An older person's daily activities may affect his health, and his health problems may, in turn, threaten his ability to function independently.

- Ask the patient if he has decreased his activities recently; inactivity increases the risk of osteoporosis. Also ask him to describe his usual diet. Older people commonly have an inadequate calcium and vitamin intake, which can cause osteoporosis and muscle weakness.
- Because the patient's eating habits may suggest other significant lines of questioning, find out how much of an appetite he usually has, how he prepares his food (how much salt he uses, for instance), and how much fluid he usually consumes. You can put this information into a chart, showing which foods he eats at what times during the day.
- Ask about mobility. Can the patient move around at home easily and safely? Can he handle his basic food, clothing, and shelter needs? Does he drive to the supermarket, use public or Elder Services transportation, or rely on a friend or relative to drive him?
- Ask if he expects to be able to continue his normal routine after being discharged from the hospital.
- To gain further information about the patient's psychosocial status and to identify any problems that might call for further evaluation, you can use assessment tools such as the Short Michigan Alcohol Screening Test—Geriatric Version and the Mini-Cog, discussed in chapter 2, as well as the Geriatric Depression scale. (See *Using the Geriatric Depression Scale*.)
- Evaluate how safe the patient's environment is for performing ADLs to determine if he needs to modify his home to accommodate his physical changes. For example, ask about stairs and the location of bathrooms. Does

his home have adequate lighting, heating, and air conditioning as well as secured carpeting, smoke alarms, enough telephones, and safe electrical wiring? Tools that you can use to assess and document ADLs include the Katz Index, the Lawton Instrumental Activities of Daily Living Scale, and the Barthel Index. (See *The Katz index*, page 58, *The Lawton Instrumental Activities of Daily Living scale*, page 59, and *The Barthel index*, pages 60 and 61.)

The physical assessment

The second part of the health assessment, the physical examination, works with the health history to identify and evaluate the patient's strengths, weaknesses, capabilities, and limitations. It also helps you validate the subjective data you gathered during the health history. Use inspection, palpation, percussion, and auscultation to collect objective patient data.

THE PHYSICAL: PREPARING AND PLANNING

Organization and planning are the keys to a successful physical examination. Because an older person may tire easily during the examination, make sure you have the necessary equipment within easy reach and in proper working order so no time is wasted. Also, be ready to modify the examination and provide further comfort measures as necessary to meet the patient's needs. Keep the following points in mind:

- Respect the patient's need for modesty; make sure that the examination area is private, and explain how to put on the gown and drape. Ask him if he needs any help changing into the gown.
- Ensure the patient's comfort throughout the examination; have pillows and blankets available for added warmth and assistance in positioning.

(*Text continues on page 62.*)

USING THE GERIATRIC DEPRESSION SCALE

The Geriatric Depression scale allows you to screen older patients for depression. To administer this test, read each question to the patient and ask him to answer "yes" or "no," choosing the answer that best fits how he felt during the past week.

To score the test, count the number of "no" answers for items marked with an asterisk and the number of "yes" answers for items that are *not* marked with an asterisk. Your total is the patient's final score. A score of 0 to 9 is considered normal (no depression), a score of 10 to 19 indicates mild depression, and a score of 20 to 30 indicates severe depression.

Question	Yes	No
1. Are you basically satisfied with your life? *	Yes	No
2. Have you dropped many of your activities and interests?	Yes	No
3. Do you feel that your life is empty?	Yes	No
4. Do you often get bored?	Yes	No
5. Are you hopeful about the future? *	Yes	No
6. Are you bothered by thoughts you can't get out of your head?	Yes	No
7. Are you in good spirits most of the time? *	Yes	No
8. Are you afraid that something bad is going to happen to you?	Yes	No
9. Do you feel happy most of the time? *	Yes	No
10. Do you often feel helpless?	Yes	No
11. Do you often get restless and fidgety?	Yes	No
12. Do you prefer to stay at home, rather than going out and doing new things?	Yes	No
13. Do you frequently worry about the future?	Yes	No
14. Do you feel you have more problems with memory than most?	Yes	No
15. Do you think it is wonderful to be alive now? *	Yes	No
16. Do you often feel downhearted and blue?	Yes	No
17. Do you feel pretty worthless the way you are now?	Yes	No
18. Do you worry a lot about the past?	Yes	No
19. Do you find life very exciting? *	Yes	No
20. Is it hard for you to get started on new projects?	Yes	No
21. Do you feel full of energy? *	Yes	No
22. Do you feel that your situation is hopeless?	Yes	No
23. Do you think that most people are better off than you are?	Yes	No
24. Do you frequently get upset over little things?	Yes	No
25. Do you frequently feel like crying?	Yes	No
26. Do you have trouble concentrating?	Yes	No
27. Do you enjoy getting up in the morning? *	Yes	No
28. Do you prefer to avoid social gatherings?	Yes	No
29. Is it easy for you to make decisions? *	Yes	No
30. Is your mind as clear as it used to be?*	Yes	No

Adapted from Yesavage J.A., et al., "Development and Validation of a Geriatric Depression Screening Scale: A Preliminary Report," *Journal of Psychiatric Research* 17:37-49, 1983. Used with permission of Elsevier.

THE KATZ INDEX

The Katz index, shown below, allows you to assess a patient's ability to perform six basic activities of daily living.

Evaluation Form   Name _____   Date _____

For each area of functioning listed below, check the description that applies.

Indicates Independence (1 point)	Indicates Dependence (0 points)
Bathing: Sponge bath, tub bath, or shower. ❑ Receives no assistance; or only needs help with one area; gets into and out of tub, if tub is usual means of bathing.	❑ Receives assistance in bathing more than one part of the body or getting into or out of the tub or shower. Cannot bathe self.
Dressing: Gets outer garments and underwear from closets and drawers and uses fasteners, including suspenders, if worn. ❑ Gets clothes and gets completely dressed without assistance. May need assistance tying shoes.	❑ Receives assistance in getting clothes or in getting dressed or stays partly or completely undressed.
Toileting: Goes to the room termed "toilet" for bowel movement and urination, cleans self afterward, and arranges clothes. ❑ Goes to toilet room, cleans self, and arranges clothes without assistance. May use object for support, such as cane, walker, or wheelchair, and may manage night bedpan or commode, emptying it in the morning.	❑ Doesn't go to toilet room for the elimination process or needs help in cleaning self or arranging clothes after elimination.
Transfer ❑ Moves into and out of bed and chair without assistance. May use object, such as cane or walker, for support.	❑ Doesn't get out of bed on own or needs assistance.
Continence ❑ Controls urination and bowel movement completely by self.	❑ Supervision helps keep control of urination or bowel movement, or catheter is used, or is incontinent.
Feeding ❑ Feeds self without assistance. Food may be prepared by someone else.	❑ Receives assistance in feeding or is fed partly or completely through tubes or by I.V. fluids.

Evaluator: _____

Overall points: _____

6 points = independence
0 points = very dependent

Adapted from Katz, S., et al. "Progress in the Development of the Index of ADL," *The Gerontologist* 10(1):20-30, 1970. Copyright © The Gerontological Society of America. Used with permission of the publisher.

THE LAWTON INSTRUMENTAL ACTIVITIES OF DAILY LIVING SCALE

This scale evaluates more sophisticated functions than does the more basic Katz index. It's most useful in identifying how a patient is currently functioning and then tracking changes in functioning over time. The patient or caregiver can complete the form within 15 minutes by circling the number (0 or 1) next to the description that most closely resembles his highest functional level.

The scale measures eight domains. Women are scored in all eight areas; men usually aren't scored in food preparation, housekeeping, or laundering. All patients are scored according to their highest level of functioning in each domain. For women, scores can range from 0 (low function) to 8 (high function); for men, scores typically range from 0 (low function) to 5 (high function).

Name .... **Rated by** .... **Date** ....

Telephone Usage

1. Operates telephone on own initiative; looks up and dials numbers 1
2. Dials a few well-known numbers 1
3. Answers telephone, but doesn't dial 1
4. Doesn't use telephone at all 0

Shopping

1. Takes care of all shopping needs independently 1
2. Shops independently for small purchases 0
3. Needs to be accompanied on any shopping trip 0
4. Completely unable to shop 0

Food Preparation

1. Plans, prepares, and serves adequate meals independently 1
2. Prepares adequate meals if supplied with ingredients 0
3. Heats and serves prepared meals, or prepares meals but doesn't maintain adequate diet 0
4. Needs to have meals prepared and served 0

Housekeeping

1. Maintains house alone with occasional assistance (heavy work) 1
2. Performs light daily tasks, such as dishwashing and bed-making 1
3. Performs light daily tasks but can't maintain acceptable level of cleanliness 1
4. Needs help with all home maintenance tasks 1
5. Doesn't participate in any housekeeping tasks 0

Laundry

1. Does personal laundry completely 1
2. Launders small items (rinses socks, stockings, etc.) 1
3. Needs others to do all laundry 0

Transportation

1. Travels independently on public transportation or drives own car 1
2. Arranges own travel by taxi, but doesn't otherwise use public transportation 1
3. Travels on public transportation when assisted or accompanied by another 1
4. Travel limited to taxi or automobile with assistance of another 0
5. Doesn't travel at all 0

Medications

1. Is responsible for taking medication in correct dosages at correct time 1
2. Takes responsibility if medication is prepared in advance in separate dosages 0
3. Isn't capable of dispensing own medication 0

Finances

1. Manages financial matters independently (budgets, writes checks, pays rent and bills, goes to bank); collects and keeps track of income 1
2. Manages day-to-day purchases, but needs help with banking, major purchases, etc. 1
3. Incapable of handling money 0

Adapted from Lawton, M.P., and Brody, E.M. "Assessment of Older People: Self-Maintaining and Instrumental Activities of Daily Living," *The Gerontologist*, 9(3)179-186, 1969. Copyright © The Gerontological Society of America. Used with permission of the publisher.

THE BARTHEL INDEX

The Barthel index, shown below, is used to assess a patient's ability to perform 10 activities of daily living. It can be used by various health care team members to document findings and track any improvement or decline in the patient's progress.

Date _____

Patient's name _____

Evaluator _____

Action	Unable	With help	Independent
Feeding (if food needs to be cut = help)	0	5	10
Moving from wheelchair to bed and return (includes sitting up in bed)	0	5 to 10	15
Personal toilet (wash face, comb hair, shave, clean teeth)	0	0	5
Getting on and off toilet (handling clothes, wipe, flush)	0	5	10
Bathing self	0	0	5
Walking on level surface (or, if unable to walk, propelling wheelchair)	0	0	5 or 15
Ascending and descending stairs	0	5	10
Dressing (includes tying shoes, fastening fasteners)	0	5	10
Controlling bowels	0	5	10
Controlling bladder	0	5	10

Definition and Discussion of Scoring

A person scoring 100 is continent, feeds himself, dresses himself, gets up out of bed and chairs, bathes himself, walks at least a block, and can ascend and descend stairs. This doesn't mean that he's able to live alone; he may not be able to cook, keep house, or meet the public, but he's able to get along without attendant care.

Feeding

10 = Independent. The person can feed himself a meal from a tray or table when someone puts the food within his reach. He must be able to put on an assistive device, if needed, cut the food, use salt and pepper, spread butter, and so forth. Also, he must accomplish these tasks in a reasonable time.

 5 = The person needs some help with cutting food and other tasks, as listed above.

 0 = Unable

Moving from Wheelchair to Bed and Return

15 = The person operates independently in all phases of this activity. He can safely approach the bed in his wheelchair, lock brakes, lift footrests, move safely from bed, lie down, come to a sitting position on the side of the bed, change the position of the wheelchair, if necessary, to transfer back into it safely, and return to the wheelchair.

10 = Either the person needs some minimal help in some step of this activity, or needs to be reminded or supervised for safety in one or more parts of this activity.

 5 = The person can come to a sitting position without the help of a second person but needs to be lifted out of bed, or needs a great deal of help with transfers.

 0 = Unable to sit with balance

Handling Personal Toilet

5 = The person can wash hands and face, comb hair, clean teeth, and shave. He may use any kind of razor but he must be able to get it from the drawer or cabinet and plug it in or put in a blade without help. A woman must put on her own makeup, if she uses any, but need not braid or style her hair.

0 = Needs assistance with grooming

Getting On and Off Toilet

10 = The person is able to get on and off the toilet, unfasten and refasten clothes, prevent soiling of clothes, and use toilet paper without help. He may use a wall bar or other stable object for support, if needed. If he needs to use a bed pan instead of toilet, he must be able to place it on a chair, use it competently, and empty and clean it.

 5 = The person needs help to overcome imbalance, handle clothes, or use toilet paper.

 0 = Dependent

THE BARTHEL INDEX (*continued*)

Bathing Self

5 = The person may use a bath tub or shower or give himself a complete sponge bath. Regardless of method, he must be able to complete all the steps involved without another person's presence.
0 = Dependent

Walking on a Level Surface

15 = The person can walk at least 50 yards without help or supervision. He may wear braces or prostheses and use crutches, canes, or a walkerette, but not a rolling walker. He must be able to lock and unlock braces, if used, get the necessary mechanical aids into position for use, stand up and sit down, and dispose of the aids when he sits. (Putting on, fastening, and taking off braces is scored under Dressing).
10 = Walks with assistance of one person more than 50 yards.
5 = If the person can't ambulate but can propel a wheelchair independently, he must be able to go around corners, turn around, maneuver the chair to table, bed, toilet, and other locations. He must be able to push a chair at least 150′ (45.7 m). Don't score this item if the person receives a score for walking.
0 = Unable to walk.

Ascending and Descending Stairs

10 = The person can go up and down a flight of stairs safely without help or supervision. He may and should use handrails, canes, or crutches when needed, and he must be able to carry canes or crutches as he ascends or descends.
5 = The person needs help with or supervision of any one of the above items.
0 = Unable

Dressing and Undressing

10 = The person can put on, fasten, and remove all clothing (including any prescribed corset or braces) and tie shoe laces (unless he requires adaptations for this). Such special clothing as suspenders, loafers, and dresses that open down the front may be used when necessary.
5 = The person needs help in putting on, fastening, or removing any clothing. He must do at least half the work himself and must accomplish the task in a reasonable time. Women need not be scored on use of a brassiere or girdle unless these are prescribed garments.
0 = Dependent

Controlling Bowels

10 = The person can control his bowels without accidents. He can use a suppository or take an enema when necessary (as in spinal cord injury patients who have had bowel training).
5 = The person needs help in using a suppository or taking an enema or has occasional accidents.
0 = Incontinent

Controlling Bladder

10 = The person can control his bladder day and night. Spinal cord injury patients who wear an external device and leg bag must put them on independently, clean and empty the bag, and stay dry, day and night.
5 = The person has occasional accidents, can't wait for the bed pan or get to the toilet in time, or needs help with an external device.
0 = Incontinent or catheterized

The total score is less significant or meaningful than the individual items because these indicate where the deficiencies lie. Any applicant to a long-term care facility who scores 100 should be evaluated carefully before admission to see whether admission is indicated. Discharged patients with scores of 100 shouldn't require further physical therapy but may benefit from a home visit to see whether any environmental adjustments are needed.

© Adapted with permission from Mahoney, F.I., and Barthel, D. W. "Functional Evaluation: The Barthel Index," *Maryland State Medical Journal* 14:62, 1965.

- Anticipate problems with mobility or strength that might require help from another person, use of alternative positions, or changes in the usual examination sequence.

THE GENERAL SURVEY: TAKING IT ALL IN

Begin the physical examination with a general, head-to-toe observation to gain an overall impression of the patient's status. The survey should include observations about:

- overall appearance, including skin, hygiene, grooming, and body build
- general mobility status
- LOC, affect, and mood
- any overt signs of distress.

VITAL SIGNS: SETTING THE BASELINE

Before taking the patient's vital signs, make sure he has had a chance to rest for about 10 minutes. If you take measurements, especially the pulse and respiratory rates, right after physical exertion, you may get elevated readings.

Temperature

- Obtain a temperature orally or tympanically, depending on your facility's policy. If the patient is a mouth breather or dyspneic, use the tympanic, axillary, or rectal route instead of the oral route.
- Normal temperature in an older adult can range from 96° to 98.6° F (35.5° to 37° C), although normal body temperature decreases with age. In adults over age 75, temperatures range from 96.9° to 98.3° F (36.1° to 36.8° C) orally and 98° to 99° F (36.7° to 37.2° C) rectally. However, the aging process alters temperature regulation, making temperature an unreliable sign of infection. The older adult is at high risk for infection because of age-related changes in immunity and increased

incidence of hospitalization, which can lead to nosocomial infections. Yet even with a clinical infection, an older person may register no fever. Hypothermia, however, is a medical emergency and calls for immediate evaluation.

Pulse

- To obtain the most accurate pulse rate, count the apical pulse for 1 full minute. Measure all pulses for rate, rhythm, strength, and equality.
- The resting pulse rate remains fairly constant through old age, ranging from 60 to 100 beats/minute. However, after exercise, an older person's pulse rate may take longer to return to the baseline.
- The incidence of arrhythmias increases with age. Immediately report any irregular rhythm.

Respirations

- Assess the patient's respiratory rate. Also assess the depth, rhythm, and quality of respirations. In an older adult, respiratory rate, rhythm, and quality remain constant during rest, but a period of apnea followed by deep breaths may occur during sleep. With exercise, the patient's respiratory rate will increase and take longer to return to the baseline.
- Keep in mind that the respiratory rate may be a more reliable sign of infection and heart failure in an older patient, especially if the resting respiratory rate is tachypneic.

Blood pressure

- Measure the patient's blood pressure in both arms. Changes may reflect typical physiologic, age-related changes: a gradual increase in systolic and diastolic values, widening pulse pressure influenced by an increase in arterial rigidity and a decrease in vessel resiliency, and a tendency to develop orthostatic hypotension. Or changes may stem from a pathologic cause, such as hypertension.

HEIGHT AND WEIGHT: THE TALL AND THE SHORT OF IT

- The best way to determine an older adult's height is to use a tape measure, measuring from the crown to the rump and then from the rump to the heels. This technique accounts for changes in the curvature of the spine such as senile kyphosis (widow's hump). Height usually decreases about 2″ to 3″ (5 to 7.5 cm) with age. Remember that a person can be slightly shorter in the afternoon than in the morning from settling of the spine.
- Obtain the patient's weight, noting whether it's with shoes or without. For accurate comparison, make sure the patient uses the same scale at the same time of day and is clothed in the same way for subsequent weight checks.
- Sudden or profound weight changes aren't a normal result of aging. However, a gradual weight gain over the years may occur if the person continues to consume the same amount of calories as when he was younger and more active. Certain diseases, such as heart failure and depression, may produce weight gain. Weight loss of more than 10% of the person's typical weight in a short period, such as 6 months, calls for follow up; it may indicate depression, a physiologic disorder, or a mechanical problem with eating.

REVIEW OF SYSTEMS: EACH IN ITS TURN

The next part of the physical examination is a complete assessment of body systems. As with the patient history, you'll need to keep in mind that an older adult typically presents differently than a younger adult. The following assessment guidelines use the major body systems

approach; you can use a head-to-toe approach for your assessments if you prefer.

Skin

- Begin your body system assessment by inspecting the skin of the scalp, head, neck, trunk, and limbs. Note color, temperature, texture, tone, turgor, thickness, and moisture.
- Depending on the patient's race, skin color can vary from whitish pink to ruddy olive or yellow tones, to shades of brown from light to blue-black. Areas such as the knees or elbows may appear relatively darker because of sun exposure, and callused areas may appear yellow.
- Disease may change skin color. Typical discolorations include redness, pallor, jaundice, ashen gray color, cyanosis, and bronze or brawny color. Brawny discoloration of the legs typically signifies chronic venous insufficiency. Ecchymosis and petechiae can occur from vitamin C deficiency.
- Skin temperature can be described as cold, cool, warm, or hot. Use the ball of your hand to get an accurate assessment and to feel for symmetrical changes in temperature. Unilateral changes along with other clinical findings suggest a problem.
- Skin typically becomes thicker with age. If corns occur, they usually appear on the dorsal portion of the small toes. Aging skin also becomes translucent, friable, and more susceptible to breakdown from trauma. The gradual decrease in total body water and sebum production leads to dry skin, particularly of the legs.
- Skin texture may be smooth or rough. Many older people experience increased dryness with flaking and scaling, particularly on their extremities.
- Skin turgor may not reliably reflect hydration in older people because of the reduced

IDENTIFYING AGE-RELATED SKIN CHANGES

The chart below shows some common skin changes that occur with aging, along with their causes.

ASSESSMENT FINDINGS	CAUSE
Lines around eyes (crow's feet), mouth, and nose	• Loss of subcutaneous fat • Thinning dermis • Decreased collagen and elastin • Decline in cell replacement
Slowed wound healing, with tendency toward infection	• Decreased rate of skin cell replacement • Less efficient immune system
Dry mucous membranes	• Decrease in sweat gland output and in the number of active sweat glands
Difficulty regulating body temperature	• Loss of subcutaneous fat (combined with decreased size, number, and function of sweat glands)
Development of brown spots (senile lentigo)	• Decreased melanocyte production, along with localized proliferations of melanocytes
Thinning and graying hair	• Decreased pigment

amount of subcutaneous tissue. Check turgor by pinching the subcutaneous tissue at the forehead or over the xiphoid process and watching for a quick return to baseline.

• Look for normal, age-related skin changes, such as lines around the eyes. Keep in mind that the declining skin function that occurs with aging leaves older patients more prone to skin disease, infection, problems with wound healing, and tissue atrophy. (See *Identifying age-related skin changes.*)

• Inspect the skin for tears, lacerations, scars, lesions, and ulcerations. Keep in mind older patients are more prone to pressure ulcers because they have less of the protective subcutaneous tissue and fat padding between the outer layer of the skin and the underlying bone. Look for early signs of ulcers such as local redness over pressure sites. Stasis ulcers of the legs, also common in older people, usually reflect chronic venous insufficiency.

• **Culture** Redness in a darker-skinned patient may not be a reliable early sign of a pressure ulcer. Try using

palpation, noting changes in temperature and firmness.

• Look for the common benign skin lesions found in older people, taking care to differentiate these from precancerous or malignant lesions. Note the size, pattern of distribution, shape, color, consistency, and borders and when they appeared. Any suspicious lesion warrants further evaluation. (See *Recognizing common skin lesions in the older adult.*)

Hair and nails

• Inspect and palpate the patient's hair, noting color, quantity, distribution, and texture (fine, silky, or coarse). You may notice lighter or gray hair, the result of a normal decline in melanocyte function, and drier hair follicles from a decrease in sebaceous gland function. Hair growth—including body hair growth—also declines. You can readily note hair thinning and sparseness around the axilla and symphysis pubis. Diseases, such as hypothyroidism, hyperthyroidism, and chronic renal

RECOGNIZING COMMON SKIN LESIONS IN THE OLDER ADULT

The photographs below show some common skin disorders that can occur in older adults.

Cherry Angiomas
These small, raised spots vary in size and can occur almost anywhere on the body, but they usually develop on the trunk.

Senile or Actinic Purpura
These lesions commonly occur in elderly individuals after some minor, often unrecognized, trauma.

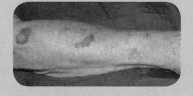

Spider Angioma
This lesion, which is a cluster of telangiectasias, may occur in healthy people but occurs more commonly in those with liver disease.

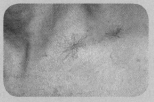

Solar Lentigines
These tan macules appear on sun-exposed areas during middle age.

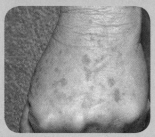

Venous Lake
These lesions typically occur in adults older than age 50 who have a history of chronic sun exposure.

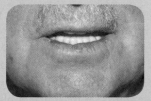

Seborrheic Keratosis
These common, noncancerous lesions tend to run in families.

disease, as well as nutritional deficiencies can also produce changes in hair texture and distribution.

- Note whether the patient is balding. Genetically predetermined balding occurs in many people, particularly men, as a normal result of aging.
- Inspect the patient's fingernails and toenails, noting color, shape, thickness, presence of lesions, and capillary refill. With age, nail growth slows as nails become brittle and thin, and longitudinal ridges in the nail plate become much more pronounced, making the nail prone to splitting. Also, the nails lose their luster and become yellowed.

- Examine any distortions in the nails. Some distortion of the normal flat or slightly curved nail surface is normal, but other changes in color, shape, or angle may indicate a disorder. For example, people with anemia usually have pale nail beds and slow capillary refill. Thick, hooked, clawlike nails signal hypertrophy of the nails, a common clinical condition. Thickened, friable, yellowed nails commonly result from a fungal infection. Ingrown nails typically cause infection and mobility problems for older adults. Redness, possibly with heat, drainage, and (in severe cases) bulging at the nail base, may indicate an infection of the nail bed.

Cyanotic nail beds and clubbing of the fingers may point to respiratory distress or heart disease.

Head and face

- Inspect the head, noting size, contour, and symmetry. The size and shape of the skull shouldn't change with age. Soft tissue swelling or bulging of the cranium may indicate recent head trauma.
- Palpate the skull, noting tenderness, masses, or lesions. Point tenderness or localized enlargement of the cranium requires further evaluation.
- Inspect the patient's face and neck area for color and proportion. His face and neck should have evenly distributed color, and he should have facial features in proportion to his head size.
- Observe the patient's facial expression and movements. He should look alert and interested, with smooth, expressive movements. A masklike or blank face commonly accompanies Parkinson's disease and certain psychiatric disorders.

Nose and mouth

- Examine the external portion of the nose, noting any asymmetry or abnormality such as a structural deformity. Inspect the internal mucosa, noting color and any discharge, swelling, bleeding, or lesions. The area should be pink and moist with clear mucus, and without crusting or lesions.
- Palpate the frontal and maxillary sinuses for tenderness, an abnormal finding.
- Inspect the mouth, beginning with the lips. Note color, symmetry, lesions or ulcerations, and hydration status. Dry, parched lips indicate dehydration.
- Note the presence of any dental appliances. Inspect the mouth with the appliance in

place, noting the fit and observing for sores or abscesses that may occur from friction. Poorly fitting dentures may produce fissures or cracks at the corners of the mouth (called *cheilosis*); vitamin B complex deficiencies produce cheilosis with reddened lips.

- Inspect the mucosa, noting color, texture, hydration status, odor, and any exudate. Poor oral hygiene can cause a white exudate that coats the mucosa or tongue.
- Palpate for lesions or nodules, looking for tenderness, pain, or bleeding. Inspect the gums for color, inflammation, lesions, and bleeding. They should be pink and moist. If the patient has his natural teeth, note the number and condition.
- Observe the tongue, noting its color, size, texture, and coating. It should look pink to red and smooth, and shouldn't move involuntarily. If the patient is experiencing extrapyramidal adverse effects from psychotropic drugs, you may see such involuntary movements as lip smacking, tongue protrusion, and slow rhythmic movements of the tongue, lips, or jaws. If the patient has hypothyroid disease, he may have an enlarged tongue.
- Assess the tongue's position. Deviation to the right or left suggests a neurologic disorder. Sublingual varicosities may result from iron deficiency anemia. (See *Recognizing sublingual varicosities*.)
- Observe the pharynx for signs of inflammation, discoloration, exudate, and lesions. The area should appear pink to pale pink, without discharge or lesions.

Eyes

- When you examine an older person's eyes, keep in mind that ocular signs of aging can affect the appearance of the entire eye. You may see that the eyes sit deeper in the bony orbits, a normal finding that results from age-induced fatty tissue loss. Check eyebrow symmetry and distribution of hair.

- Compare the color of the patient's eyelids to his facial skin color; the lid should be free from color changes such as redness. Check for lesions or edema, and note the direction of the eyelashes. Determine whether the upper eyelid partially or completely covers the pupil, indicating ptosis, an abnormal finding. Common conditions affecting the eyelids in older people include entropion and ectropion (in which the edges turn inward or outward, respectively) and ptosis. (See *Identifying eyelid changes*, page 68.)

- Inspect the lacrimal apparatus, noting any discharge, redness, edema, excessive tearing, or tenderness. Aging can affect the lacrimal apparatus in several ways. For example, the delicate canaliculi and nasolacrimal ducts may become plugged or kinked, resulting in constantly watering eyes. Conversely, these blockages can also reduce tear production and cause burning, dry, or irritated eyes (known as *keratitis sicca*).

- Examine the sclera and conjunctiva. The sclera usually appears creamy white. Because of the presence of fat, however, the sclera and conjunctiva may appear yellow. One common observation in older people is a yellow-tinged thickening of the bulbar conjunctiva, triangular in shape and occurring on the inner and outer margins of the cornea.

- When you inspect the conjunctiva, be aware that its luster may appear dimmed, and it may be drier and thinner than in a younger person. This dryness may trigger frequent episodes of conjunctivitis.

RECOGNIZING SUBLINGUAL VARICOSITIES

The small, purplish or blue-black round swellings shown here may appear under the tongue with aging. Although these dilations of the lingual veins usually have no clinical significance, they may be evidence of iron deficiency anemia.

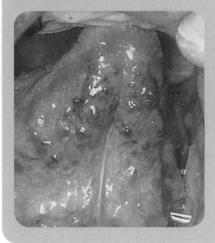

- When you inspect the corneas, you may note lipid deposits on the periphery, known as *arcus senilis*. In people who are age 50 or older, these deposits usually have no pathologic effect. The cornea also flattens with age, sometimes causing astigmatism. (See *Recognizing arcus senilis*, page 69.)

- Inspect the pupils. Note and compare pupil size, shape, and reaction to light. Both pupils should respond equally. An older adult's pupils may be abnormally small if he's taking medication to treat glaucoma. If the patient had an intraocular lens implanted in the pupillary space after cataract removal, his pupil may have an irregular shape. Cataracts readily appear as opacification in the pupil and may obscure the transmission of light to the macula.

IDENTIFYING EYELID CHANGES

The following eyelid changes may occur at any time, but they're more common in adults older than age 60.

Ectropion

Ectropion is the outward turning (eversion) of the eyelid. Involutional ectropion— the most common form— usually results from an age-related weakness in the lid. This condition results from loss of tone and usually affects the entire lower lid, although it can also affect the upper lid. Ectropion increases the risk of dry eye and infections; in severe cases, the patient may require corrective surgery.

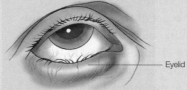

Eyelid turns inward

Ptosis

In ptosis, the eyelid losses elasticity, resulting in a droopy appearance. The condition can affect one or both eyes, and can result in loss of vision, headaches, and eyebrow strain. As the problem progresses, the patient may have to lift his eyelid manually to see out from under the drooping lid. The patient may need corrective surgery to relieve the uncomfortable symptoms.

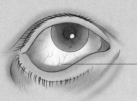

Weakness in the eyelid causes the outward turning of the eyelid

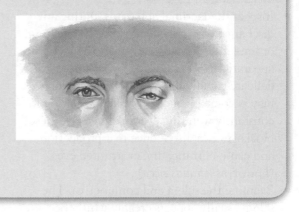

Entropion

Entropion is the inward turning (inversion) of the eyelid. It may occur in one or both eyes and in either the upper or lower eyelid. Like ectropion, it occurs more commonly in the lower eyelid. Entropion can cause redness and pain around the eye and increased sensitivity to light and wind. This increased sensitivity can cause excessive tearing, which can diminish vision. The sagging of the skin about the eye can be corrected with surgery if the symptoms are uncomfortable or if the patient is at increased risk for infection from continual eye irritation.

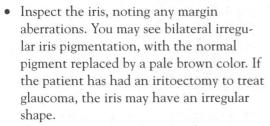

- Inspect the iris, noting any margin aberrations. You may see bilateral irregular iris pigmentation, with the normal pigment replaced by a pale brown color. If the patient has had an iritoectomy to treat glaucoma, the iris may have an irregular shape.
- Test visual acuity with and without corrective lenses, noting any differences.
- Perform an ophthalmoscopic examination to inspect internal eye structures. You may have trouble seeing these structures in a patient with senile miosis; to improve visualization, use a bright light in a dimly lit room. During the examination, observe for larger, dark red veins; small, bright red arteries; a yellowish, oval optic disk; and an avascular macula. You may also see background eye changes, characteristic of diseases common in older people. When you examine the macula with the ophthalmoscope, you may note that the foveal reflex isn't as bright as in younger patients, a normal finding.

Ears

- Inspect the auricle, observing for color and temperature changes, discharge, or lesions, and palpate for tenderness. Inspect the internal ear structures with an otoscope. Examine the external canal and tympanic membrane and watch for the light reflex. Note any lesion, bulging of the tympanic membrane, cerumen accumulation, or (in an older male) hair growth.
- Inspection and palpation of the auricles and surrounding areas should yield the same findings as in younger adults, with the exception of the normally hairy tragus in older men. Examination with the otoscope should yield similar results. Remember that the eardrum in some older adults may normally appear dull and retracted instead of pearl gray, but this can also be a clinically significant sign. Cerumen buildup may make otoscopic examination impossible until the ears are cleaned.
- To detect hearing loss early in an older person, always perform the Weber's and Rinne tuning fork tests. The Rinne test is normal if the patient hears the air-conducted tone twice as long as the bone-conducted tone, with air conduction about equal in both ears. Weber's test is normal if the patient hears the tone equally well in both ears. If the patient has hearing loss in one ear, the tone will sound louder in that ear because bone conducts the tone to the ear.
- Evaluate the patient's ability to hear and understand speech, in case you need to recommend rehabilitative therapy.
- If the patient wears a hearing aid, inspect it carefully for proper functioning. Check how well the aid fits. Examine the ear-piece, sound tube, and any connecting tubing for cracks and for the presence of dust, cerumen, or other sound-obstructing

RECOGNIZING ARCUS SENILIS

In older adults, arcus senilis, caused by lipid deposits deep along the edge of the cornea, may appear as a gray arc around the cornea. This condition is considered a normal part of aging; it isn't necessarily related to high cholesterol, and it doesn't affect vision or require treatment.

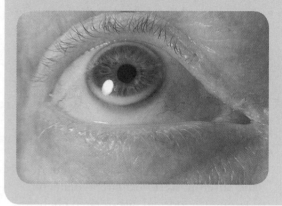

matter. Make sure the batteries are installed correctly. If the patient tells you that sounds are fluttery or garbled when he uses the hearing aid, the aid may not be functioning properly.

- Suspect presbycusis if an older adult complains of gradual hearing loss over many years but has no history of ear disorders or severe generalized disease. The patient's family or friends may report that he doesn't listen and that they frequently have to repeat themselves. In most people, the physical examination shows no abnormalities of the ear canal or eardrum.
- If the patient has a history of vertigo, ear pain, or nausea, suspect some condition other than presbycusis. Any hearing or vestibular function abnormality requires immediate referral for audiometric testing.

Neck

- Inspect the neck, looking for scars, masses, and asymmetry. If you see any evident masses, gently palpate them, noting consistency, size, shape, mobility, and tenderness. Repeat this for the lymph nodes.

• Check the trachea for alignment. The trachea is normally located midline at the suprasternal notch. Note displacement and the presence of masses.

• Inspect the thyroid gland while the patient takes a sip of water. Note masses or bulging. Normally, the thyroid is invisible. Next, try to palpate the thyroid, which normally isn't palpable. Note any masses, nodules, or enlargement.

Chest and respiratory system

• Inspect the chest's shape and symmetry anteriorly and posteriorly. Examine the anteroposterior-to-lateral diameter. Despite the normal, age-related change in anteroposterior-to-lateral diameter, an older patient's thorax should be symmetrical.

• Look for rib retraction along the intercostal spaces as the patient inhales deeply, and see if the intercostal spaces bulge as he exhales. An older patient with asthma or emphysema, secondary to chronic obstructive pulmonary disease, will typically show intercostal retraction or bulging. During respirations, listen for inspiratory or expiratory wheezes, which may be audible from the oral airways.

• Palpate the anterior and posterior chest for tenderness, masses, or lumps. Localized tenderness over the costochondral junctions suggests costochondritis, a common cause of chest pain in older patients. Palpating for diaphragmatic excursion may be difficult because of loose skin covering the older adult's chest, so when you position your hands, slide them toward his spine, raising loose skin folds between your thumbs and the spine. Excursion should be symmetrical,

but lung expansion may be reduced in an older patient because of decreased elasticity of the rib cage.

• Palpate the anterior and posterior chest symmetrically for tactile fremitus: it's usually most evident near the tracheal bifurcation. Percuss each of the patient's lung fields anteriorly and posteriorly, from apex to base. Make sure you percuss symmetrically for comparison. Normal lung fields will sound resonant, and bony prominences, organs, or consolidated tissue will sound dull. When you percuss the chest, remember that loss of elastic recoil capability in an older person stretches the alveoli and bronchioles, producing hyperresonance. Auscultate each lung from apex to base, both anteriorly and posteriorly. Make sure you assess the right middle lobe as well. Ask the patient to take deep breaths, in and out, with his mouth open.

• During auscultation, carefully observe how well the patient tolerates the examination. He may tire easily because of low tolerance or oxygen deficits. Also, taking deep breaths during auscultation may produce light-headedness or syncope faster than in a younger person, so advise the patient to take breaths slowly. You may hear diminished sounds at the lung bases because the alveoli of an older adult have lost their elasticity, causing them to collapse during normal breathing. Consequently, the lungs only partially inflate at rest. You may also hear rales due to the collection of fluid resulting from this collapse. These moist breath sounds shouldn't be mistaken as a sign of congestive heart failure. Bronchial or tubular breath sounds may also be heard over the trachea, especially in a debilitated or bedridden patient.

• In the absence of disease, crackles at the bases can be attributed to reduced mobility.

If you hear crackles, ask the patient to cough. Crackles secondary to heart failure won't clear with coughing, but crackles caused by physical immobility may clear. An older adult with pulmonary fibrosis or interstitial lung disease commonly exhibits "Velcro-type" crackles. Rhonchi or wheezes signify bronchospasm and require further evaluation.

- If the patient shows evidence of adventitious breath sounds with dullness on percussion, check for consolidation, and then check for egophony to help confirm consolidation.

- During your assessment, keep in mind that older adults have a greater risk of developing respiratory disorders than do younger adults. Also, they may not experience the same signs and symptoms as younger people. (See *Recognizing respiratory disorders in the older adult*.)

Cardiovascular system

- Inspect and palpate the point of maximal impulse (PMI). In a young person, the PMI is located around the fifth or sixth left intercostal space at the midclavicular line. In an older person, the PMI may be displaced downward to the left.

- Using the ball of your hand, palpate over the aortic, pulmonic, and mitral areas for thrills, heaves, or vibrations. You may detect a palpable thrill in a person with valvular heart disease.

- Auscultate the heart over the aortic, pulmonic, tricuspid, and mitral areas as well as Erb's point. Listen for S_1 and S_2 over each area, noting the intensity and splitting of S_1. Also listen for extra diastolic heart sounds, S_3 and S_4, which you may be able to detect in an older adult. An S_3 heart sound occurs between S_1 and S_2, usually at the lower sternal border, and indicates ventricular

> ### RECOGNIZING RESPIRATORY DISORDERS IN THE OLDER ADULT
>
> Because chest muscles normally weaken with age, older adults typically have more trouble clearing secretions. As a result, they're at increased risk for developing pneumonia, tuberculosis, and other respiratory diseases. Adults who smoked for several years are at even greater risk.
>
> When you assess older adults for respiratory disorders, keep in mind that they may present with different signs and symptoms than younger adults. For instance, older adults with pneumonia may not have an increase in temperature. Instead, primary signs might be confusion and a slightly increased respiratory rate. Similarly, the classic signs of tuberculosis—a positive skin test, fever, night sweats, and hemoptysis—usually don't appear in older adults with the disease. Instead, they may experience weight loss and anorexia, signs easily mistaken for a GI disorder or cancer.

decompensation. In an older adult, S_3 isn't a reliable indicator of heart failure; it may be physiologic or it may occur in response to an increased diastolic flow. An S_4 heart sound occurs after S_2 and before S_1; it's most audible over the heart's apex.

- Auscultate for cardiac murmurs, keeping in mind that a murmur doesn't necessarily indicate an abnormality. If you hear one, note where it sounds the loudest.

- Listen to the heart over the apex, counting for 1 full minute and noting the rate and rhythm. You may note atrial fibrillation, a common rhythm abnormality exhibited as an irregular rhythm, or such other abnormal findings as bradycardia or tachycardia. Widespread variations in rhythm are common among older people.

- Assess the vessels of the head, neck, trunk, and extremities. Palpate the carotid arteries one at a time, pressing lightly to avoid obliterating the carotid pulse. Don't palpate both at once; doing so could cause bradycardia. Because of increased baroreceptor sensitivity, as well as atherosclerotic changes in the vessels, palpating the carotid arteries can cause the arterial lumen to narrow (the pulse may be more difficult to palpate). Note the rate, rhythm, strength, and equality of both pulses.

- Auscultate each carotid artery for bruits, high-pitched sounds that indicate a narrowing of either the arterial or venous lumen.
- Assess for jugular vein distention. To do so, identify the level of venous pulsation and measure its height in relation to the sternal angle. A height exceeding 1¼″ (3 cm) is considered abnormal and indicates right-sided heart failure.
- Palpate the peripheral arteries, paying attention to the rate, rhythm, strength, and equality of pulses. Also note the presence of any bruits. In the older adult, expect arteries to be tortuous and appear kinked; they also may feel stiffer than those of a young person. Even so, the pulses should be symmetrical in strength.
- Inspect the patient's legs, noting color, temperature, presence or lack of hair, edema, trophic changes of the toes, and varicosities. Tight, shiny skin (without edema) and demarcated hair loss—possibly combined with pain, pallor, pulselessness, decreased temperature, paresthesia, or paralysis—may indicate arterial insufficiency. Note any color variations, including pallor, erythema, or pink, red, mottled, cyanotic, or brawny discoloration. If you see pallor with cyanotic or mottled discoloration, the patient may have arterial insufficiency. Brawny discoloration points to long-standing chronic venous insufficiency. The patient shouldn't have any significant color deterioration that's attributable to age alone.
- Using the ball of your hand, assess the temperature of the extremities; it should

feel equal bilaterally. A feeling of heat may indicate thrombosis, but this response may be reduced in an older adult.
- Assess for edema over bony prominences or the sacrum. It's typically more pronounced in the most dependent body areas. Ascertain if the edema is pitting or nonpitting, and grade the degree. If you do find edema, the patient will need further evaluation to determine the cause.

GI system

- Begin your assessment of the older adult's GI system as you would any other person's assessment: Inspect the abdomen, noting shape, symmetry, scars, masses, pulsations, distention, or striae. The abdomen contour may be obese, scaphoid, or distended.
- Auscultate all four quadrants for bowel sounds. Listen over the abdominal aorta and renal arteries for bruits with the bell of your stethoscope.
- Percuss the abdomen to determine the presence of air or fluid, liver size, and bladder distention. Air in the large bowel will sound tympanic; fluid will sound dull. Keep in mind that bowel obstruction can occur secondary to long-standing fecal impaction. On percussion, this presents as a distended and tympanic abdomen. If the bowel is impacted, percussion will reveal dullness.
- Percuss the liver. The normal liver size at the midclavicular line is 2¼″ to 4¾″ (5.7 to 12 cm) in diameter. Also, percuss over the symphysis pubis toward the umbilicus, noting any change in percussion. Dullness in this area may indicate bladder distention.
- Palpate the belly, noting masses or tenderness on light or deep palpation. Watch for peritoneal signs, such as rigidity or rebound tenderness. Masses in the lower quadrants may be impacted stool. Try to palpate the liver; normally it isn't palpable. If you notice

tenderness in the epigastric region, the patient may have gastroesophageal reflux disease or a hiatal hernia.

- Palpate the abdomen—usually easier and more accurate than palpating the belly in an older patient because his abdominal wall is typically thinner (from muscle wasting and loss of fibroconnective tissue) and his muscle tone more relaxed. A rigid abdomen occurs less commonly in elderly patients; abdominal distention is more common.

Genitourinary system

- Use the same basic assessment techniques to assess an older adult's genitourinary system as you would with a younger patient. Keep in mind that, because of degenerative changes affecting body functions, an older person is more susceptible to certain renal disorders than a younger adult. Susceptibility to infection, for example, increases with age, and kidney infection from obstruction is a common cause of hospitalization in older adults. An immobilized older person is especially vulnerable to infection from urinary stasis or poor personal hygiene. A urinary tract infection in an older adult is typically asymptomatic, or the symptoms are vague and ill defined; if untreated, it may progress to renal failure.
- Assess for the combination of frequent urination, urgency, incontinence, urine retention, and infection in an older woman. These may point to cystocele, which can result from poor musculature from childbearing and from aging. Obstruction in older women may result from uterine prolapse or pelvic cancer.
- Assess both men and women for urinary frequency, dysuria, and hematuria, signs of bladder cancer. Remember that older adults have a higher cancer risk and that bladder

is more common after age 50 and more prevalent in men than in women.

- Assess the older male patient for obstructed urine flow, which can result from the prostate gland enlarging enough to compress the urethra and sometimes the bladder. Almost all men over age 50 have some degree of prostatic enlargement, but obstructed urine flow can signal benign prostatic hyperplasia (BPH) or possibly advanced prostatic cancer. Untreated BPH can impair renal function, causing urinary hesitancy, intermittence, straining, and a reduction in the urine stream's diameter and force. Continued enlargement of the gland causes increased urinary frequency and nocturia, possibly with hematuria. Keep in mind these signs and symptoms may also result from another urinary system disorder, and some commonly used medications, such as OTC diphenhydramine (Benadryl), can also decrease the flow of urine in men.
- Inspect the older male patient's genitalia, including the pubic hair, glans of the uncircumcised penis, penile shaft, and scrotum. Look for bulging masses, lesions, inflammation, edema, or discoloration. Palpate lesions, noting size, shape, consistency, and tenderness. Pubic hair becomes sparse and gray with age.
- Palpate the male patient's testes for size, shape, consistency and tenderness. In an older adult, the testes are usually slightly smaller than adult size. They should be equal, smooth, freely movable, and soft without nodules. Inspect and palpate the inguinal canal; bulging is abnormal and needs further evaluation.
- When assessing the genitalia of a female patient, inspect the perineum for rash, lesions, or nodules. Examine the area for color, size, and shape. Inspect the vaginal

orifice and observe for bulging of tissues or organs.

- Perform an internal pelvic examination on a female patient, if qualified. Take care to maximize the patient's comfort, because the atrophic changes of the vaginal mucosa in the older female increase her discomfort during the pelvic examination. When you begin, remember to use a small speculum because of the decreased vaginal size in an older woman. To facilitate insertion, dampen the speculum with warm water; don't use a lubricant because it may alter Papanicolaou (Pap) test results. Proceed slowly; abrupt insertion of the speculum can damage sensitive degenerating tissue. When you perform the bimanual examination, remember that the ovaries usually regress with age, and you may not be able to palpate them. Obtain a Pap test to screen for cervical cancer.
- To examine the rectum, place the female patient in a side-lying position and ask the male patient to bend over. Inspect the anus and overall skin surface characteristics. The area should be smooth and uninterrupted, with coarse skin and slightly increased pigmented areas around the anus. Note masses, nodules, lesions, or hemorrhoids.
- To palpate the rectum, use a gloved, lubricated finger, noting muscle tone. After withdrawing the finger, test any stool for blood. For males, assess the prostate gland. Note the size, consistency, shape, surface, and symmetry, and record any tenderness. Slide the gloved, lubricated finger down the center of the walnut-shaped gland and then out to each side, feeling for any fullness or hard nodular areas. The gland should feel firm, not boggy, to the touch and should be round, soft, nontender, free from

masses, and about ¾" to 1½" (2 to 4 cm) in diameter.

Musculoskeletal system

- When assessing the older patient's musculoskeletal system, note any limitations in the patient's range of motion (ROM), difficulty ambulating, and diffused or localized joint pain. Throughout the assessment, remember that an older patient may need more time or assistance with tests, such as ROM or gait assessment, because of weakness and decreased coordination. Watch for signs of motor and sensory dysfunction, including weakness, spasticity, tremors, rigidity, and various types of sensory disturbances. Keep in mind that an uncertain gait and balance problems may cause damaging falls. Make sure you differentiate gait changes caused by joint disability, pain, or stiffness from those caused by neurologic impairment or another disorder.
- Observe the patient's walk, noting gait and posture. Gait reflects the integration of reflexes as well as motor function. An older adult tends to take smaller steps, reduce the height of his steps, reduce his arm swing, and flex his elbows and knees. Gait disorders may occur if the patient limps or drags a foot from paresis. Posture may reveal kyphotic changes of the spine. To avoid injury, the patient with this condition must compensate by tilting his head back.
- Assess static balance and station by gently pushing on the patient's shoulders while he's standing. The normal response includes bending at the waist, knees, ankles, and shoulders to create a forward flexion of the body. An abnormal response, in which the patient falls forward without bending, may indicate musculoskeletal or neurologic dysfunction.

- Observe the patient's tandem walking for exaggerated ataxia, and to observe the position of the head and neck in relation to the shoulders and legs. Note whether the patient turns quickly and whether his head, neck, and shoulders move as one unit or separately.
- To assess calf and ankle muscles for weakness, have the patient walk on his toes and then on his heels. Observe his spine from the side. Assess the height of the hips; hips should be equally aligned. People who have had hip fractures or hip surgery may have a shortened leg.
- Elicit Romberg's sign to evaluate posture and balance; it's positive if the patient sways. Inspect the joints of the hands, wrists, elbows, shoulders, neck, hips, knees, and ankles. Note joint enlargement, swelling, tenderness, crepitus, temperature changes, or deformities. A person with degenerative joint disease will complain of pain with motion and have enlarged joints from bone changes, ROM stiffness, tenderness, crepitus, joint deformities, and palpable osteophytes.
- Assess the foot for common deformities. These include hallux valgus, prolapsed metatarsals, and hammer toes.
- Inspect each muscle group for atrophy, fasciculations, involuntary movements, and tremor. Move the joints through passive ROM exercises, and palpate the muscles for tone and strength. Note any crepitus during the ROM exercises. Resistance to passive ROM indicates hypertonicity, whereas flaccidity indicates hypotonicity.
- Assess for rigidity and spasticity. You can most easily detect rigidity in the wrist or elbow joint. Cogwheel rigidity typically occurs secondary to diseases involving the basal ganglia and as an adverse effect of certain neuroleptic drugs.
- Throughout the physical examination, ask the patient to show you how he buttons or zips his clothing, allowing you to directly observe his ability to perform selected ADLs. Observe him grasping items, such as a doorknob or water faucet.

Neurologic system

- Use the same techniques for a neurologic examination of an older adult as you would for a younger adult. However, keep in mind that you'll usually detect an alteration in one or more senses in an older patient. Your examination should include assessment of the following: LOC or awareness level, affect and mood, cognition, orientation, speech, general knowledge, memory, reasoning, object recognition and higher cognitive functions, cranial nerves, motor and sensory systems, and reflexes.
- Begin by observing the patient's general appearance, including mood, affect, and grooming. Note whether he's appropriately dressed, responds appropriately to questions, and is oriented to time, place, and person. Changes in the environment, such as admission to an acute care facility, can cause marked confusion in an older person who was previously alert and oriented.
- Note the patient's affect. A flat affect signals a disorder of the basal ganglia such as Parkinson's disease. An older patient who seems depressed may require further evaluation; several assessment tools are available, including the Geriatric Depression Scale. (See *Using the Geriatric Depression Scale*, page 57.)
- Note the patient's speech. Speech disorders usually occur in response to circulatory

disorders; you can readily detect them during casual conversation.

- Assess vocabulary and general knowledge level by discussing current news items or family events.
- Assess the patient's memory—his immediate, recent, and remote recall. Assess immediate recall by naming a certain number of objects or reciting a group of numbers and having the patient repeat them back immediately. To elicit recent memory, ask the patient about events that occurred in the past 24 to 48 hours. For remote memory, ask the patient to recall significant events that occurred many years ago.
- Assess the patient's ability to reason. Ask him questions requiring judgment, insight, and abstraction.
- Assess object recognition. Point to two objects and ask the patient to identify each. The response is graded as normal or agnosia (the inability to name objects). Several screening tools assess an older adult's cognitive status, including the Mini-Cog test (discussed in chapter 2), a quick screening tool that tests attention, recall, and language.

Cranial nerves

Assess each cranial nerve sequentially, beginning with cranial nerve I and progressing to cranial nerve XII. Few changes occur among older adults as a normal byproduct of aging, except for the following:

- Olfactory nerve (I)—progressive loss of smell
- Optic nerve (II)—decreased visual acuity, presbyopia, and limited peripheral vision
- Facial nerve (VII)—decreased perception of taste, particularly sweet and salty; drooping or relaxation of the muscles in the forehead and around the eyes and mouth

- Auditory nerve (VIII)—presbycusis or loss of high-tone hearing, later generalized to all frequencies
- Glossopharyngeal nerve (IX)—sluggish or absent gag reflex
- Hypoglossal nerve (XII)—unilateral tongue weakness (may also be caused by malnutrition or structural malformation of the face).

Motor and sensory systems

- Evaluate muscle and joint function. Also assess for rapid, rhythmic, alternating movements, which determine coordination. Observe the patient for his ability to repeat maneuvers and for smoothness in execution. Expect an older person to have a reduced response speed.
- Check the patient's ability to perceive pain by using the sharp and dull end of a safety pin; temperature by using hot and cold substances; touch by using a light touch of the hand; and vibration by using a vibrating tuning fork. Also evaluate two-point discrimination and position sense. The patient should have accurate, symmetrical perception.

Reflexes

- Assess an older adult's reflexes the same way as you would for other age-groups.
- Assess the patent's plantar and Babinski's reflexes to look for indications of upper motor neuron disease. Hyperactive, diminished, or asymmetrical responses are abnormal.

Hematologic and immune systems

- Assess hematologic and immune function as you would for a younger adult. However, when obtaining certain diagnostic tests, be alert to the possibility of changes related to normal aging.

- When evaluating vital signs, remember that an older patient will have a diminished febrile response to infection.

Endocrine system

- When assessing an older patient's endocrine system, keep in mind that many endocrine disorders cause signs and symptoms in older people that resemble normal changes from aging, making endocrine disorders easily overlooked.
- Look for a combination of changes in mental status and physical deterioration, including weight loss, dry skin, and hair loss. These may point to hypothyroidism, although they may be normal changes that occur with aging.
- Determine if the patient is anxious, depressed, or apathetic; any may signal hyperthyroidism and call for further evaluation. Anxiety is the more common symptom, but hyperthyroidism can also cause depression and apathy (known as apathetic hyperthyroidism of elderly patients) in older patients.

- If the patient has signs and symptoms of heart failure or atrial fibrillation, suspect hyperthyroidism in an older patient; such a patient is more likely to initially have these signs and symptoms rather than the classic signs that typically occur in younger adults.

Accurate Assessments: A Healthy Payoff

Mastering the skills and knowledge needed to assess older patients allows you to recognize the normal changes that occur with aging. More importantly, it helps you to spot developing problems early on, when intervention can do the most good for your older patients. Understanding how the body and mind age and what signs to look for not only lets you perform thorough, accurate assessments of your older patients, it also gives you the chance to help those patients remain as healthy as possible well into their senior years.

Nutrition: The Food Factor

"Life expectancy would grow by leaps and bounds if green vegetables smelled as good as bacon."

—DOUG LARSON

How and what we eat plays a crucial role in our overall health. Eat too little, and we don't have the fuel to function. Eat too much, and we put on extra weight. Eat the wrong kinds of things, and we may not only put on extra weight, but not have the right kind of fuel for good health.

We each learn certain patterns of eating as we grow up. But by early adulthood, our bodies have finished the job of growing and maturing. At that point, we need to shift from eating to grow and become healthy adults, to eating to maintain a healthy body. We need to sustain a healthy weight and physical fitness, avoid excess weight gain, and retain or build strength.

One significant change in how people should eat as they age is in how many calories they should consume. Adults need fewer calories than growing young people, and older adults typically need even fewer calories, although general caloric requirements for adults depend on activity levels.

According to the *Dietary Guidelines for Americans 2005,* for adults ages 19 to 50 years, a sedentary man requires 2,200 to 2,600 cal/day; a moderately active man, 2,400 to 2,800 cal/day; and an active man, 2,800 to 3,000 cal/day. A sedentary woman in this age range requires 1,800 to 2,000 cal/day; a moderately active woman, 2,000 to 2,200 cal/day;

⧗ Timeline *Nutrition: Food development in the United Sta*

Over the 20th century and into the 21st, every aspect of the foods we eat has gone through changes—from food safety and regulations to how food is grown or engineered, harvested, packaged, and cooked. This timeline highlights some of the food developments that have taken place starting in the early 1900s.

1900 38% of U.S. workforce employed in agriculture

1902 Fannie Farmer opens up cooking school in Boston

1906 Food & Drugs Act and Meat Inspection Act authorize regulation of safety and quality of food

1906 Kellogg's begins manufacturing cornflakes

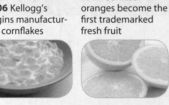

1915 A gallon of milk costs 36 cents

1916 First electric refrigerators sell for $900

1919 Sunkist oranges become the first trademarked fresh fruit

1920 Prohibition begins banning sale of alcoholic beverages

1924 Clarence Birdseye organizes first frozen food company

1926 Beef grading standards introduced by the United States Department of Agriculture

1928 Sliced bread introduced

1933 First sit-down strike in the United States held at Hormel meat packing plant in Minnesota

1936 Shopping cart invented

1942 Wartime food rationing (sugar, coffee, processed foods, meats, canned fish, cheese, canned milk, fats) begins

1945 Microwave oven patented

1900   10   20   30   40

and an active woman, 2,200 to 2,400 cal/day. As discussed later in this chapter, older adults typically require fewer calories.

What we consume also affects illness. Between ages 40 and 60, such chronic illnesses as heart disease, hypertension, arthritis, and diabetes commonly begin to develop, with more than 80% of adults over age 65 suffering from one or more of these ailments. Establishing healthy food and exercise habits, such as reducing total fat intake, eating more fruits and vegetables, and maintaining a balance of food intake and physical activity to stabilize weight, can decrease the risk of developing such chronic illnesses in later years, decrease the severity of disease when it does develop, and speed recovery time. With the increased life expectancy in the United States—more than 80% of Americans live past age 65 today compared with fewer than 50% in the early 1900s—maintaining a healthy diet over a lifetime becomes crucial.

1950 Pillsbury introduces first boxed cake mix

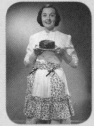

1957 Idaho overtakes Maine as the largest producer of potatoes in the United States

1959 Congress passes law enacting food stamps

1963 Irradiation introduced to sterilize fruits and vegetables

1964 Diet Pepsi debuts

1966 Ingredients list required on all packaged food items

1967 First plastic milk bottles used

1974 First bar-code checkout scanner installed in a supermarket; package of Wrigley's chewing gum first product scanned

1981 Artificial sweetener aspartame approved by the Food and Drug Administration

1982 First genetically engineered crop (tomato) developed

1990 Campbell's Soup produces 20 billionth can of tomato soup

2005 USDA confirms first domestic case of mad cow disease

2006 Fresh spinach determined to be the cause of a nationwide outbreak of *Escherichia coli* food poisoning

2008 Governor of California signs a bill banning trans fat use in California restaurants and retail food establishments

50   60   70   80   90   2000

Changing Bodies, Changing Lives—and Changing Diets

Nutritional needs change as adults grow older, largely because their tissues and organ systems are aging. Many older adults also take medications for chronic illness, which can affect nutritional needs. Changes that occur naturally in the body as it ages as well as changes from the outside, such as economic and social changes, affect nutritional needs and the older adult's ability to meet those needs.

Focus on the physical

Even after a person reaches physical adulthood at age 20, the body continues to change. For instance, the body typically continues to gradually lose lean body mass and gain adipose tissue. Some of these changes can be offset through strength training and aerobic exercise; some can't.

GI SYSTEM

Several GI changes that can occur with aging can impair an older adult's nutritional status.

- Loss of dentition, periodontal disease, and jawbone deterioration can make chewing difficult.
- Although saliva production doesn't significantly decrease in healthy older adults, dry mouth, or *xerostomia*, commonly occurs as an adverse effect of the medications that many older people take. Up to 38% of older adults experience xerostomia.
- Oral mucosa loses elasticity, epithelial cells atrophy, and blood supply to connective tissue diminishes with aging. As a result, an older person's oral mucosa becomes more friable and susceptible to infection and ulceration, especially when combined with xerostomia and vitamin deficiencies.
- Secretion of gastric digestive enzymes falls off as a person ages, making it more difficult to digest certain foods. Poor lactase secretion, for example, makes it hard to digest milk products.
- Delayed gastric emptying may cause early satiety and hunger suppression in older adults.
- Loss of lower esophageal sphincter muscle tone increases the incidence of esophageal reflux and heartburn.
- Nutrient absorption decreases as the blood supply to the intestines decreases and gastric mucosa degenerates.
- In the small intestine, muscle fibers and mucosal surfaces atrophy with age. The number of lymphatic cells decreases, the small intestine slowly loses weight, and the villi shorten and widen, ending up being more like parallel ridges than fingerlike projections. Although these changes may affect immune function and absorption of some nutrients, such as calcium and vitamin D, they don't significantly affect small intestine motility or transit time.
- In the large intestine, mucus secretion decreases and the rectal wall loses elasticity.

The older adult's perception of rectal wall distention also diminishes, which can lead to constipation because the older adult needs more volume in his large intestine before he feels the need to defecate.

METABOLISM

Metabolic rate decreases with age, but because lean body mass also decreases, the overall metabolic rate doesn't significantly decrease. However, an older adult's glucose metabolism may develop problems, resulting in glucose intolerance.

CENTRAL NERVOUS SYSTEM

Common central nervous system conditions that can prevent an older adult from eating a balanced diet include tremors, slowed reaction time, short-term memory loss, cognitive deterioration (from Alzheimer's and similar diseases), and depression.

RENAL SYSTEM

Kidneys decrease in size as an adult grows older, and by age 70, they lose about a third of their efficiency and lack functional reserve. Despite this reduction in size and efficiency, they can still maintain adequate waste removal to maintain normal blood levels. However, as blood flow decreases and new renal tissue fails to generate, the kidneys begin to lose their ability to clear nitrogenous and other waste products from the body; many older adults also develop urinary incontinence from loss of sphincter tone.

SENSES

Although some people experience more loss of sense function than others, all adults lose some sense function as they age.

- Loss of visual acuity, especially in low-light settings, begins around age 40; this can lead to an older adult not seeing well enough to prepare food or see that food is spoiled.

- The sense of smell, or olfactory function, gradually decreases.
- Taste changes occur from olfactory function loss and the loss of taste buds and saliva. Sweet and salty tastes go first, followed by bitter and sour.
- The sense of thirst becomes less acute with age, leaving older adults at risk for dehydration. Signs of dehydration in older adults include confusion and lethargy.

Looking beyond the body

Although changes in physiologic function have a profound effect on an older adult's nutritional status, don't overlook other factors during a nutritional assessment. The alterations in economic status and social situation that can occur with aging can greatly affect nutrition.

MONEY MATTERS

Many older adults live on fixed incomes, with about 20% of people over age 65 living in poverty. Such economic hardship can limit the ability to eat a well-balanced diet. For instance, an older adult who needs to watch his spending may cut meat and dairy products out of his diet because of cost, even though these foods provide protein and other important nutrients, such as iron, B vitamins, and zinc.

An older adult who relies on just social security or a pension has a greater risk for malnutrition. Some of these adults qualify for assistance but don't like to ask for help, leaving them with too little money for proper nutrition.

THE SOCIAL SCENE

The decrease in mobility, loss of sensory acuity, and development of other functional limitations that can occur with aging can all lead to social isolation. Older people also face losses as members of their peer group begin to die. Many older people in such situations may lose interest in eating, affecting their nutritional status.

Social isolation has other effects on nutrition, too. For instance, an older person who lives alone and can't drive to the store or who can't stand up long enough to prepare a meal can't maintain an adequate diet.

The situation can be even worse for institutionalized patients, who no longer have control over the quality or preparation of the food they eat and who may have more debilitating illnesses than those still living at home. Institutional food may not taste like what they're used to at home, especially for patients who are used to an ethnic diet. Even though nursing homes try to meet residents' dietary preferences and eating schedules, sometimes they can't. A patient may also be on a restricted diet or have another medical problem that limits food choices.

Encouraging family members of such residents to bring favorite foods (as allowed) when they visit and offering frequent, small meals may help increase intake for these patients. In an Alzheimer's unit, having finger foods available at all times has improved intake for patients who can't sit still long enough to eat a regular meal.

MEALS ON WHEELS

One program in particular helps address the nutritional needs of older adults who face difficulties meeting their nutritional needs at home. The Meals On Wheels Association of America operates throughout the United States, delivering one meal each weekday to older people who can't shop or prepare their own food.

According to Meals On Wheels, over 5 million senior citizens (11.4% of all senior citizens) have experienced some form of food insecurity. Of these, about 2.5 million were at risk of hunger, and about 750,000 suffered from

MODIFIED MyPyramid FOR OLDER ADULTS

Use this food pyramid, designed specifically for older adults, to choose the right kinds and right amounts of foods each day.

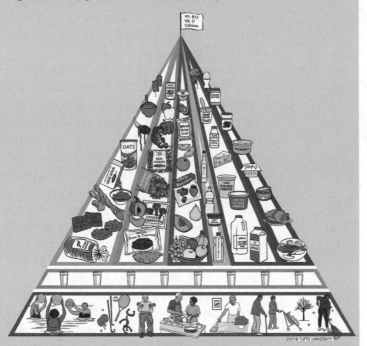

Used with permission. © 2007, Tufts University.

limited mobility, concerns about safety, or lack of money. Projections estimate that by 2025, 9.5 million older Americans will experience some form of food insecurity, 3.9 million will be at risk of hunger, and 1 million will suffer from hunger.

Meeting nutritional needs

The *Dietary Guidelines for Americans 2005* includes recommendations for older adults. Not surprisingly, nutritional requirements change as a person ages, with older adults having some different requirements for calories, protein, carbohydrates, fat, vitamins, and minerals than younger adults.

COUNTING CALORIES

As the body ages, caloric needs diminish and lean muscle mass decreases, although nutrient requirements may stay the same. A particular older adult's exact calorie requirements depend on his degree of mobility, overall health, level of fitness, and any illnesses he may have.

According to the *Dietary Guidelines for Americans 2005* for adults age 51 and older, a sedentary man requires 2,000 to 2,200 cal/day; a moderately active man, 2,200 to 2,400 cal/day; and an active man, 2,400 to 2,800 cal/day. A sedentary woman in this age range requires 1,600 cal/day; a moderately active woman, 1,800 cal/day; and an active woman, 2,000 to 2,200 cal/day. (See *Modified MyPyramid for older adults*.)

hunger because of financial constraints. Those at greater risk for hunger included people with limited incomes, those under age 70, African-Americans, Hispanics, people who had never married, renters, and people living in the South.

Despite these statistics, keep in mind that hunger occurs at all income levels and in all ethnic groups. Living in a rural area increases the risk for malnutrition, for instance. But an older adult in the city may live right across the street from a grocery store and still not shop there because of

PROTEIN: THE POWER SOURCE

Protein helps maintain muscle strength, fight infections, and renew the body's cells. An older adult typically has the same need for protein as a younger adult; he may even need slightly more protein to compensate for the loss of lean body tissue. The recommended daily allowance (RDA) for protein in a healthy adult is 0.8 g/kg body weight/day. An adult over age 65 typically needs slightly more—1.0 g/kg body weight/day—to maintain a positive nitrogen balance.

Good sources of dietary protein include poultry four times a week, fish twice a week, and red meat once or twice a week. Eggs, cheese, and legumes (including peas, beans, and lentils) provide alternative sources of protein. Up to 14% of an older adult's total calories should come from proteins.

If an older patient has trouble chewing, suggest adding protein supplements—such as instant breakfast drinks, peanut butter, yogurt, or health food store supplements or commercial supplemental products such as Ensure—to the diet. A patient with impaired GI tract functioning or who takes medications that interfere with amino acid and micronutrient absorption may also need more protein.

CARBOHYDRATES: ENERGY BOOSTERS

The body's main source of energy, carbohydrates should compose 55% to 60% of an older adult's daily calories. Carbohydrates can be simple or complex; indigestible fiber is also a type of complex carbohydrate. A diet high in complex carbohydrates and fiber helps lower cholesterol; those with diabetes in particular benefit from a high-fiber, high–complex carbohydrate diet.

Simple carbohydrates

Simple carbohydrates (sucrose) come from white sugar, fruit sugar, and lactose in milk. Although the body can easily break down simple carbohydrates as a ready source of energy, they're typically calorie-dense, making them a less healthy choice than complex carbohydrates.

Complex carbohydrates

Complex carbohydrates must be broken down by the body into simple sugars before the body can use them, a process that takes time and energy. Complex carbohydrates are found in vitamin- and mineral-rich vegetables and grains, making them a good dietary choice.

Fiber

Dietary fiber is an indigestible complex carbohydrate present in certain foods. Older adults should consume between 25 and 30 grams of fiber each day. Fiber-rich foods combined with regular activity and adequate water intake help older adults maintain normal bowel function; too little dietary fiber may contribute to the development of large-bowel cancer.

For an older adult who doesn't have much fiber in his diet, suggest a gradual increase in fiber intake because a sudden increase can cause diarrhea, cramps, flatulence, or constipation. Keep in mind that an older adult's intestines may not readily tolerate rough fiber such as nuts. Recommend instead vegetables, fruits, and whole-grain cereals, which he's more likely to tolerate. To readily increase fiber in the diet, especially bulk-forming fiber, suggest switching from white to whole-grain breads and eating high-fiber cereal for breakfast.

Nutrition A Guide to Types of Fat

The chart below lists the types of fat found in foods. It can serve as a guide to making healthier food choices.

Type of fat	Source	Examples
Saturated fatty acids	Animal fats and some vegetable oils (usually solid at room temperature)	Meat, poultry, butter, and palm oil
Trans fatty acids	Vegetable oils that have been processed into margarine or shortening	Margarines and shortening, baked goods, snack foods
Monounsaturated fatty acids	Vegetable oils (usually liquid at room temperature)	Olive, peanut, and canola oils
Polyunsaturated fatty acids	Seafood and vegetable oils (soft or liquid at room temperature)	Corn, sunflower, safflower, canola, and linolic oils
Omega-3 fatty acids	Fatty fish	Tuna, salmon, herring, and mackerel

FAT: A LITTLE GOES A LONG WAY

Like carbohydrates, dietary fats provide energy. Fats also help absorb fat-soluble vitamins and essential fatty acids, add flavor to food, and provide a sense of fullness (satiation) to a meal. The potential drawback: Fats have twice as many calories per gram as carbohydrates.

Fats are categorized by their source. Saturated fats come from animals, and eating too much can lead to high serum cholesterol levels. Polyunsaturated and monounsaturated fats come from vegetables, and omega-3 fatty acids come from fatty fish. Although unsaturated fats are a better dietary choice than saturated fats, fat intake still should range only from 10% to 30% of an older adult's daily calorie intake. (See *A guide to types of fat*.)

VITAMINS: THE GREAT FACILITATORS

Although vitamins are organic compounds, they can also be produced synthetically. Vitamins don't provide energy themselves, but they play a crucial role in how the body uses major nutrients, such as protein, carbohydrates,

and fats. The body itself can't produce enough vitamins for proper functioning, so the rest must come from food. The body absorbs fat-soluble vitamins (A, D, E, and K) in different portions of the small intestine and water-soluble vitamins (B, C, biotin, folic acid, and pantothenic acid) throughout the GI tract. (See *Guide to vitamins*.)

An older adult with a vitamin deficiency—for instance, a person whose food choices fall short of the ideal—can develop a variety of problems, such as night blindness from a lack of vitamin A. Such a person may benefit from taking a daily multivitamin. If the older adult is also a member of a special population, such as a smoker, he may need further supplementation. (See *Vitamin deficiencies in the older adult*, page 88, and *Vitamin supplementation for older adults and special populations*, page 88.)

MINERALS: BUILDING AND BALANCING

Unlike vitamins, which are organic, minerals are simple inorganic substances widely

GUIDE TO VITAMINS

Good health requires intake of adequate amounts of vitamins to meet the body's metabolic needs. A vitamin excess or deficiency, although rare, can lead to various disorders. The chart below reviews major functions and food sources of vitamins.

VITAMINS	MAJOR FUNCTIONS	FOOD SOURCES
Water-soluble Vitamins		
Vitamin B_1 (thiamine)	Appetite stimulation, blood building, carbohydrate metabolism, circulation, digestion, growth, learning ability, muscle tone maintenance	Meat, fish, poultry, pork, molasses, brewer's yeast, brown rice, nuts, wheat germ, whole and enriched grains
Vitamin B_2 (riboflavin)	Antibody and red blood cell (RBC) formation; energy metabolism; cell respiration; epithelial, ocular, and mucosal tissue maintenance	Meat, fish, poultry, milk, molasses, brewer's yeast, eggs, fruit, green leafy vegetables, nuts, whole grains
Vitamin B_3 (niacin)	Circulation, cholesterol level reduction, growth, hydrochloric acid production, metabolism (carbohydrate, protein, fat), sex hormone production	Eggs, lean meat, milk products, organ meat, peanuts, poultry, seafood, whole grains
Vitamin B_6 (pyridoxine)	Antibody formation, digestion, deoxyribonucleic acid and ribonucleic acid synthesis, fat and protein utilization, amino acid metabolism, hemoglobin production	Meat, poultry, bananas, molasses, brewer's yeast, desiccated liver, fish, green leafy vegetables, peanuts, raisins, walnuts, wheat germ, whole grains
Vitamin B_{12} (cobalamin)	Blood cell formation, cellular and nutrient metabolism, iron absorption, tissue growth, nerve cell maintenance	Beef, eggs, fish, milk products, organ meat, pork
Vitamin C (ascorbic acid)	Collagen production, digestion, fine bone and tooth formation, iodine conservation, healing, RBC formation, infection resistance	Fresh fruits and vegetables, especially citrus fruits and green leafy vegetables
Biotin	Cell growth, fatty acid production, metabolism, vitamin B utilization, skin, hair, nerve, and bone marrow maintenance	Egg yolks, legumes, organ meats, whole grains, yeast, milk, and seafood
Folate (folic acid)	Cell growth and reproduction, hydrochloric acid production, liver function, nucleic acid formation, protein metabolism, RBC formation	Citrus fruits, eggs, green leafy vegetables, milk products, organ meat, seafood, whole grains
Pantothenic acid	Antibody formation, cortisone production, growth stimulation, stress tolerance, vitamin utilization, conversion of carbohydrates, fats, and protein	Eggs, legumes, mushrooms, organ meats, salmon, wheat germ, whole grains, fresh vegetables, yeast
Fat-soluble Vitamins		
Vitamin A (retinol)	Body tissue repair and maintenance, infection resistance, bone growth, nervous system development, cell membrane metabolism and structure	Fish, green and yellow fruits and vegetables, milk products
Vitamin D (calciferol)	Calcium and phosphorus metabolism (bone formation), myocardial function, nervous system maintenance, normal blood clotting	Bonemeal, egg yolks, organ meat, butter, cod liver oil, fatty fish
Vitamin E (tocopherol)	Aging retardation, anticoagulation, diuresis, fertility, lung protection (antipollution), male potency, muscle and nerve cell membrane maintenance, myocardial perfusion, serum cholesterol reduction	Butter, dark green vegetables, eggs, fruits, nuts, organ meat, vegetable oils, wheat germ
Vitamin K (menadione)	Liver synthesis of prothrombin and other blood-clotting factors	Green leafy vegetables, safflower oil, yogurt, liver, molasses

---

🍎 *Nutrition* | Vitamin Deficiencies in the Older Adult

The chart below details the signs and symptoms of deficiencies of important vitamins and the effect of such deficiencies on the body's ability to function.

Deficient Vitamin	Signs and Symptoms	Effect on Body Functioning
A	• Dry skin • Poor wound healing • Night blindness	Abnormal visual adaptation to darkness, and decreased resistance to infections
B_6	• Nausea • Vomiting • Loss of appetite • Dermatitis • Motor weakness • Dizziness • Depression • Sore tongue	Neurologic and immunologic difficulties
B_{12}	• Vomiting • Fatigue • Constipation • Anemia • Decreased memory • Depression	Neurologic changes that affect sensation, balance, and memory
C	• Weakness • Dry mouth • Skin changes	Delayed tissue healing
D	• Weakness • Gait disturbance • Pain	Excessive bone demineralization or osteoporosis

---

VITAMIN SUPPLEMENTATION FOR OLDER ADULTS AND SPECIAL POPULATIONS

Even though vitamin supplements can't compete with the array of vitamins, minerals, and fibers found in foods, many older patients may benefit from vitamin supplements. If an older patient is also part of a special population—for instance, if he also smokes—he may need additional supplements.

Older Patients

Older patients may have an increased need for vitamins because of chronic disease, adverse effects of medication, illness, poor chewing and swallowing, physical limitations, or a decreased sense of smell or taste. Absorption of vitamin B_{12} and synthesis of vitamin D decrease with ageing. Research has shown that a multivitamin and mineral supplement may improve immune function.

Alcoholics

Alcohol alters vitamin absorption, metabolism, and excretion. Nutrients that may be affected include riboflavin, niacin, thiamine, folate, and pantothenic acid.

Smokers

Smokers require more vitamin C than nonsmokers. If these patients don't consume enough vitamin C in their diet, they may need a supplement.

Dieters and Particular Eaters

People who consume less than 1,200 calories a day have difficulty getting the necessary nutrients for a healthy diet. Those who eliminate specific food groups from their diet, such as vegans and people with food intolerances or allergies, also may not take in the needed nutrients.

Nutrition — Dietary Reference Intakes for Adults Age 51 and Older

The Dietary Reference Intakes (DRIs), which are repacing the Recommended Daily Allowances (RDAs), have higher reference values for older adults for several nutrients and vitamins.

Nutrient	Men		Women	
	51 to 70 years	>70 years	51 to 70 years	>70 years
Calcium (mg/d)	1,200	1,200	1,200	1,200
Phosphorus (mg/d)	700	700	700	700
Magnesium (mg/d)	420	420	320	320
Fluoride (mg/d)	3.8	3.8	3.1	3.1
Vitamin D (µg/d)	10	15	10	15
Thiamin (mg/d)	1.2	1.2	1.1	1.1
Riboflavin (mg/d)	1.3	1.3	1.1	1.1
Niacin (mg/d)	16	16	14	14
Vitamin B_6 (mg/d)	1.7	1.7	1.5	1.5
Folate (µg/d)	400	400	400	400
Vitamin B_{12} (µg/d)	2.4	2.4	2.4	2.4

Adapted from "Position of the American Dietetic Association: Nutrition, Aging, and the Continuum of Care," *Journal of the American Dietetic Association* 100(5):580-95, May 2000. Used with permission of Elsevier.

distributed in nature. They play a role in promoting growth and maintaining health.

Calcium

Calcium is normally retained in bones, with a small amount found in the tissues and blood. With aging and immobility, bones tend to lose calcium, resulting in osteoporosis. In certain diseases, calcium leaves the bones and enters the bloodstream, causing hypercalcemia. Signs and symptoms include confusion, abdominal pain, muscle pain, weakness, and anorexia.

For older adults, the more common risk is taking in too little calcium, which has been linked to colon cancer and hypertension in addition to osteoporosis. The RDA of calcium for adults age 51 and older is 1,200 mg, but many older adults don't meet the dietary reference intake (DRI) for calcium. (See *Dietary reference intakes for adults age 51 and older*.)

To help prevent osteoporosis, suggest to your older patients that they consume 3 cups of low-fat or fat-free milk—or an equivalent amount of low-fat or fat-free yogurt or low-fat cheese (1½ oz of cheese equals 1 cup of milk)—every day. If they're lactose intolerant, recommend lactose-free milk products, yogurt, and cheese. If they can't or don't drink milk, suggest calcium-fortified foods and beverages. Tell your older patients who don't meet the DRI for calcium that they should take calcium supplements.

Iron

Although older adults have a lower physiologic requirement for iron, they may still be at risk for iron deficiency because of decreased absorption of iron. Causes include antacid interference, decreased stomach acid secretion, blood loss from disease (such as GI ulcers) or medication use (such as aspirin), and the inability to eat enough iron-rich foods. Leading sources of iron in the American diet include ready-to-eat cereals and red meat. However, red meat is expensive, carries other health risks such as too much fat, and may be difficult to eat for some older people who have trouble chewing or swallowing.

Sodium

Sodium ions play a crucial role in several bodily functions, including acid-base balance, fluid balance, nerve impulses, and muscle contraction. Most salt in the body comes from eating processed foods—such as frozen dinners, chips, and canned soups—or adding salt to food either during cooking or at the table.

Because the sense of taste decreases with age, many older adults tend to use too much salt to flavor to their food. Let your older patients know that too much sodium (hypernatremia) leads to fluid retention and edema. Explain that older adults should have no more than 1,500 mg of sodium each day—about ¾ tsp of salt. Tell those with hypertension, renal failure, or heart conditions that they need to take extra care to limit their sodium intake.

Magnesium

Magnesium is needed for bone and tooth formation, nerve activity, glucose metabolization, and fat and protein synthesis. A large percentage of adults age 70 and older, however, don't meet the DRI for magnesium (420 mg/day for men and 320 mg/day for women).

Compounding the problem, many older adults may not fully absorb the magnesium they do consume because of genitourinary disorders, chronic alcoholism, or diabetes. Signs of magnesium deficiency include personality changes (irritability, aggressiveness), vertigo, muscle spasms, weakness, and seizures.

In contrast, some older patients take in too much magnesium, typically from such medications as magnesium-based antacids and cathartics. Signs of magnesium toxicity include diarrhea, dehydrations, and impaired nerve activity.

Potassium

The intracellular ion potassium helps maintain acid-base balance and interacts with sodium to promote fluid exchange through cell membranes. Potassium deficiency (hypokalemia) occurs more commonly in older adults because many take antihypertensives and diuretics, which can deplete the body's potassium supply. Signs and symptoms include muscle weakness and cramping, anorexia, apprehension, depression, and disorientation.

Poor nutrition: Recognizing the risks

Researchers estimate that up to two-thirds of older adults are at risk for nutritional deficits. Those at greatest risk include older people with limited education or income and those who live alone. Limited mobility because of chronic disease also increases the malnutrition risk, and admittance to a health care facility such as a nursing home greatly increases the risk. Despite these risks, overall, just 3% to 6% of the elderly population actually suffers from malnutrition.

However, several factors can have a particular effect on older adults' nutritional status. Many older adults take several medications, and some of these can interfere with nutrient absorption. Wounds, burns, and infection—all risks for the elderly—increase nutrient needs. Depression can rob an older adult of his appetite, and cultural food preferences also affect nutrition.

MULTIPLYING MEDICATIONS

Many older adults suffer from chronic illness, often from more than one, and need to take several medications. In fact, the average number of prescriptions per older adult in the United States has risen from 19.6 per year in 1992 to 28.5 per year in 2000; by 2010, the number is projected to rise to 38.5 prescriptions, per year, per older adult. And that increases the risk of drug-induced malnutrition.

Medications can affect nutrition in several ways. Some drugs can alter the taste of food, and taking multiple medications each day—either prescription or over-the-counter drugs— can decrease the sense of hunger. Taking several medications also increases the potential for drug interactions. Taking five or more different medications a day leads to a 50% chance of interaction, and taking eight or more medications leads to an almost 100% chance of interaction.

Here are some of the drug and food interactions that can occur:

- Grapefruit juice can increase the absorption of drugs such as statins and calcium channel blockers, leading to a higher-than-intended dosage of the drug.
- Antihypertensives may decrease the body's potassium supply; an older patient taking an antihypertensive should have his serum potassium checked and, if necessary, take a potassium supplement.
- The aluminum hydroxide contained in some antacids can bind to phosphorus in food, preventing bone from absorbing and

using phosphorus. Over time, this can result in phosphorus depletion.
- Laxatives cause food to move rapidly through the body, which decreases the absorption of many vitamins and minerals and can lead to poor nutrient absorption.
- Some anticonvulsants can decrease folate absorption.
- Some cholesterol-lowering medications reduce cholesterol by removing bile acids, which the body needs to absorb the fat-soluble vitamins A, D, E, and K, possibly leading to a reduced absorption of these vitamins.
- Large amounts of aspirin can lead to an increased loss of folate.
- Some anticonvulsant medications can cause the liver to increase the removal of vitamin D from the body.

EXTRA FUEL FOR HEALING

Wounds, burns, and infection affect nutrition by increasing the body's need for nutrients to heal. The body must have increased protein for both the inflammatory response and to form collagen for wound healing. Even short periods of low protein intake can delay healing and lead to wounds with poor tensile strength. In fact, the amount of protein a body requires for healing actually doubles.

Without essential amino acids such as arginine, growing new blood vessels (called *angiogenesis*), fibroblast proliferation, collagen synthesis, and scar remodeling won't occur. The body also needs enough amino acids to support the immune response and produce collagen. If the body doesn't have the carbohydrates it needs, it will instead break down protein for use, which can delay healing.

Vitamins also play a vital role. The body needs extra A, C, K, and B-complex vitamins as well as zinc and iron for healing. B-complex vitamins are coenzymes in a number of metabolic functions involved in wound healing, particularly in energy release from carbohydrates. Vitamin C aids collagen synthesis by helping form the bonds between strands of collagen fiber. Vitamin K helps form thrombin, and vitamin A aids in the cross-linking of collagen and the proliferation of epithelial cells. Zinc assists in protein synthesis. Iron plays a role in the synthesis of adenosine triphosphate, the fuel the body runs on.

A DEPRESSING SITUATION

Depression can lead to poor nutrition in an older adult, generally by decreasing appetite. Although depression isn't a normal part of aging, many caregivers and 58% of older adults unfortunately think it is. And several life changes that occur with aging can lead to depression, including changes in a person's living situation, the death of a spouse, and declining health.

You can help your older patients cope with depression by teaching them how and why it occurs and by giving them a chance to openly discuss it. Keep in mind that only 38% of people over age 65 believe depression is a health problem, yet about 15% of assisted-living residents and as many as 25% of nursing home patients have signs and symptoms of the disorder. Older adults also have a much higher suicide risk: 50% higher than the risk for young people and the nation as a whole.

THE CULTURE CONNECTION

A person's cultural and ethnic background can affect both food choices and food preparation. For example, some Hispanic people believe that illness results from an imbalance between hot and cold foods, so they select foods to cure illness based on this belief.

Cultural dietary choices don't usually harm an older adult's health. But someone with hypertension or diabetes whose cultural diet includes foods high in sodium or sugar may aggravate his condition. (See *Cultural influences on eating patterns*.)

Nutritional Status: Keeping Things in Balance

Every person, from growing child to aging adult, should try to maintain a healthy, balanced diet, with intake, or nutrient supply, matching the body's needs, or demand. Both overnutrition (in which supply exceeds demand) and undernutrition (in which demand exceeds supply) lead to imbalance.

To evaluate a person's nutritional status and detect any nutritional imbalances, you'll first need to perform a complete nutritional assessment. Information from the assessment allows the health care team to set appropriate goals and determine nutritional interventions to correct any imbalances, whether actual or potential. Interventions may include a diet lower in overall calories, fat, cholesterol, or sodium. Or the patient may need vitamin or mineral supplements to correct an imbalance.

The nutritional assessment: All the ingredients

The nutritional assessment provides the essential information for determining appropriate nutritional interventions. A complete assessment includes a nutritional screening, a diet history, physical findings, and laboratory results.

NUTRITIONAL SCREENING: SURVEYING THE SITUATION

Several screening surveys allow you to assess an older patient's nutritional status. The questionnaire and checklist developed by the Nutrition Screening Initiative and the Mini Nutritional Assessment are two such tools.

⚑ *Culture*   Cultural Influences on Eating Patterns

An older person's culture or religion can affect how he eats. Although cultural influences don't typically harm a patient's nutritional status, it helps to understand how different cultures can influence diet.

African-Americans
- "Soul food" common, particularly in the southern United States
- Common main courses: wild game, fried fish and poultry, pork, and all parts of pig
- Common vegetables and side dishes: corn, rice, okra, greens, legumes, tomatoes, hot breads, and sweet potatoes
- Methods of food preparation: stewing, barbequing, and frying with lard or saltpork
- Low consumption of milk (possibly due to lactose intolerance)
- Low calcium intake

Asian-Americans
- Common foods: rice, wheat, pork, eggs, chicken, soybean products, and a variety of vegetables
- Methods of food preparation: stir-frying with lard, peanut oil, or sesame oil; seasoning with ginger, soy sauce, sesame seeds, and monosodium glutamate
- Beverages: green tea, rare use of milk products because lactose intolerance is common

Hispanics
- Common main courses: eggs, tacos, chicken, corn, tortillas, and pinto or calico beans

- Common vegetables and side dishes: rice, corn, squash, bread, and tomatoes
- Methods of food preparation: frying with lard; seasoning with garlic, onions, and chili powder
- Beverages: herbal teas, carbonated soda, and milk in hot beverages

Native Americans
- Many obtain foods from their natural environment (fish, roots, fruits, berries, wild greens, and wild game)
- May rely on nonperishable foods because of lack of refrigeration
- May depend on commodity foods provided by U.S. Department of Agriculture
- May be influenced by tribal culture
- May have limited use of dairy products because of lactose intolerance

Religious Influences
- Some groups of Jews follow prescribed rules for preparing and serving foods (e.g., they eat only kosher meat and poultry and don't eat shellfish or pork products).
- Mormons don't drink tea, coffee, or alcohol.
- Hindus are vegetarians.
- Seventh Day Adventists are lacto-ovovegetarians.
- Roman Catholics don't eat meat on Ash Wednesday or Good Friday.

From Miller, C. *Nursing for Wellness in Older Adults*, 5th ed. Philadelphia: Lippincott Williams & Wilkins, 2009. Used with permission

Nutrition Screening Initiative checklist

The Nutrition Screening Initiative, formed by the American Academy of Family Physicians, the American Dietetic Association, and the National Council on Aging, has developed a useful nutritional questionnaire and checklist you can use to help determine an older patient's nutritional status. It was originally developed as a tool to increase consumers' nutrition awareness and consists of a questionnaire—a 10-item, yes-or-no–style form that you can give to older patients or their family members or caregivers to fill out and score themselves—and a checklist that uses the acronym DETERMINE to highlight nutritional risks. If the questionnaire indicates that the patient is at risk for poor nutrition, he can receive further screening. (See *Determine your nutritional health*, pages 94 and 95.)

Mini Nutritional Assessment

The Mini Nutritional Assessment is an easy tool for screening and assessing an older patient for malnutrition. It takes about 20 minutes to complete both the screening and assessment sections of this 18-item survey. The tool incorporates several anthropometric measurements, dietary intake questions, and health and functional status questions. A patient found to be at risk on the screening portion of the tool should then receive the assessment portion. The tool includes four components: anthropometric measurements (body mass index [BMI], self-reported weight loss), global assessment (lifestyle, medications, mobility), dietary assessment (number of meals, protein and fluid intake), and subjective assessment (self-rated health and nutritional status). (See *Mini Nutritional Assessment*, page 96.)

DIET HISTORY: YOU ARE WHAT YOU ATE

You may have trouble obtaining an adequate diet history unless the patient's family members and friends are available to give you additional information. But try to gather as much information as you can because a thorough diet history can offer insight into the patient's social and economic situation—such as what kind of access he has to a grocery store—as well as his cognitive status.

DETERMINE YOUR NUTRITIONAL HEALTH

The warning signs of poor nutritional health are often overlooked. Use this checklist to find out if you or someone you know is at nutritional risk.

Read the statements below. Circle the number in the "yes" column for those that apply to you or someone you know. For each "yes" answer, score the number in the box. Total your nutrition score.

	Yes
I have an illness or condition that made me change the kind and/or amount of food I eat.	2
I eat fewer than 2 meals per day.	3
I eat few fruits or vegetables or milk products.	2
I have 3 or more drinks of beer, liquor, or wine almost every day.	2
I have tooth or mouth problems that make it hard for me to eat.	2
I don't always have enough money to buy the food I need.	4
I eat alone most of the time.	1
I take 3 or more prescribed or over-the-counter drugs a day.	1
Without wanting to, I have lost or gained 10 pounds in the last 6 months.	2
I am not always physically able to shop, cook, and/or feed myself.	2
	Total

Total your nutrition score. If it's:

0-2	**Good!** Recheck your nutrition score in 6 months.
3-5	**You are at moderate nutrition risk.** See what can be done to improve your eating habits and lifestyle. Your office on aging, senior nutrition program, senior citizens center, or health department can help. Recheck your nutrition score in 3 months.
6 or more	**You are at high nutritional risk.** Bring this checklist the next time you see your doctor, dietitian, or other qualified health or social service professional. Talk with them about any problems you may have. Ask for help to improve your nutritional health.

DETERMINE YOUR NUTRITIONAL HEALTH (*continued*)

The nutrition checklist is based on the warning signs described below. Use the word *DETERMINE* to remind yourself of the warning signs.

Disease

Any disease, illness or chronic condition which causes you to change the way you eat, or makes it hard for your to eat, puts your nutritional health at risk. Four out of five adults have chronic diseases that are affected by diet. Confusion or memory loss that keeps getting worse is estimated to affect one out of five or more of older adults. This can make it hard to remember what, when, or if you've eaten. Feeling sad or depressed, which happens to about one in eight older adults, can cause big changes in appetite, digestion, energy level, weight, and well-being.

Eating Poorly

Eating too little and eating too much both lead to poor health. Eating the same foods day after day or not eating fruit, vegetables, or milk products daily will also cause poor nutritional health. One in five adults skip meals daily. Only 13% of adults eat the minimum amount of fruit and vegetables needed. One in four older adults drink too much alcohol. Many health problems become worse if you drink more than one or two alcoholic beverages per day.

Tooth Loss/Mouth Pain

A healthy mouth, teeth, and gums are needed to eat. Missing, loose, or rotten teeth or dentures which don't fit well or cause mouth sores make it hard to eat.

Economic Hardship

As many as 40% of older Americans have incomes less than $6,000 per year. Having less—or choosing to spend less—than $25–$30 per week for food makes it very hard to get the foods you need to stay healthy.

Reduced Social Contact

One-third of all older people live alone. Being with people daily has a positive effect on morale, well-being, and eating.

Multiple Medicines

Many older Americans must take medicines for health problems. Almost half of older Americans take multiple medicines daily. Growing old may change the way we respond to drugs. The more medicines you take, the greater the chance for side effects such as increased or decreased appetite, change in taste, constipation, weakness, drowsiness, diarrhea, nausea, and others. Vitamins or minerals, when taken in large doses, act like drugs and can cause harm. Alert your doctor to everything you take.

Involuntary Weight Loss/Gain

Losing or gaining a lot of weight when you are not trying to do so is an important warning sign that must not be ignored. Being overweight or underweight also increases your chance of poor health.

Needs Assistance in Self-Care

Although most older people are able to eat, one of every five have trouble walking, shopping, buying, and cooking food, especially as they get older.

Elder Years Above Age 80

Most older people lead full and productive lives. But as age increases, risk of frailty and health problems increase. Checking your nutritional health regularly makes good sense.

Reprinted with permission from The Nutrition Screening Initiative, a project of the American Academy of Family Physicians, the American Dietetic Association, and the National Council on Aging and by a grant from Ross Products Division, Abbott Laboratories.

MINI NUTRITIONAL ASSESSMENT

The Mini Nutritional Assessment can help you screen your older adult patients for malnutrition. The forms has two parts: screening and assessment. If the patient scores 11 points or less on the screening portion, the second part of the tool is completed to provide a more detailed assessment.

Last name: _____   First name: _____   Sex: _____   Date: _____

Age: _____   Weight (kg): _____   Height (cm): _____   I.D. number: _____

SCREENING

A Has food intake declined over the past 3 months due to loss of appetite, digestive problems, chewing, or swallowing difficulties?
0 = severe loss of appetite
1 = moderate loss of appetite
2 = no loss of appetite   ☐

B Weight loss during the last 3 months
0 = weight loss greater than 3 kg (6.6 lbs)
1 = does not know
2 = weight loss between 1 and 3 kg (2.2 and 6.6 lbs)
3 = no weight loss   ☐

C Mobility
0 = bed or chair bound
1 = able to get out of bed or chair but does not go out
2 = goes out   ☐

D Has suffered psychological stress or acute disease in the past 3 months
0 = yes
2 = no   ☐

E Neuropsychological problems
0 = severe dementia or depression
1 = mild dementia
2 = no psychological problems   ☐

F Body Mass Index (BMI) (weight in kg)/(height in m^2)
0 = BMI less than 19
1 = BMI 19 to less than 21
2 = BMI 21 to less than 23
3 = BMI 23 or greater   ☐

Screening score subtotal
(max. 14 points)   ☐☐
12 points or greater = Normal (not at risk, no need to complete assessment)
11 points or below = Possible malnutrition (continue assessment)

ASSESSMENT

G Lives independently (not in a nursing home or hospital)
0 = no   1 = yes   ☐

H Takes more than 3 prescription drugs per day
0 = yes   1 = no   ☐

I Pressure sores or skin ulcers
0 = yes   1 = no   ☐

J How many full meals does the patient eat daily?
0 = 1 meal
1 = 2 meals
2 = 3 meals   ☐

K Selected consumption markers for protein intake
● At least one serving of dairy products (milk, cheese, yogurt) per day?
yes ☐   no ☐
● Two or more servings of legumes or eggs per week?
yes ☐   no ☐
● Meat, fish, or poultry every day?
yes ☐   no ☐
0.0 = 0 or 1 yes
0.5 = 2 yes
1.0 = 3 yes   ☐.☐

L Consumes two or more servings of fruits or vegetables per day?
0 = no   1 = yes   ☐

M How much fluid (water, juice, coffee, tea, milk…) is consumed per day?
0.0 = less than 3 cups
0.5 = 3 to 5 cups
1.0 = more than 5 cups   ☐.☐

N Mode of feeding
0 = unable to eat without assistance
1 = self-fed with some difficulty
2 = self-fed without any problem   ☐

O Self view of nutritional status
0 = views self as being malnourished
1 = is uncertain of nutritional state
2 = views self as having no nutritional problem   ☐

P In comparison with other people of the same age, how does the patient consider his or her health status?
0.0 = not as good
0.5 = does not know
1.0 = as good
2.0 = better   ☐.☐

Q Mid-arm circumference (MAC) in cm
0.0 = MAC less than 21
0.5 = MAC 21 to 22
1.0 = MAC 22 or greater   ☐.☐

R Calf circumference (CC) in cm
0 = CC less than 31
1 = CC 31 or greater   ☐

Assessment score subtotal
(max. 16 points)   ☐☐.☐

Screening score subtotal	☐☐
Assessment score subtotal	☐☐.☐
Total score (max. 30 points)	☐☐.☐

Malnutrition indicator score
17 to 23.5 points =
    at risk of malnutrition   ☐
Less than 17 points =
    malnourished   ☐

A typical diet history includes

- the number of snacks and meals a person eats each day
- chewing or swallowing difficulties
- GI issues or symptoms that affect eating
- history of disease or surgery
- oral health and denture use
- medication use
- appetite
- activity level
- need for assistance preparing or eating meals
- allergies
- food preferences
- food aversions.

Make sure that the patient or caregiver answering your questions understands portion size so that you get an accurate diet history. For instance, you might explain that 4 oz of meat is about the size of a pack of playing cards, and a serving of vegetables is about ½ cup. You can use the patient's food recall to help determine how many calories he consumes in a day, how much protein he eats, and whether he has any problematic food intake patterns, such as eating too many salty or starchy foods or too few fruits and vegetables.

Formal diet history tools you can use include the 24-hour food recall and the food frequency record. These examine how much, what, and how often a person typically eats to determine nutritional status.

24-hour food recall

A quick, easy method for evaluating a person's intake, the 24-hour food recall requires a person to recount all the types and amounts of foods and beverages he consumed during a 24-hour period. He can choose either the previous 24 hours or a typical 24-hour period.

To help your patient identify portion sizes, you can use food models or pictures of typical food portions. You may need to gather spe-

cific details in some situations, such as food preparation (e.g., frying versus dry-roasting meat). Open-ended questions also reveal more information than typical yes-or-no questions. Once completed, the food recall can indicate whether the patient's diet is meeting his nutritional needs.

Food frequency record

The food frequency record consists of a checklist of particular foods that lets the patient indicate what he eats and how often he eats that item. It typically lists foods in one column. Another column allows the patient to mark off how often he eats that food (such as once or more per day, per week, or per month), or if he eats a food frequently, seldom, or never. The checklist typically doesn't include the serving size, and it may only include specific foods or nutrients that may be deficient or excessive in the diet. You can instead use a questionnaire that organizes food items by food groups, with the patient recording how often he consumes each type of food.

Either checklist provides a more complete dietary picture when used in conjunction with the 24-hour food recall. These tools help identify deficiencies or excesses, allowing the development of goals to meet the patient's nutritional and educational needs.

Psychosocial factors

The diet history may also reveal other factors that influence that patient's nutritional habits, including:

- illiteracy
- a language barrier
- a lack of knowledge about nutrition and food safety
- social isolation
- cultural or religious influences
- low or limited income
- limited access to transportation

OVERCOMING HEIGHT MEASUREMENT PROBLEMS

Getting an accurate height for an older patient who is confined to a wheelchair or one who can't stand because of scoliosis poses a challenge. You can get an approximate height measurement by measuring the patient's arm span or by using his knee height.

To measure the patient's arm span, have him hold his arms straight out from the sides of his body. Then measure from the tip of one middle finger to the tip of the other. This distance is the patient's approximate height.

To use knee height, measure the distance from the patient's heel to the top of the knee and then use this formula:

- Women = $(1.83 \times \text{knee height in cm}) - (0.24 \times \text{age}) + 84.88$
- Men = $(2.02 \times \text{knee height in cm}) - (0.04 \times \text{age}) + 64.19$

Regardless of the method used, note any evidence of diminished height in an older patient. A decrease in height may stem from osteoporotic changes and calls for further investigation

- physical inactivity or illness
- inadequate cooking resources (such as a lack of major kitchen appliances or no kitchen access)
- use of tobacco or recreational drugs
- limited community resources.

PHYSICAL FINDINGS: THE BODY BASICS

A physical assessment of the patient's height, weight, BMI, and overall physical appearance—including the condition of the patient's mouth and teeth—can help determine the patient's health status and identify illness. Some findings may stem from an alteration in the patient's nutritional status or malnutrition, but keep in mind that height and weight findings typically reflect chronic changes in nutritional status rather than acute processes. Ongoing height and weight measurements can reveal trends.

You may have difficulty assessing an older patient's height and weight, especially if the patient is bedridden or obese. If you find that the patient has gained or lost 10 lb (4.5 kg) or more in the previous 6 months, make sure you ask him about it.

Height

To measure height, use a fixed measuring stick against a wall. Ask the patient to stand as straight as possible, without shoes, with his back against the measuring stick. You may need to adapt your method if the patient can't stand or isn't able to cooperate. (See *Overcoming height measurement problems*.)

Weight

Measure weight using a beam-balance scale or a bed scale if the patient is bedridden. If possible, weigh the patient on the same scale at the same time of day that he's been weighed before (typically before breakfast and after voiding), in the same amount of clothing, and without shoes.

Body mass index

A measurement of weight in relationship to height, BMI can be calculated using conventional pounds and inches or using the metric system (kilograms and centimeters). (See *Calculating BMI.*) You can also estimate BMI without doing any calculations (See *Determining BMI.*)

Using BMI to evaluate body weight requires little skill. The major disadvantage is that BMI works on the assumption that excess weight results from excess fat; it doesn't allow for such other reasons as edema or large muscle mass.

A person with a BMI:

- of less than 18.5 is underweight.
- between 18.5 and 24.9 has a normal weight for his height.

CALCULATING BMI

Use one of the formulas below to calculate your patient's body mass index (BMI).

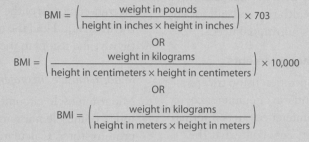

$$BMI = \left(\frac{\text{weight in pounds}}{\text{height in inches} \times \text{height in inches}} \right) \times 703$$

OR

$$BMI = \left(\frac{\text{weight in kilograms}}{\text{height in centimeters} \times \text{height in centimeters}} \right) \times 10,000$$

OR

$$BMI = \left(\frac{\text{weight in kilograms}}{\text{height in meters} \times \text{height in meters}} \right)$$

DETERMINING BMI

Body mass index (BMI) measures weight in relation to height. The BMI ranges shown here are for adults. They aren't exact ranges for healthy or unhealthy weights; however, they show that health risks increase at higher levels of overweight and obesity. To use the graph below, find your patient's weight along the bottom and then go straight up until you come to the line that matches his height. The shaded area indicates whether your patient is healthy, overweight, or obese.

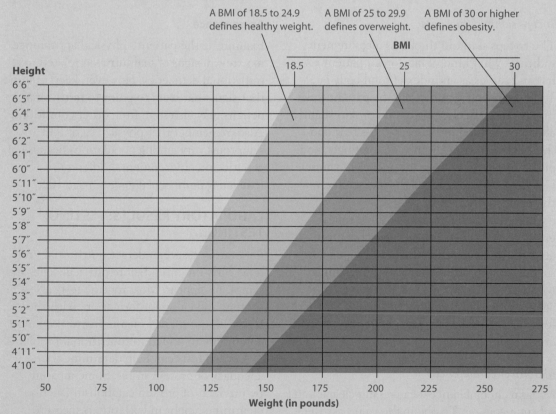

Adapted from *Nutrition and Your Health: Dietary Guidelines for Americans,* 5th ed. (Home and Garden Bulletin No. 232.) Washington, D.C.: U.S. Department of Agriculture, U.S. Department of Health and Human Services, 2000.

- between 25.0 and 29.9 is overweight.
- of 30.0 or more is obese.

All measures other than normal place the patient at a higher health risk and call for further assessment of his nutritional needs.

Body composition measurements

Measuring body composition using triceps skinfold thickness, midarm circumference, or midarm muscle circumference offers information not about weight, but about what the body contains: fat or muscle tissue. You can compare measurements to reference standards or use them to evaluate changes over time. If a patient's measurements fall below 90% of the reference value, he needs nutritional intervention.

Triceps skinfold thickness

The triceps skinfold thickness measurement indicates what kind of fat stores a patient has and serves as an index of total body fat. To measure the skinfold, tell the patient to let his arm hang freely, grasp a fold of skin slightly above the midpoint between the elbow and shoulder with your thumb and forefinger, and pull the skin away from the underlying muscle. Use the calipers and read the measurement to the nearest millimeter.

Take the reading a total of three times, either at the same site or at other appropriate sites (biceps, calve, thigh, subscapular, or suprailiac skinfold). Then add the readings together and divide by 3 to arrive at an average. For men, 11.3 mm is 90% of standard and for women, 14.9. (See *Taking anthropometric arm measurements.*)

Midarm circumference

Midarm circumference measures muscle mass and subcutaneous fat. To obtain this value, ask the patient to flex the forearm of his nondominant arm 90 degrees. Then place the arm in a dependent position, wrap a measuring tape around the middle of the upper arm between the top of the acremonium process of the scapula and olecranon process of the ulna, and measure from the midpoint. Hold the tape firmly, but not too tightly, and record to the nearest millimeter.

Midarm muscle circumference

Midarm muscle circumference provides an index of muscle mass and indicates somatic protein stores. Calculate this value by multiplying the triceps skinfold measurement by 3.14 and then multiply that value by the midarm circumference measurement. Record the value in centimeters. This value isn't affected much by edema and provides a quick estimation.

Appearance

Examining the patient's physical appearance may reveal signs of malnutrition related to a nutritional deficiency. However, keep in mind that signs that seem to point to nutritional deficits may also stem from other conditions. Also, remember that physical signs and symptoms vary among populations because of genetic and environmental differences. (See *Evaluating nutritional disorders*, page 102.)

LABORATORY RESULTS: TESTING, TESTING...

Laboratory tests can detect nutritional problems early on, often before physical signs and symptoms appear. Most routine tests assess protein and calorie information, with the serum albumin level measurement used most commonly to screen for nutritional problems.

Several tests can help determine the adequacy of protein stores. Some measure by-products of protein catabolism (such as creatinine height index); others measure the products of protein metabolism (such as albumin level, transferrin level, hemoglobin

TAKING ANTHROPOMETRIC ARM MEASUREMENTS

Follow the steps below to determine triceps skinfold thickness, midarm circumference, and midarm muscle circumference.

Triceps Skinfold Thickness

1. Find the midpoint circumference of the arm by placing the tape measure halfway between the axilla and the elbow. Grasp the patient's skin with your thumb and forefinger, about ⅜″ (1 cm) above the midpoint, as illustrated below.
2. Place calipers at the midpoint and squeeze for 3 seconds.
3. Record the measurement to the nearest millimeter.
4. Take two more readings and use the average.

Midarm Circumference and Midarm Muscle Circumference

1. Measure the midarm circumference at the midpoint, as illustrated below. Record the measurement in centimeters.
2. Calculate the midarm muscle circumference by multiplying the triceps skinfold thickness (measured in millimeters) by 3.14.
3. Subtract this number from the midarm circumference.

Recording the Measurements

Record all three measurements as a percentage of the standard measurements (see chart below), using this formula:

$$\frac{\text{Actual measurement}}{\text{Standard measurement}} \times 100\%$$

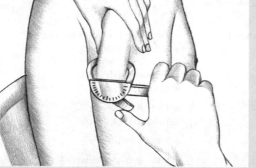

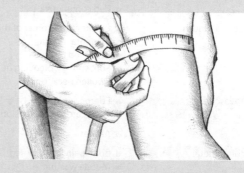

After taking and recording the measurements above, consult the chart at right to determine your patient's caloric status. A measurement less than 90% of the standard indicates caloric deprivation. A measurement over 90% indicates adequate or more than adequate energy reserves.

Measurement	Standard	90%
Triceps skinfold thickness	Men: 12.5 mm Women: 16.5 mm	Men: 11.3 mm Women: 14.9 mm
Midarm circumference	Men: 29.3 cm Women: 28.5 cm	Men: 26.4 cm Women: 25.7 cm
Midarm muscle circumference	Men: 25.3 cm Women: 23.3 cm	Men: 22.8 cm Women: 20.9 cm

EVALUATING NUTRITIONAL DISORDERS

This chart can help you interpret nutritional assessment findings. Body systems are listed below with signs and symptoms and the implications for each.

BODY SYSTEM OR REGION	SIGN OR SYMPTOM	IMPLICATIONS
General	• Weakness and fatigue • Weight loss	• Anemia or electrolyte imbalance • Decreased calorie intake, increased calorie use, or inadequate nutrient intake or absorption
Skin, hair, and nails	• Dry, flaky skin • Dry skin with poor turgor • Rough, scaly skin with bumps • Petechiae or ecchymoses • Sore that won't heal • Thinning, dry hair • Spoon-shaped, brittle, or ridged nails	• Vitamin A, vitamin B-complex, or linoleic acid deficiency • Dehydration • Vitamin A deficiency • Vitamin C or K deficiency • Protein, vitamin C, or zinc deficiency • Protein deficiency • Iron deficiency
Eyes	• Night blindness; corneal swelling, softening, or dryness; Bitot's spots (gray triangular patches on the conjunctiva) • Red conjunctiva	• Vitamin A deficiency • Riboflavin deficiency
Throat and mouth	• Cracks at the corner of the mouth • Magenta tongue • Beefy, red tongue • Soft, spongy, bleeding gums • Swollen neck (goiter)	• Riboflavin or niacin deficiency • Riboflavin deficiency • Vitamin B_{12} deficiency • Vitamin C deficiency • Iodine deficiency
Cardiovascular	• Edema • Tachycardia, hypotension	• Protein deficiency • Fluid volume deficit
GI	• Ascites	• Protein deficiency
Musculoskeletal	• Bone pain and bow leg • Muscle wasting	• Vitamin D or calcium deficiency • Protein, carbohydrate, and fat deficiency
Neurologic	• Altered mental status • Paresthesia	• Dehydration and thiamine or vitamin B_{12} deficiency • Vitamin B_{12}, pyridoxine, or thiamine deficiency

level, hematocrit, prealbumin level, and total lymphocyte count).

Serum albumin level

The serum albumin level indicates protein levels in the body, an important indicator of nutritional status. Albumin makes up more than 50% of total proteins in the blood and affects the cardiovascular system by helping to maintain osmotic pressure. Keep in mind that albumin production requires functioning liver cells and an adequate supply of amino acids, the building blocks of protein.

The serum albumin level is decreased in those with serious protein deficiency and loss of blood protein from burns, malnutrition, liver or renal disease, heart failure, major surgery, infections, or cancer.

Creatinine height index

The creatinine height index involves a 24-hour urine collection to measure urinary excretion of creatinine. The test helps define body protein mass and evaluate protein depletion. The results are interpreted by using a formula to compute the patient's results, then comparing that with the expected results for a person of that height.

Increased values may indicate decreased protein stores. However, keep in mind that creatinine values decrease with age because of a normal decrease in lean muscle mass. This test also has limited value because not only age, but also exercise, stress, and severe illness can all greatly alter results.

Transferrin level

Synthesized mainly in the liver, transferrin is a carrier protein that transports iron. Transferrin levels decrease along with protein levels, so a drop indicates a depletion of protein stores. The serum transferrin level reflects the patient's current protein status more accurately than albumin because of transferrin's shorter half-life.

A normal transferrin level is more than 200 mg/dl; a decreased level may indicate protein malnutrition. It may also indicate inadequate protein production from liver damage, protein loss from renal disease, acute or chronic infection, or cancer. An elevated level may indicate severe iron deficiency.

Hemoglobin level

Hemoglobin (Hb) is the main component of red blood cells (RBCs), which transport oxygen. Its formation requires an adequate supply of protein in the form of amino acids. Hb values help assess the blood's oxygen-carrying capacity and are useful in diagnosing anemia, protein deficiency, and hydration status.

Decreased Hb suggests iron deficiency anemia, protein deficiency, excessive blood loss, or overhydration. Increased Hb suggests dehydration or polycythemia. Normal Hb values vary with age and the type of blood sample tested.

Hematocrit

The hematocrit (HCT) level reflects the proportion of blood occupied by RBCs. This test helps diagnose anemia and dehydration. Decreased values suggest iron deficiency anemia or excessive fluid intake or blood loss. Increased values suggest severe dehydration or polycythemia Normal HCT values reflect age, sex, sample type, and the laboratory performing the test.

Prealbumin

Because prealbumin has a much shorter half-life than albumin (only 2 days), it serves as a more sensitive test. Prealbumin also isn't as affected by liver disease and hydration status as albumin; however, the test is more expensive to perform. A normal prealbumin value ranges from 19 to 38 mg/dl; an abnormal value helps diagnose protein-calorie malnutrition, a condition found in more than 30% of hospitalized patients in which the body breaks down muscle, fat, and protein.

Total lymphocyte count

A lymphocyte is a type of white blood cell, the main cells responsible for fighting infection. A total lymphocyte count can help indicate nutritional status because malnutrition decreases the total number of lymphocytes, which, in turn, impairs the body's ability to fight infection.

The total lymphocyte count evaluates the health of the patient's immune system and helps evaluate protein stores, and decreased lymphocytes may indicate malnutrition when no other cause for the decreased value is apparent. Keep in mind, though, that decreased values can also indicate other medical conditions, such as infection, leukemia, and tissue necrosis, limiting the test's value for evaluating nutritional status.

Food for Thought: A Final Word

For many older adults, maintaining proper nutrition isn't easy. Changing nutritional needs as bodies age, changing living circumstances, decreased mobility from chronic disease, fixed incomes—all can conspire to make the seemingly simple task of eating the right foods to stay healthy a significant challenge.

You can help them rise to the challenge. By carefully assessing older patients' nutritional status and needs, intervening where necessary, and helping your patients and their caregivers make good nutritional choices, you can help your patients live better, healthier, lives. And that's a recipe worth following. (See *Critical thinking questions: Nutrition.*)

5

Medication:
The Right Prescription

> *"Prescription: A physician's guess at what will best prolong the situation with least harm to the patient."*
>
> —AMBROSE BIERCE

I n the United States, four out of every five people age 65 and older suffer from one or more chronic disorders, which helps explain why older people take more drugs than any other age-group. Although adults age 65 and older make up only 12% of the U.S. population, they take 30% to 40% of prescribed drugs. That's about 400 million prescriptions a year—twice the number of prescriptions filled for those younger than age 65.

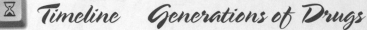

⧖ Timeline   Generations of Drugs

Most of the drugs commonly taken today were discovered within the past century. This timeline features important drug developments along with some interesting cultural and historical events.

1906 The Food and Drug Administration (FDA) is established to oversee labels and packaging information for over-the-counter drugs

1906 Alzheimer's disease first identified

1911 The term "vitamine" is introduced to define substances that prevent deficiency diseases, such as scurvy

1918 Spanish flu pandemic kills 50 to 100 million people worldwide

1922 First insulin dose given to 14-year-old boy with diabetes

1928 Penicillin discovered

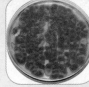

1932 Scientists split the atom

1932-1972 Tuskegee Experiment involving untreated syphilis subjects eventually leads to major changes in how patients are protected during research studies

1935 Alcoholics Anonymous founded

1938 Food, Drug, and Cosmetic Act passed

1938 LSD first synthesized; use of drug is central to 1960's counterculture movement

1945 First computer (ENAIC) built

1945 United Nations founded

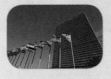

1900   10   20   30   40

Aging Bodies: Handle with Care

Drug therapy for older adults presents a special set of problems rooted in age-related changes. Physiologically, aging alters body composition and triggers changes in the digestive system, liver, and kidneys. These changes affect drug metabolism, absorption, distribution, and excretion, which may lead to the need for altered drug dosages and administration techniques. Such changes also potentiate adverse reactions to drugs and may interfere with therapeutic compliance.

An older patient may also have difficulty complying with his drug regimen because of poor hearing and vision deficits, forgetfulness, the need for multidrug therapy, poor understanding of dosages and directions, and various socioeconomic factors (such as poverty and social isolation). To ensure compliance, such a patient needs family members and other caregivers, physicians, pharmacists, and other health care professionals to supervise the situation; he also needs teaching about his medications.

Even when an older adult receives the optimum drug dosage, he's still at risk for adverse

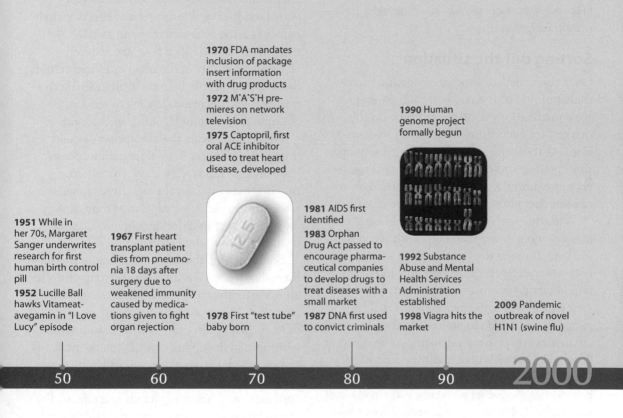

1970 FDA mandates inclusion of package insert information with drug products

1972 M*A*S*H premieres on network television

1975 Captopril, first oral ACE inhibitor used to treat heart disease, developed

1990 Human genome project formally begun

1951 While in her 70s, Margaret Sanger underwrites research for first human birth control pill

1952 Lucille Ball hawks Vitameatavegamin in "I Love Lucy" episode

1967 First heart transplant patient dies from pneumonia 18 days after surgery due to weakened immunity caused by medications given to fight organ rejection

1978 First "test tube" baby born

1981 AIDS first identified

1983 Orphan Drug Act passed to encourage pharmaceutical companies to develop drugs to treat diseases with a small market

1987 DNA first used to convict criminals

1992 Substance Abuse and Mental Health Services Administration established

1998 Viagra hits the market

2009 Pandemic outbreak of novel H1N1 (swine flu)

50   60   70   80   90   2000

drug reactions. Ongoing physiologic changes, poor compliance with the drug regimen, and greater drug consumption contribute to older adults experiencing twice as many adverse drug reactions as younger patients. In fact, about 40% of the people who experience adverse drug reactions are older than age 65.

The snowball effect

Signs and symptoms of adverse drug reactions in older patients (such as confusion, weakness, and lethargy) are typically blamed on disease. If the adverse reaction isn't recognized or is misidentified, the patient will probably continue taking the drug. To compound the problem, if the patient has multiple physical dysfunctions or adverse drug reactions, or both, he may consult several physicians or specialists who—unknown to one another—may prescribe more drugs. If the patient's drug history remains uninvestigated and if the patient takes even more nonprescription drugs to relieve common complaints (such as indigestion, dizziness, and constipation), he may innocently fall into a pattern of inappropriate and excessive drug use. Known as *polypharmacy*, this pattern imperils the patient's safety and the drug regimen's effectiveness.

Although many drugs can cause adverse reactions, most serious reactions in older adults result from relatively few drugs: diuretics, anticoagulants, antihypertensives, cardiac glycosides, corticosteroids, sleeping aids, and nonprescription drugs.

Sorting out the situation

Over time, medications are becoming increasingly tailored to the needs of each patient. New medications continue to come on the market, for everything from cancer to depression. At the same time, drug companies market their products to consumers, making consumers more aware of products and more likely to request them from their health care providers.

With the plethora of drugs available and with patients more aware than ever of what's on the market, choosing the right drugs for an older patient's specific medical condition and health requirements becomes much trickier. To play your part in managing medications for older patients, you'll need to understand the pharmacokinetics and pharmacodynamics of aging, what drugs older patients commonly use, and what kinds of adverse effects and interactions—with other drugs, herbal supplements, even food—can occur. You'll also have to take into account the physical changes of aging on I.M. drug administration. Finally you should have a firm grasp on how and what to teach older patients and their caregivers about their medications.

Pharmacokinetics: The Body's Effect

Pharmacokinetics examines what the body does to drugs—specifically, how the body absorbs, distributes, metabolizes, and excretes drugs. Pharmacokinetics change as the body ages, often significantly affecting how an older person responds to a drug.

Absorption

Although drug absorption in the GI tract doesn't usually change significantly with aging, pharmacokinetic studies on drug absorption reveal varied results. Possible age-related effects include reduced gastric acid secretion and gastric emptying, reduced blood flow, and reduced absorptive capacity of the small intestine; certain diseases can contribute to these changes. Active transport also decreases, leading to reduced absorption of vitamin B_{12}, iron, and calcium.

Aging also affects the absorption of oral drugs. For instance, if an older patient doesn't have enough fluids to swallow an oral drug, the drug may not pass through his esophagus. Other drugs, including aspirin, certain antibiotics, potassium chloride, vitamin C, and iron, can irritate the esophagus.

Some administration routes, such as the sublingual route, bypass the gastric system entirely, allowing a drug to enter systemic circulation directly. Changes such as dry mouth—a common occurrence in older adults—can interfere with normal dissolving of a sublingual medication. Conversely, an older patient's body may systemically absorb intranasal, ophthalmic, and auricular drugs, resulting in adverse effects. For example, systemic absorption of the glaucoma drug timolol (Timoptic) can reduce pulse rate and blood pressure.

The increase in body fat and decrease in lean body mass that typically occur as a person ages can also interfere with absorption. Make sure you use the correct needle length and technique to administer subcutaneous and I.M. injections into the correct space, and keep in mind that an older person may not absorb some I.M. drugs as efficiently.

Distribution

Age-related changes affect drug distribution more than absorption. Body composition changes as people age, with a progressive decrease in total body water and lean body mass, and an increase in body fat. Illness, poor nutrition, and inadequate hydration—all possible in older patients—can also affect drug distribution.

The amount of drug that binds to plasma proteins determines how much unbound drug is left over and free to exert its effect on the body. The pH of a particular drug determines the particular receptor site, with acidic drugs binding to albumin and basic drugs binding to α1-acid glycoprotein.

Acute illness and poor nutrition, both common in older adults, decreases plasma albumin levels. As a result, an older adult experiencing acute illness or poor nutrition who receives an acidic drug may end up with more unbound drug in his system than intended. This can result in increased pharmacologic and adverse effects as well as an increased risk of toxicity. Common acidic medications include diazepam, phenytoin (Dilantin), warfarin (Coumadin), and aspirin.

In contrast, acute illness, cancer, and arthritis in older adults can lead to an increase in α1-acid glycoprotein, the protein basic drugs bind to. This can lead to a reduced effect from such basic drugs such as lidocaine (Xylocaine) and propranolol.

Dehydration and the normal decrease in total body water that occurs with aging increase the serum concentration of such water-soluble drugs as gentamicin, digoxin, ethanol (Ethamolin), theophylline, and cimetidine (Tagamet). As a result, an older patient may need a decreased loading dose of a drug such as digoxin.

Keep in mind, too that lipid-soluble drugs have a prolonged half-life in older patients because of their decrease in lean body mass. Lipid-soluble drugs such as diazepam will have a prolonged effect.

 Keep in mind that a malnourished or dehydrated older

patient has an increased risk for a change in drug distribution; monitor dehydrated patients and those with decreased serum albumin levels for signs of drug toxicity.

Metabolism

How age-related changes in metabolism affect different drugs depends on the administration route and metabolism of a specific drug. Metabolism of a drug can take place in several sites in the body, but the process typically occurs in the liver. Many oral drugs, for instance, are absorbed by the small intestine into the venous network known as the *portal system*. The venous network then carries this drug to the liver, where it may undergo first-pass metabolism before entering systemic circulation.

In an older patient, age-related changes such as decreased liver size and hepatic blood flow can affect this process—for instance, by resulting in decreased first-pass metabolism of a drug. An older patient taking propranolol, labetalol, or another drug that undergoes extensive first-pass metabolism may experience an increased effect of the drug because he has more of the free-acting drug in his system.

Other drugs, including such angiotensin-converting enzyme (ACE) inhibitors as enalapril (Vasotec) and perindopril (Aceon), must pass through the liver to become activated. An older patient with reduced liver size and hepatic blood flow may have a slowed or reduced first-pass activation of these drugs.

Medication Alert An older patient may have an extended half-life of long-acting benzodiazepines and tricyclic antidepressants because of reduced hepatic clearance.

Older patients who take several drugs may also experience a change in normal metabolism of these drugs from drug-drug, drug-metabolite, or drug-food interactions. In normal metabolism, about 50 isoenzymes that make up the

THE ROLE OF ENZYMES IN SOME COMMON DRUG INTERACTIONS

A *substrate* is a drug that's metabolized by an enzyme. An *inducer* is a drug that increases the enzyme's ability to metabolize the substrate. An *inhibitor* is a drug that prevents the enzyme from metabolizing the substrate. The table below lists some common substrates and their inducers and inhibitors.

SUBSTRATE	INDUCER	INHIBITOR
Caffeine	Rifampin	Amiodarone
Ibuprofen	Carbamazepine	Amiodarone
Naproxen	None	Cimetidine
Alprazolam	Carbamazepine	Erythromycin
Codeine	Dexamethasone	Fluoxetine
Ondansetron	Omeprazole	Cimetidine
Lovastatin	Verapamil	St. John's wort

cytochrome P-450 system metabolize most drugs. But another drug, its metabolites, or even food may interact with this system, interfering with normal metabolization of a drug. Grapefruit juice, for instance, inhibits a specific isoenzyme called CYP3A3/4, resulting in reduced metabolism of calcium channel blockers such as amlodipine (Norvasc) and leading to increased action of the drug. (See *The role of enzymes in some common drug interactions.*)

Excretion

Renal function varies greatly in older patients, but aging kidneys usually remove waste products—including the byproducts of medications—less effectively. The kidneys' decreased effectiveness, coupled with circulatory changes (such as those from diabetes, renovascular occlusive disease, and heart failure) that reduce blood flow to the kidneys, means that more of a drug remains in an older patient's bloodstream. This can lead to elevated drug levels and possible drug toxicity.

One reason the kidneys are less effective is that the glomerular filtration rate also declines with age. This decline in glomerular filtration rate affects the clearance of many drugs,

including water-soluble antibiotics, diuretics, digoxin, water-soluble beta-adrenergic blockers, lithium, and nonsteroidal anti-inflammatory drugs (NSAIDs).

The danger to the patient of such a reduction in renal excretion depends on the toxicity of the drug. Those drugs with a narrow therapeutic index, such as aminoglycoside antibiotics, digoxin, and lithium, will more likely have serious adverse effects, even if they accumulate only marginally more than intended. Because of this, older patients with reduced renal function should receive lower doses of such drugs.

You can estimate a patient's glomerular filtration rate by finding out his creatinine clearance. The Cockcroft-Gault formula allows you to estimate creatinine clearance based on a patient's serum creatinine level, age, and weight. An older patient who has a creatinine clearance of less than 50 ml/minute is at risk for drug-related problems. Keep in mind, though, that an older patient's decrease in kidney function is typically accompanied by a decrease in lean body mass. This can result in a constant serum creatinine level, which can mask the patient's declining kidney function. (See *The Cockcroft-Gault formula.*)

THE COCKCROFT–GAULT FORMULA

A low creatinine clearance may indicate renal dysfunction, which affects a renally excreted drug's metabolism and appropriate dosage. For men, calculate creatinine clearance using the following formula. For women, use the following formula and multiply the answer by 0.85.

$$\frac{(140 - \text{age in years}) \times \text{lean body weight in kg}}{\text{serum creatinine in mg/dL} \times 72}$$

Pharmacodynamics: The Drug's Effect

Pharmacodynamics examines what drugs do to the body: how drugs act in the body and interact with body tissues. As an adult ages, pharmacodynamics change significantly. Age-related changes in tissue sensitivity to drugs can enhance some drug effects, and receptor sites on target organs may respond with either more or less sensitively to drugs. A receptor site may even respond normally to one drug, but not to another. When receptor sites become less sensitive to a drug, an older patient will need a higher dosage to achieve the same therapeutic effect. Older adults' brain receptors can become especially sensitive, resulting in a strong response to psychotropic drugs. (See *Common pharmacodynamic changes with aging.*)

Drugs that have a narrow margin of safety, such as psychoactive medications, warfarin, and digoxin, pose a particular risk. Physical changes in older patients that affect pharmacodynamics can make it very difficult to find the right dosage to achieve a therapeutic effect with minimal adverse effects and without risking toxicity. (See *Age-related changes that can affect pharmacodynamics*, page 112.)

Commonly Used Drugs: Adjust for Age

Several drugs that older adults commonly take often work differently in older adults than they do in younger patients. The examples on the next page detail some of those differences. Keep in mind, however, that a particular patient's response to a medication can vary depending on several factors.

COMMON PHARMACODYNAMIC CHANGES WITH AGING

Several drugs work differently in older patients because of normal changes that occur with aging. This table lists the pharmacodynamic effect in older patients of several commonly used drugs.

DRUG	PHARMACODYNAMIC EFFECT	AGE-RELATED CHANGE
Adenosine	Minute ventilation and heart rate	No change
Aspirin	Acute gastroduodenal mucosal damage	No change
Diazepam	Sedation	Increased
Diltiazem	Antihypertensive effect	Increased
Furosemide	Latency and size of peak diuretic response	Decreased
Heparin	Activated partial thromboplastin time	No change
Isoproterenol	Chronotropic effect	Decreased
Morphine	Analgesic effect	Increased
Verapamil	Acute antihypertensive effect	Increased
Warfarin	Prothrombin time	Increased

AGE-RELATED CHANGES THAT CAN AFFECT PHARMACODYNAMICS

This table shows common age-related physiological changes that can alter the pharmacodynamic response. Keep in mind that such changes can have a dramatic effect on the uptake, movement, binding, and interaction of drugs in an older patient's system.

BODY COMPOSITION	
Body fat	Increased
Lean body mass	Decreased
Total body water	Decreased
CARDIOVASCULAR FUNCTION	
Resting heart rate	Decreased
Stroke volume	Slightly decreased
Cardiac output	Slightly decreased
CENTRAL NERVOUS SYSTEM FUNCTION	
Blood supply to brain	Diminished
REFLEX RESPONSE	
Baroreceptor reflex activity	Diminished
RENIN-ANGIOTENSIN-ALDOSTERONE SYSTEM	
Plasma rennin level	Diminished
Urine aldosterone level	Diminished
Sympathetic innervation to juxtaglomerular cells	Diminished

Adapted from Hammerlein, A., et al. "Pharmacokinetic and Pharmacodynamic Changes in the Elderly: Clinical Implications," *Clinical Pharmacokinetics* 35(1):49-64, July 1998.

ACE inhibitors

ACE inhibitors reduce blood pressure by interrupting the renin-angiotensin activating system. Most ACE inhibitors are excreted through the kidney by glomerular filtration and tubular secretion. Renal impairment increases plasma concentration of the drug, so an older patient may need an adjusted dosage, especially a patient with a creatinine clearance below 30 ml/minute. Newer ACE inhibitors, such as benazepril (Lotensin) and fosinopril (Monopril), are also eliminated by the biliary route, which puts less stress on the kidneys.

Antibiotics

Because aging kidneys have a decreased ability to eliminate drugs, an older patient may need a dosage adjustment of an antibiotic. Antibiotics may also lead to *Clostridium difficile*–associated diarrhea, with a risk for fatal colitis.

The antibiotics ciprofloxacin (Cipro), ofloxacin (Floxin), levofloxacin (Levaquin), and other fluoroquinolones can increase the risk of tendinitis and tendon rupture in all ages, but patients older than 60 years; those taking corticosteroids; and those who have received kidney, heart, or lung transplants are at even greater risk. This risk starts during therapy and continues for several months, even after therapy stops. Using a corticosteroid along with antibiotics also increases this risk.

Anticholinergics

Anticholinergics (also called cholinergic blockers) interrupt parasympathetic nerve impulses in the central nervous system and autonomic nervous system. They also prevent acetylcholine from stimulating cholinergic receptors.

These drugs can affect older patients in several ways. As people age, the receptor density of muscarinic acetylcholine receptors in the brain decreases, contributing to a decrease in memory. Anticholinergics (especially muscarinic antagonists) can further impair an older patient's memory.

Effects in older patients from anticholinergic drugs can range from mild to severe. Early effects include dry mouth. These can progress to increased thirst, urinary retention, and agitation as well as more serious effects, such as delirium, hallucinations, cognitive impairment, seizures, and cardiac arrhythmias.

Anticholinergics can also increase intraocular pressure in older patients with closed-angle glaucoma and increase the risk of heatstroke in older patients by inhibiting diaphoresis. Toxicity is also more likely to occur if the patient takes two or more anticholinergic drugs when he's in a very warm environment.

Drugs that can produce anticholinergic effects include antiparkinsonian drugs that have atropine-like activity, tricyclic antidepressants (TCAs), phenothiazines, and antihistamines. Sometimes, an older adult is intentionally given an anticholinergic for a disorder such as an overactive bladder, a common occurrence in older adults.

Rx *Medication Alert* If a patient taking an acetylcholinesterase inhibitor (such as donepezil [Aricept] for Alzheimer's disease) is also prescribed a drug that has anticholinergic properties, monitor the patient closely. Anticholinergics are the pharmacologic opposites of acetylcholinesterase inhibitors and may decrease their effects.

Anticoagulants

Older adult patients taking anticoagulants have an increased risk for bleeding, especially if they take NSAIDs at the same time, which commonly happens. Because older patients are at an increased risk for falling, patients taking anticoagulants also have a greater risk for bleeding and bruising from falling. Watch such patients for bruising and bleeding; they also need their international normalized ratio (a test used to monitor anticoagulant therapy) carefully monitored.

Antidepressants

As the name implies, antidepressants are generally prescribed to treat depression. Examples include TCAs, selective serotonin reuptake inhibitors (SSRIs), and selective serotonin norepinephrine reuptake inhibitors (SSNRIs). Older patients can react differently to these drugs than younger adults; prescribers need to select carefully to find a drug that alleviates the patient's signs and symptoms with minimal adverse effects.

In some cases, a side effect can help a patient. An older patient who needs an antidepressant and is experiencing increased sleepiness may benefit from the stimulating effect of a drug such as sertraline (Zoloft), an SSRI, or venlafaxine (Effexor), an SSNRI.

TCAS

The oldest class of antidepressants, TCAs work by preventing the reuptake of norepinephrine or serotonin (or both) into the presynaptic nerve endings, which results in increased synaptic concentrations of these neurotransmitters. These drugs can be effective, but they produce significant adverse effects. For instance, some TCAs have anticholinergic effects, which, as discussed above, can cause problems for older adults. Some TCAs, such as imipramine (Tofranil) and doxepin (Sinequan), produce more anticholinergic activity than others, such as nortriptyline (Pamelor) and desipramine (Norpramin).

TCAs cause a gradual loss in the number of beta-adrenergic receptors. And because of the effect of TCAs on cardiac conduction, an overdose may be lethal. An older patient with a preexisting cardiac condition is more likely to experience cardiac toxicity. TCAs also have the potential to slow intraventricular conduction, producing heart block. Ventricular arrhythmias can result from a TCA's proar-rhythmic activity; when this does occur, it's often early in the course of treatment. The use of the TCA amitriptyline has been linked to sudden death in patients with a history of cardiac disease.

Because TCAs have high lipid solubility, the changes in pharmacokinetics that occur with aging typically lead to an increased volume of distribution. And, although phar-macokinetics varies extensively from patient to patient, older adults receiving typical dosages of TCAs tend to have higher plasma drug levels and metabolites than younger patients; elimination of TCAs also slows with aging.

Orthostatic hypotension, the result of adrenoreceptor antagonist activity, can be a potentially serious adverse effect in older patients. A drop in orthostatic blood pressure of 10 to 15 mm Hg or more before the start of TCA therapy is linked to an increased risk of symptomatic orthostatic hypotension.

TCAs can also produce antihistamine effects and sedation in older adults, contribut-ing to daytime somnolence. Such an effect can sometimes be helpful in a depressed patient with insomnia.

SSRIs

Often prescribed for depression in older adults, SSRIs inhibit the central nervous system's neuronal reuptake of the neurotransmitter serotonin. SSRIs don't have significant anticholinergic, hypotensive, or cardiac effects but, because they're typically nonsedating, they may cause insomnia until depression improves.

Rx *Medication Alert* An SSRI taken with St. John's wort, a herbal remedy for depression, places the patient at high risk for developing serotonin syndrome, which causes mental, autonomic, and neuromuscular changes.

Antihypertensives

For many older adults, antihypertensives may do their job too well, lowering blood pressure rapidly enough to cause insufficient blood flow to the brain. Possible results include dizziness, fainting, even stroke. Light-headedness and fainting can result from the atherosclerosis and decreased elasticity of blood vessels common in older adults. The decrease in baroreflex sensitivity that occurs with aging and hyper-tension can lead to such adverse reactions to antihypertensives as orthostatic hypotension, postprandial hypotension, syncope, and falls.

Because of such risks, older patients need carefully individualized dosages and treatments and often benefit from slower, less aggressive treatment of hypertension. Many older patients even need two drugs to control hypertension.

Any comorbidities the patient may have influence what hypertensive therapy he should receive. A patient with diabetes, for instance, may benefit from a thiazide-type diuretic and ACE inhibitor or angiotensin II receptor blocker because of the kidney damage diabetes can cause.

The older adult on antihypertensive therapy needs monitoring for orthostatic hypotension and hypotension after meals to prevent falls. Home blood pressure readings throughout the day can help determine if the patient needs any adjustment in medication and allow you to time his medication with his blood pressure pattern. Most, but not all, older patients have different blood pressure readings in the morning and at night, with lower blood pressure at night. Those that don't experience this drop in blood pressure at night are at higher risk for cardiovascular mortality. Other patients whose blood pressure drops much lower at night have a greater risk of falling. These daily fluctuations call for further study, but they highlight the importance of individualizing hypertensive therapy in older patients. **℞ Medication Alert** Before a patient on hypertensive therapy receives a new antihypertensive, assess him for any conditions or drug interactions—including interactions from caffeine, NSAIDs, and nasal decongestants—that could contribute to an inadequate response to his current therapy.

Antipsychotics

Antipsychotics can control psychotic symptoms such as delusions, hallucinations, and thought disorders that can occur with schizophrenia, mania, and other psychoses. Typical antipsychotics work by blocking the dopamine receptors, but they can produce such adverse effects as tardive dyskinesia and extrapyramidal signs and symptoms. Atypical antipsychotics, such as risperidone (Risperdal), olanzapine (Zyprexa), and quetiapine (Seroquel), also block the dopamine receptors, but not as much as typical antipsychotics, resulting in far fewer extrapyramidal adverse effects. Because of the pharmacokinetic and pharmacodynamic changes associated with aging, antipsychotics used in older patients can produce both anticholinergic effects (dry mouth, constipation, blurred vision, urinary retention, and cognitive impairment) and extrapyramidal signs and symptoms (bradykinesia, stiffness, cogwheel rigidity, akinesia, and akathisia).

Although it's an off-label use, antipsychotics are sometimes prescribed for older patients to help manage behaviors associated with dementia, such as paranoia, agitation, hallucinations, and delusions. However, these drugs can further impair cognitive function in these patients, most likely secondary to anticholinergic effects that further impact an already impaired cholinergic system. **℞ Medication Alert** Older patients are more likely to experience extrapyramidal effects from antipsychotics than younger patients, and these effects continue for a longer time after discontinuing the drug.

Other adverse effects of antipsychotics include excessive sedation, orthostatic hypotension, and an increased risk of falls and hip fractures. Many antipsychotics can also produce cardiac arrhythmias. All these adverse effects occur more commonly in older patients and at lower dosages than are typically used in younger patients.

Benzodiazepines

Benzodiazepines are a type of antianxiety agent that help relieve nervousness, tension, and other symptoms of anxiety by slowing the central nervous system. Examples include alprazolam (Xanax), chlordiazepoxide (Librium), diazepam (Valium), and lorazepam (Ativan). These drugs have less effect on the respiratory system and a larger therapeutic range than barbiturates, which are also used to treat anxiety. Barbiturates also have a low margin of safety in older adults and often produce significant sedation, increasing the risk for falls. Older patients using benzodiazepines, however, can also experience adverse effects, including dependence, cognitive impairment, and an increased risk for falls.

Benzodiazepines are categorized according to their half-lives, which are determined by their lipid solubility and the presence or absence of active metabolites. The older benzodiazepines, such as diazepam, chlordiazepoxide, and flurazepam (Dalmane), are highly lipid-soluble, and because adipose tissue stores typically increase with age, these drugs have an increased volume of distribution. The half-lives of these drugs can increase four-fold in an 85-year-old patient compared with a younger adult, with the half-life of diazepam sometimes exceeding 80 hours. Lower lipid-soluble benzodiazepines, such as lorazepam and oxazepam, have half-lives of less than 8 hours and therefore have less risk for accumulation and toxicity in older patients. However, because all benzodiazepines undergo hepatic degradation, the decreased hepatic function that occurs with aging can increase their half-lives.

Alternatives for controlling anxiety in older patients include zolpidem (Ambien) and buspirone (BuSpar). Zolpidem, once thought to be a good choice for older patients because of its shorter half-life, has a potential to cause confusion in older adults. Buspirone helps control anxiety in older patients without many of the adverse effects of benzodiazepines.

Beta-adrenergic blockers

Beta-adrenergic blockers are used for long-term prevention of angina and are one of the main types of drugs used to treat hypertension. They work by decreasing blood pressure and blocking beta-adrenergic receptor sites in the heart muscle and conduction system. This decreases heart rate and reduces the force of the heart's contractions, resulting in a lower demand for oxygen.

In older adults, sympathetic nervous system activity increases, which results in decreased myocardial sensitivity to catecholamines (epinephrine). This activity also reduces sensitivity to beta-adrenergic blockers. However, beta-adrenergic blockers may still be effective in an older adult after a myocardial infarction,

with some medications in this group more effective than others. Commonly prescribed beta-adrenergic blockers include bisoprolol (Zebeta), carvedilol (Coreg), and metoprolol (Lopressor).

Both albuterol and propranolol (Inderal) show reduced responses when used in older patients because of impaired beta-receptor function. Atenolol (Tenormin) and metoprolol are cardioselective beta-adrenergic blockers better tolerated by older adults.

R₂ Medication Alert Normal changes from aging, coupled with the effects of a beta-adrenergic blocker, limit the ability of the older patient's cardiovascular system to respond to shock. As a result, an older adult patient with superimposed shock may appear stable, possibly without an initial increase in pulse rate.

Calcium channel blockers

Calcium channel blockers prevent the passage of calcium ions across the myocardial cell membrane and vascular smooth muscle cells. This causes dilation of the coronary and peripheral arteries, which in turn decreases the force of the heart's contractions, reduces the heart's workload, and decreases blood pressure. By preventing arterioles from constricting, calcium channel blockers also reduce afterload, decreasing the heart's demand for oxygen. Some calcium channel blockers, such as diltiazem (Cardizem) and verapamil (Calan), also reduce heart rate by slowing conduction though the sinoatrial and atrioventricular nodes. A slower heart rate also reduces the heart's need for oxygen.

In older adults, verapamil has less effect on cardiac conduction and a greater effect on blood pressure and heart rate. Older adults may also be more sensitive to the negative inotropic and vasodilator effects of verapamil as well as have diminished baroreceptor sensitivity.

Cardiac glycosides

Cardiac glycosides are a group of drugs derived from digitalis, a substance that occurs naturally in foxglove plants. The most commonly used cardiac glycoside is digoxin (Lanoxin).

Digoxin inhibits an enzyme that regulates the amount of sodium and potassium in cells. It acts on the central nervous system to enhance vagal tone, slowing contractions through the sinoatrial and atrioventricular nodes and providing an antiarrhythmic effect.

As the body ages and renal function and rate of excretion decline, an older patient on digoxin therapy may have a buildup of digoxin in his blood that can reach the point of causing nausea, vomiting, diarrhea and, most seriously, cardiac arrhythmias. Early signs of inotropic toxicity include appetite loss, confusion, and depression.

Because an older patient is likely to have a prolonged peak plasma concentration of digoxin, he should receive a reduced loading dose. Systemic clearance of digoxin also decreases with age because the body clears digoxin mainly through the kidneys, with digoxin clearance proportional to creatinine clearance. A patient's clearance of digoxin—along with renal function and body weight—determines what maintenance dosage he should receive.

Corticosteroids

An older patient taking a corticosteroid may experience short-term reactions, including fluid retention and psychological effects ranging from mild euphoria to acute psychotic reactions. In older patients who have been taking prednisone or related steroidal compounds for months or even years, long-term toxic effects such as osteoporosis can be especially severe. To prevent serious toxicity, the patient on long-term therapy needs careful monitoring for subtle changes in appearance, mood, and mobility; impaired healing; and fluid and electrolyte disturbances.

Diuretics

Diuretics trigger the excretion of water and electrolytes from the kidneys, making these a primary choice for treating renal disease, edema, hypertension, and heart failure.

Because total body water content decreases with age, a normal dosage of a thiazide diuretic such as hydrochlorothiazide (Microzide) or a loop-diuretic such as furosemide (Lasix) may result in fluid loss and even dehydration in older patients. These diuretics may also deplete an older patient's potassium level, making him feel weak, and they may raise blood uric acid and glucose levels, complicating gout and diabetes mellitus.

Decreased sympathetic innervation of the juxtaglomerular cells of the kidneys occurs as the body ages, resulting in lower levels of plasma renin and aldosterone. As a result, diuretics have a more potent effect on older patients. The risk for dehydration in older adults—a risk compounded by decreased appetite, decreased thirst, and reduced kidney function, which can lead to fluid and electrolyte imbalance—calls for careful dosage selection.

NSAIDs

Used as antipyretics, anti-inflammatories, and analgesics, NSAIDs are lipid-soluble drugs with strong protein binding. They work by inhibiting an enzyme, which results in the suppression of the inflammatory response and pain. Many older adults use NSAIDs to help manage chronically painful conditions, such as osteoarthritis. The drugs are also used for both inflammatory musculoskeletal disorders and noninflammatory conditions.

Older adults taking NSAIDs may have a higher concentration of unbound drug in their systems because of the increased stores of adipose tissue and reduced plasma protein that typically occurs in older adults. The decreased renal clearance found in many older adults also increases the potential for excessive drug levels and toxicity.

NSAIDs can also affect the GI system—both directly through topical injury and systemically by inhibiting prostaglandin synthesis—resulting in peptic ulcers and GI bleeding. They can also produce renal insufficiency.

NSAIDs can interfere with other drugs. For instance, they blunt the effects of antihypertensive agents, especially beta-adrenergic blockers and ACE inhibitors. Specific NSAIDs can also result in adverse effects that are particularly dangerous for older patients. Naproxen (Aleve) may interfere with renal blood flow and glomerular filtration rate, worsening heart failure and elevating blood pressure. Ketorolac is toxic to the gastric mucosa and poses a risk for patients with renal impairment.

Because of the potential for common adverse reactions in older patients, NSAID use for pain management calls for careful consideration of the risks and benefits for each patient. An older patient on an NSAID should have his renal function monitored. Some patients on NSAID therapy may benefit from also taking misoprostol (Cytotec), a synthetic prostaglandin analogue, which can reduce the risk of GI adverse effects.

For those patient's who shouldn't take NSAIDs, alternatives include acetaminophen, tramadol (Ultram), corticosteroids, and opioids. Acetaminophen can help control chronic pain from osteoarthritis, but it must be used cautiously in older patients with hepatic disease and in those who use alcohol. Tramadol, a nonnarcotic analgesic, can also control both acute and chronic pain, and it doesn't have a great degree of plasma protein binding, doesn't elevate blood pressure or worsen heart failure, and has no potential for GI toxicity. However, it can cause nausea, vomiting, and unsteadiness.

Opioid agonists

An opioid is any derivative of the opium plant or any synthetic drug that imitates natural narcotics. Opioid agonists (also called narcotic agonists) include opium derivatives and synthetic drugs with similar properties. They decrease or relieve pain without causing a loss of consciousness; some also have antitussive and antidiarrheal effects.

Opioid agonists reduce pain by binding to opiate receptor sites in the peripheral and central nervous systems. When these drugs stimulate the opiate receptors, they mimic the effects of endorphins (naturally occurring opiates that are part of the body's own pain relief system). This receptor-site binding produces the therapeutic effects of analgesia and cough suppression as well as adverse reactions, such as respiratory depression and constipation.

Opioids generally safe for older adults include morphine (Avinza), oxycodone (Roxicodone), hydrocodone, and hydromorphone (Dilaudid). Underweight older patients should use transdermal fentanyl (Duragesic) with caution because absorption occurs through body fat. I.V. fentanyl may have reduced clearance and a greatly prolonged half-life in older adults. Older patients shouldn't take meperidine (Demerol) because it converts to the toxic metabolite normeperidine, which accumulates in renal failure and may lead to central nervous system excitation. This metabolite also produces confusion, psychosis, and seizure activity.

RECOGNIZING COMMON ADVERSE REACTIONS IN OLDER ADULTS

Common signs and symptoms of adverse reactions to medications include hives, impotence, incontinence, stomach upset, and rashes. Older adult patients are especially susceptible and may experience more serious adverse reactions, such as orthostatic hypotension, dehydration, and altered mental status.

Orthostatic Hypotension

Marked by lightheadedness or fainting and unsteady footing, orthostatic hypotension occurs as a common adverse effect of antidepressant, antihypertensive, antipsychotic, and sedative medications.

To prevent accidents such as falls, warn the patient not to sit up or get out of bed too rapidly. Instruct him to call for help walking if he feels dizzy or faint.

Dehydration

If the patient is taking diuretics such as hydrochlorothiazide, be alert for dehydration and electrolyte imbalances. Monitor the patient's blood levels, and provide potassium supplements, as ordered.

Oral dryness results from many medications. If anticholinergic medications cause dryness, suggest sucking on sugarless candy for relief.

Altered Mental Status

Agitation or confusion may follow ingestion of alcohol or anticholinergic, antidiuretic, antihypertensive, antipsychotic, and antidepressant medications. Paradoxically, depression is a common adverse effect of antidepressants.

Anorexia

This is a warning sign of toxicity—especially from digitalis glycosides, bronchodilators, and antihistamines. That's why physicians typically prescribe very low initial dosages.

Blood Disorders

If the patient takes an anticoagulant such as warfarin (Coumadin), watch for signs of easy bruising or bleeding (such as excessive bleeding after toothbrushing). Easy bruising or bleeding may be a sign of other problems, such as blood dyscrasias or thrombocytopenia. Drugs that may cause these reactions include several antineoplastic agents (such as methotrexate), antibiotics (such as nitrofurantoin), and anticonvulsants (such as valproic acid and phenytoin). A patient who bruises easily should report this sign to his physician immediately.

Tardive Dyskinesia

Characterized by abnormal tongue movements, lip pursing, grimacing, blinking, and gyrating motions of the face and extremities, this disorder may be triggered by psychotropic drugs, such as haloperidol (Haldol) or chlorpromazine.

Adverse Reactions: The Wrong Response

A patient's desired reaction to a drug is called the expected therapeutic response. An adverse reaction (also called a side effect), on the other hand, is a harmful, undesirable response. Adverse drug reactions can range from mild reactions that disappear when the patient stops taking the drug to debilitating, chronic conditions. Adverse reactions can appear shortly after starting a new drug; they often become less severe with time.

Several drugs can cause adverse reactions in older patients. Benzodiazepines and antianxiety drugs, prescribed to help relieve nervousness and tension, can cause depressive symptoms. Metoclopramide (Reglan), prescribed as an antiemetic, and tacrine (Cognex), prescribed for Alzheimer's disease, may cause Parkinson-like tremors from their antidopaminergic and cholinergic effects. A TCA may trigger syncope or arrhythmias. Several medications—including barbiturates, anticholinergics, antispasmodics, and muscle relaxants—can cause cognitive impairment. And chlorpromazine (Thorazine) and bupropion (Wellbutrin) can cause seizures. (See *Recognizing common adverse reactions in older adults*.)

Outside factors

Sometimes other factors influence how a patient responds to a drug. Disease processes and the physiological changes of aging can play a role in adverse reactions. Inappropriate prescribing, poor adherence to the medication regimen, and medication errors can also lead to adverse reactions, and taking an incorrect dose can result in serum drug levels over or under the therapeutic range. Keep in mind that an estimated 35% of older people experience some kind of adverse drug reaction, and almost half of these are preventable.

One of the greatest risks is failing to recognize an adverse reaction. Some adverse reactions that occur in older patients, such as anxiety, confusion, and forgetfulness, may be dismissed as behaviors typical of older adults rather than recognized as reactions to a drug. (See *Adverse reactions misinterpreted as age-related changes*, pages 122 and 123.)

Interactions

A common cause of adverse reactions in older adults is the interaction of medications with other substances. Such interactions can occur between drugs, between drugs and herbal supplements, and between drugs and foods. The more drugs a patient takes, the greater the chances that a drug or other interaction will occur. With older adults typically taking more than one medication, you'll need to be especially alert to such interactions in your older patients.

POLYPHARMACY

Using multiple medications doesn't only result in the overuse drugs—it also greatly increases the potential for adverse reactions. Polypharmacy is common in older adults, with those age 65 and older taking more drugs than any other group in the United States, including the highest proportion of prescribed medications.

Here are some of the statistics. Of all adults over age 65, 79% take some type of medication. People older than age 65 (12% of the population) consume 30% to 40% of all prescription drugs and purchase 40% of all over-the-counter (OTC) drugs. Women age 65 years and older take 10 or more medications, and 23% take at least 5 prescribed medications. If an older patient sees different health care providers for different conditions, the problem can grow worse, especially if providers don't collaborate and review all of the medications the patient takes, including OTC drugs and herbal remedies.

Many older patients also take drugs they probably shouldn't take. About 5% of older patients received at least 1 of the 11 medications classified by experts as drugs older patients should always avoid. Another 13% received at least 1 of the 8 medications that are considered rarely appropriate, and 17% received at least 1 of the 14 medications often misused (although these drugs have some indications for these patients). For example, 70% of older adults received propoxyphene, an analgesic medication considered rarely appropriate for older patients and a drug that has a long history of limited efficacy and potential for toxicity.

The problem isn't likely to go away any time soon, either. By 2040, it's estimated that baby boomers will make up 25% of the total population—and buy 50% of all prescription drugs.

Reviewing the situation

Making sure an older patient is taking the right medications requires regular review. Such a review should examine all drugs the patient is taking, evaluate dosages and monitor for toxicity, determine if the patient is taking the most appropriate drugs for his condition, and make sure the drugs he's taking are suitable for an older adult.

Any new prescription also calls for a careful assessment of what the patient already takes. And when deciding on the dosage of a new drug, the longstanding principle of "start low and go slow" should set the guidelines: starting a drug at the lowest dose and titrating upward to reach the optimal clinical benefit. If a prescription orders a higher-than-recommended starting dosage, the patient's primary health care practitioner should be consulted. A maintenance digoxin dosage of more than 0.125 mg/day, for instance, may place an older adult at risk for toxicity.

Part of a medication review includes discontinuing medications the patient no longer needs. When you perform a medication review for an older patient, make sure you compare the patient's needs with the medications available for use. The Hartford Institute for Geriatric Nursing's updated 2002 Beers criteria can serve as an appropriate screening tool for reviewing medication use in older adults. It contains 48 medications and classes of medications that the general population of adults age 65 and older shouldn't receive.

Unless the benefit of the drug outweighs the potential adverse reaction, the drug should be discontinued. For example, when prescribing warfarin, the prescriber must balance preventing a thrombotic event in a patient with atrial fibrillation with the common potential adverse reaction of increased bleeding. Keep in mind the Beers criteria doesn't identify all potential drug-related adverse reactions, nor does it indicate the possible harm of not using a potentially helpful medication. (See *The Beers criteria*, page 124.)

Reconciling medications

According to The Joint Commission, medication reconciliation is the process of comparing a patient's medication orders with an accurate list of all the medications the patient currently takes. Goals include preventing drug interactions, dosing errors, transcription errors, duplication of therapy, and omissions. When you reconcile a patient's medications, make sure you clarify any discrepancies with the physician before administering any drug.

Reconciliation should take place on both admission and discharge and whenever the patient is transferred to another setting. According to the Joint Commission's National Patient Safety Goals for reducing medication errors, the patient should also be given a complete list of medications that he'll be receiving on discharge from the health care facility.

DRUGS AND HERBAL SUPPLEMENTS

Medications can interact not just with other medications, but also with herbal supplements. Also called botanicals, herbal supplements are plant-based products that have medicinal properties. Many older adults—especially those with chronic conditions—take such supplements, viewing them as a safe because they're not actual drugs. But in older patients who also take other medications or more than one herbal supplement, interactions can occur.

Herbs with similar bioactivity to OTC or prescription drugs can potentiate the effects of those drugs, increasing the risk for adverse reactions, interactions, and drug toxicity. Glucosamine, for instance, commonly taken to maintain joint function, can decrease glucose tolerance by increasing insulin resistance, which interferes with diabetes treatment. Gingko biloba, commonly used to increase cognitive function, interacts with warfarin, a commonly prescribed anticoagulant, to increase bleeding time. (See *Herbs and medications with similar bioactivity*, page 125.)

If your patient is taking an herbal supplement, ask him some general questions, such as

(Text continues on page 125.)

℞ *Medication Alert* Adverse Reactions Misinterpreted as Age-Related Changes

In older patients, adverse drug reactions can easily be misinterpreted as the typical signs and symptoms of aging. The table below, which shows possible adverse reactions for common drug classifications, can help you avoid such misinterpretations.

Drug classifications	Agitation	Anxiety	Arrhythmias	Ataxia	Changes in appetite	Confusion	Constipation	Depression	
ACE inhibitors						●	●	●	
Alpha₁ adrenergic blockers		●					●	●	
Antianginals	●	●	●			●			
Antiarrhythmics			●				●		
Anticholinergics	●	●	●			●	●	●	
Anticonvulsants	●		●	●	●	●	●	●	
Antidepressants, tricyclic	●	●	●	●		●	●	●	
Antidiabetics, oral					●				
Antihistamines						●	●	●	
Antilipemics							●		
Antiparkinsonians	●	●	●	●	●	●	●	●	
Antipsychotics	●	●	●	●	●	●	●	●	
Barbiturates	●	●	●			●			
Benzodiazepines	●			●	●	●	●	●	
Beta-adrenergic blockers		●	●					●	
Calcium channel blockers		●	●		●		●		
Corticosteroids	●				●	●		●	
Diuretics			●			●			
NSAIDs		●				●	●	●	
Opioids	●	●				●	●	●	
Skeletal muscle relaxants	●	●		●		●		●	
Thyroid hormones		●	●		●				

	Difficulty breathing	Disorientation	Dizziness	Drowsiness	Edema	Fatigue	Hypotension	Insomnia	Memory loss	Muscle weakness	Restlessness	Sexual dysfunction	Tremors	Urinary dysfunction	Visual changes
			●		●	●	●	●				●			●
			●	●	●	●	●	●					●	●	●
			●		●	●	●	●			●	●		●	●
	●		●		●	●									
		●	●	●		●	●		●	●	●			●	●
	●		●	●	●	●	●						●		●
	●	●	●	●	●	●	●	●			●	●	●	●	●
			●			●	●			●					
		●	●	●		●							●	●	●
			●			●		●		●		●	●	●	●
		●	●	●		●	●	●		●			●	●	●
			●	●		●	●	●			●	●	●	●	●
	●	●		●		●	●				●				
	●	●	●	●		●		●	●				●	●	●
	●		●			●	●	●	●				●	●	●
	●		●		●	●	●	●					●		●
					●	●	●			●					●
			●			●	●			●				●	
			●	●	●	●		●		●					●
	●	●	●	●		●	●	●	●		●	●		●	●
			●	●		●	●	●					●		
								●					●		

THE BEERS CRITERIA

The list below identifies medications and classes of medications to avoid in older patients.

A
alprazolam (Xanax)
amiodarone (Cordarone)
amitriptyline (Elavil)
amphetamines
anorexic agents

B
barbiturates
belladonna alkaloids (Donnatal)
bisacodyl (Dulcolax)

C
carisoprodol (Soma)
cascara sagrada
chlordiazepoxide (Librium, Mitran)
chlordiazepoxide-amitriptyline
(Limbitrol)
chlorpheniramine (Chlor-Trimeton)
chlorpropamide (Diabinese)
chlorzoxazone (Paraflex)
cimetidine (Tagamet)
clidinium-chlordiazepoxide (Librax)
clonidine (Catapres)
clorazepate (Tranxene)
cyclandelate (Cyclospasmol)
cyclobenzaprine (Flexeril)
cyproheptadine (Periactin)

D
desiccated thyroid
dexchlorpheniramine (Polaramine)
diazepam (Valium)
dicyclomine (Bentyl)
digoxin (Lanoxin)
diphenhydramine (Benadryl)
dipyridamole (Persantine)
disopyramide (Norpace,
Norpace CR)
doxazosin (Cardura)
doxepin (Sinequan)

E
ergot mesyloids (Hydergine)
estrogens
ethacrynic acid (Edecrin)

F
ferrous sulfate (iron)
fluoxetine (Prozac)
flurazepam (Dalmane)

G
guanadrel (Hylorel)
guanethidine (Ismelin)

H
halazepam (Paxipam)
hydroxyzine (Vistaril, Atarax)
hyoscyamine (Levsin, Levsinex)

I
indomethacin (Indocin, Indocin SR)
isoxsuprine (Vasodilan)

K
ketorolac (Toradol)

L
lorazepam (Ativan)

M
meperidine (Demerol)
meprobamate (Miltown, Equanil)
mesoridazine (Serentil)
metaxalone (Skelaxin)
methocarbamol (Robaxin)
methyldopa (Aldomet)
methyldopa-hydrochlorothiazide
(Aldoril)
methyltestosterone (Android,
Virilon, Testred)
mineral oil

N
naproxen (Naprosyn, Anaprox,
Aleve)
neoloid
nifedipine (Procardia, Adalat)
nitrofurantoin (Macrodantin)

O
orphenadrine (Norflex)
oxaprozin (Daypro)
oxazepam (Serax)
oxybutynin (Ditropan)

P
pentazocine (Talwin)
perphenazine-amitriptyline
(Triavil)
piroxicam (Feldene)
promethazine (Phenergan)
propantheline (Pro-Banthine)
propoxyphene (Darvon) and
combination products

Q
quazepam (Doral)

R
reserpine (Serpalan, Serpasil)

T
temazepam (Restoril)
thioridazine (Mellaril)
ticlopidine (Ticlid)
triazolam (Halcion)
trimethobenzamide (Tigan)
tripelennamine

Adapted with permission from Fick, D.M., et al. "Updating the Beers Criteria for Potentially Inappropriate Medicine Use in Older Adults: Results of a U.S. Consensus Panel of Experts," *Archives of Internal Medicine* 163(22):2716-24. Table 1, p. 2720. Evidence Level VI: Expert Opinion, Copyright © 2003. American Medical Association.

HERBS AND MEDICATIONS WITH SIMILAR BIOACTIVITY

Several herbal supplements work similarly to medications, increasing the risk of an interaction. This table lists several herbal supplements and drugs that have similar bioactivity.

HERB	MEDICATION
Angelica	Calcium channel blockers
Birch bark, willow bark, wintergreen, meadowsweet	Aspirin
Black cohosh, fennel, red clover, stinging nettle	Estrogen
Dong quai, feverfew, garlic, gingko biloba, wintergreen	Anticoagulants
Ginseng, St. John's wort, yohimbe	Monoamine oxidase inhibitors
Guarana, kola nut	Caffeine
Lobelia	Nicotine
Thyme, purslane	Lithium

why he's taking the herb and how long he has been taking it. Find out if the condition he's trying to treat has been diagnosed. If so, ask if he's currently taking or has ever taken prescription or OTC drugs for the condition. (See *Potential adverse reactions associated with herbal supplements*, page 126.)

DRUGS AND FOOD

When you take an older patient's drug history, make sure you also ask about his dietary history, because even foods can alter the effect of some prescribed medications. For example, if the patient takes warfarin, he should maintain a consistent intake of the green, leafy vegetables that he normally eats because the vitamin K found in such vegetables reduces the anticoagulant effects of warfarin by increasing the synthesis of clotting factors. (See *The effects of foods on health conditions and medication use*, pages 129 to 131.)

Administering I.M. Drugs: Tailor Your Technique

The physical changes of aging significantly affect I.M. drug administration. To give an older patient an I.M. injection, you'll need to choose the right equipment and site and modify your technique.

CHOOSING A NEEDLE

Remember that most older adults have less subcutaneous tissue and less muscle mass than younger patients—especially in the buttocks and deltoids. As a result, you may need to use a shorter needle than you would for a younger adult.

SELECTING A SITE

Also remember that an older adult patient typically has more fat around the hips, abdomen, and thighs. This makes the vastus lateralis muscle and ventrogluteal area (gluteus medius and minimus, but not gluteus maximus muscles) the primary injection sites.

You should be able to palpate the muscle in these areas easily. However, if the patient is extremely thin, gently pinch the muscle to elevate it and to avoid putting the needle completely through it because that would alter the absorption and distribution of the drug.

Rx Medication Alert Never give an I.M. injection in an immobile limb because of poor drug absorption and the risk that a sterile abscess will form at the injection site.

POTENTIAL ADVERSE REACTIONS ASSOCIATED WITH HERBAL SUPPLEMENTS

Many older patients take herbal supplements to help relieve various disorders. This list includes popular supplements, why they're taken, and possible adverse reactions.

HERB	POSSIBLE REASON FOR USE	POSSIBLE ADVERSE REACTION
Black cohosh	• Relief of menopausal symptoms, (night sweats, hot flashes, irritability, sleep disturbances) • Treatment of dysmenorrhea • Relief of premenstrual syndrome	• Bradycardia • Headache • Hypotension • Joint pain • Seizures • Weight gain
Bloodroot*	• Anticancer agent • Digestive system stimulant • Emetic	• Arrhythmias • Bradycardia • Dizziness • Impaired vision • Intense thirst
Boneset	• Influenza symptom relief • Decongestant • Laxative	• Liver toxicity • Mental changes • Respiratory problems
Camomile	• Antidiarrheal • Antianxiety agent • Stomatitis relief • Relief from restlessness • Flatulence relief • Motion sickness relief • Wound healing • Treatment of hemorrhagic cystitis	• Anaphylaxis • Conjunctivitis • Contact dermatitis • Eczema • Eyelid angioedema • Nausea • Vomiting
Coltsfoot	• Asthma treatment • Bronchitis treatment • Treatment of dry, hacking cough • Laryngitis relief • Treatment of hoarseness • Relief of lung cancer symptoms • Mouth and throat irritation relief • Sore throat relief • Relief from wheezing	• Fever • Liver toxicity
Dandelion	• Mild diuretic • Cholesterol level reduction • Appetite stimulant • Treatment of minor digestive problems • Treatment of kidney and bladder stones • Treatment of liver and gallbladder problems • Urinary tract infection treatment	• Increase in concentration of lithium or potassium • Interaction with diuretics
Echinacea	• Immune system stimulant	• Allergic reaction • Fever • GI disturbances • Polyuria • Taste disturbance

POTENTIAL ADVERSE REACTIONS ASSOCIATED WITH HERBAL SUPPLEMENTS (*continued*)

HERB	POSSIBLE REASON FOR USE	POSSIBLE ADVERSE REACTION
Ephedra	<ul><li>Appetite suppressant</li><li>Asthma treatment</li><li>Treatment of respiratory tract infection</li><li>Decongestant</li><li>Relief from mild bronchospasm</li><li>Relief from chills associated with colds</li><li>Fever reduction</li><li>Headache relief</li></ul>	<ul><li>Anxiety</li><li>Dizziness</li><li>Hypertension</li><li>Insomnia</li><li>Tachycardia</li></ul>
Evening primrose oil	<ul><li>Relief from premenstrual syndrome</li><li>Cystic mastitis treatment</li><li>Neurodermatitis treatment</li><li>Mastalgia treatment</li><li>Relief from menopause symptoms</li></ul>	<ul><li>Allergic reaction</li><li>GI disturbances</li><li>Headache</li></ul>
Feverfew	<ul><li>Asthma treatment</li><li>Menstrual cramp relief</li><li>Treatment of migraine headaches</li><li>Mouthwash</li><li>Psoriasis treatment</li><li>Rheumatoid arthritis treatment</li><li>Tranquilizer</li></ul>	<ul><li>Interference with blood clotting</li></ul>
Garlic	<ul><li>Treatment for high cholesterol and triglyceride levels</li><li>Treatment for bacterial and fungal infections</li><li>Digestive problem relief</li><li>Treatment for hypertension</li><li>Prevention of atherosclerosis</li><li>Treatment for minor respiratory disorders</li></ul>	<ul><li>Asthma</li><li>Body odor</li><li>Contact dermatitis</li><li>Facial flushing</li><li>Fatigue</li><li>Flatulence</li><li>Headache</li><li>Heartburn</li><li>Hypersensitivity reactions</li><li>Inhibition of blood clotting</li><li>Insomnia</li><li>Orthostatic hypotension</li><li>Potentiation of antidiabetic drugs</li><li>Shortness of breath</li></ul>
Ginkgo biloba	<ul><li>Memory enhancer</li><li>Treatment of degenerative and vascular dementia</li><li>Treatment of peripheral artery occlusive disease</li><li>Relief of vertigo</li><li>Relief of tinnitus</li></ul>	<ul><li>Allergic reaction</li><li>Dizziness</li><li>GI disturbances</li><li>Headache</li><li>Increased anticoagulation</li><li>Palpitations</li></ul>
Ginseng	<ul><li>Energy booster for fatigue, exhaustion, stress, and convalescence</li></ul>	<ul><li>Anxiety</li><li>Asthma</li><li>Hypertension</li><li>Insomnia</li><li>Postmenopausal bleeding</li><li>Tachycardia</li></ul>

*These herbs have been declared as unsafe by the Food and Drug Administration because the plants contain poisonous components.

(continued)

POTENTIAL ADVERSE REACTIONS ASSOCIATED WITH HERBAL SUPPLEMENTS (*continued*)

HERB	POSSIBLE REASON FOR USE	POSSIBLE ADVERSE REACTION
Goldenseal	● Bladder inflammation treatment ● Arthritis treatment ● Eczema treatment ● Allergy treatment ● Relief of cold and flu symptoms ● Kidney stone treatment ● Relief of laryngitis (as a gargle) ● Sore throat relief	● Vasoconstriction
Hawthorn	● Heart failure treatment	● Hypotension
Kava	● Antianxiety agent ● Antidepressant	● Damage to skin, liver, eyes, and spinal cord from long-term use
Licorice	● Anti-inflammatory agent for upper respiratory tract ● Treatment of gastric or duodenal ulcers	● Hypernatremia ● Hypokalemia
Lobelia*	● Asthma treatment ● Treatment of chronic bronchitis ● Treatment of pneumonia ● Relief of smoking withdrawal symptoms ● Spastic colon treatment ● Treatment of spastic muscle conditions	● Vision and hearing problems
Motherwort	● Amenorrhea treatment ● Antianxiety agent ● Relief of symptoms of menopause	● Increased anticoagulation
Nettle	● Anti-inflammatory effects caused by prostaglandins ● Mild forms of benign prostatic hyperplasia ● Reduce sneezing ● Reduce itching	● Hypokalemia
Saw palmetto	● Benign prostatic hyperplasia ● Congestion from colds, bronchitis, or asthma ● Mild diuretic ● Urinary antiseptic and astringent	● Abdominal pain ● Diarrhea ● Dizziness ● Headache ● Hypertension ● Nausea ● Urine retention
Senna	● Constipation	● Potentiation of digoxin
Skullcap	● Anxiety ● Nervous tension ● Hysteria ● Convulsions ● Symptoms associated with premenstrual syndrome ● Stress-related headaches ● Anorexia nervosa ● Insomnia ● Muscle spasms ● Tension headaches ● Restless leg syndrome ● Mild Tourette's syndrome	● Drowsiness ● Potentiation of antianxiety or sedative medications

POTENTIAL ADVERSE REACTIONS ASSOCIATED WITH HERBAL SUPPLEMENTS (*continued*)

HERB	POSSIBLE REASON FOR USE	POSSIBLE ADVERSE REACTION
St. John's wort	• Depression • Anxiety • Seasonal effective disorder • Restlessness • Viral infections • Sleep problems	• Dry mouth • Dizziness • GI complaints • Fatigue • Headache • Pruritus • Neuropathies • Hypothyroidism • Delayed hypersensitivity • Photosensitivity
Valerian	• Restlessness • Mild sleep promoting agent in nervous and anxiety-related sleep disturbances	• Drowsiness • Potentiation of antianxiety or sedative medications
Yohimbe*	• Certain depressive disorders • Erectile dysfunction	• Anxiety • Hypertension • Mental changes • Tachycardia

* These herbs have been declared as unsafe by the Food and Drug Administration because the plants contain poisonous components.

THE EFFECTS OF FOODS ON HEALTH CONDITIONS AND MEDICATION USE

Many of your older patients have one or more chronic disorders and take several medications. You can use this table to teach them about the foods they should and shouldn't eat based on their health conditions and the medications they take.

FOODS AND DIETARY CONCERNS	REPRESENTATIVE FOODS
Calcium-rich foods (should be eaten by patients with hypocalcemia and post-menopausal women)	Bok choy Broccoli Calcium-fortified beverages, cereals, and breads Canned salmon Canned sardines Cheese Clams Collard greens Creamed soup Kale Milk Molasses Oysters Sardines Soy beans and other soy-based products Spinach Tofu Turnip greens Yogurt

(continued)

THE EFFECTS OF FOODS ON HEALTH CONDITIONS AND MEDICATION USE (*continued*)

FOODS AND DIETARY CONCERNS	REPRESENTATIVE FOODS
High-sodium foods (should be avoided by patients with congestive heart failure [CHF] fluid overload, or hypertension)	Beer Butter Buttermilk Canned seafood Canned soup Canned spaghetti Cookies Cured meat Fast food Pickles Prepackaged dinners Pretzels Salad dressings Sauces Sauerkraut Snack foods, such as cheese puffs, crackers, and potato chips Tomato ketchup
Iron-rich foods (should be eaten by patients who need to maintain their red blood cell levels)	Beets Cereals Dried beans and peas Dried fruit Enriched grains Leafy green vegetables Organ meats, such as heart, kidney, liver
Low-sodium foods (should be eaten by patients with CHF, fluid overload, or hypertension)	Egg yolks Fresh fruit Fresh vegetables Grits Honey Jam and jelly Lean meat Lima beans Macaroons Potatoes Poultry Pumpkin Red kidney beans Sherbet Unsalted nuts
Potassium-rich foods (should be eaten by patients taking potassium-wasting diuretics)	Avocados Bananas Broccoli Cantaloupe Dried fruit Grapefruit Lima beans Navy beans Nuts Oranges

THE EFFECTS OF FOODS ON HEALTH CONDITIONS AND MEDICATION USE (*continued*)

FOODS AND DIETARY CONCERNS	REPRESENTATIVE FOODS
Potassium-rich foods (*continued*)	Peaches Potatoes Prunes Rhubarb Spinach Sunflower seeds Tomatoes
Purine-rich foods (should be avoided by patients with gout)	Anchovies Kidneys Lentils Liver Sardines Sweetbreads
Tyramine-rich foods (should be avoided by patients taking monoamine oxidase inhibitors and some antihypertensives)	Aged cheese Avocados Bananas Beer Bologna Caffeinated beverages Chocolate Liver Pepperoni Pickled fish Red wine (Chianti) Ripe fruit Salami Smoked fish Yeast Yogurt
Urine acidifiers (helpful for excretion of some drugs)	Cheese Cranberries Eggs Fish Grains Plums Poultry Prunes Red meat
Urine alkalinizers (helpful for excretion of some drugs)	Apples Berries Citrus fruit Milk Vegetables
Vitamin K-rich foods (should be avoided or strictly limited when taking anticoagulants)	Collard greens Kale Mustard greens Parsley (raw) Spinach Swiss chard Turnip greens

CHECKING TECHNIQUE

To avoid inserting the needle in a blood vessel, pull back on the plunger and look for blood before injecting the drug. Because of age-related changes, the older adult is also at a great risk for hematomas. To check for bleeding after an I.M. injection, you may need to apply direct pressure over the puncture site for a longer time than usual. Gently massage the site to aid in drug absorption and distribution. However, avoid site massage with certain drugs given by the Z-track injection technique such as iron dextran.

Patient Teaching: Empower the Patient

When you teach an older patient about his medications, you give him the knowledge and skills he'll need to take his medications appropriately and maintain his own health. As you plan your teaching, keep in mind that discharge planning begins at admission.

To start, you'll need to understand what the patient already knows about his medications and his ability to self-administer his drugs. You'll also need to review all the drugs he takes, including prescriptions from all providers, OTC medication, and herbal remedies, and perform a medication reconciliation, as discussed earlier.

Compliance

A major potential roadblock to successful patient teaching is a lack of compliance. In fact, noncompliance in older patients is so prevalent, it's no wonder most nurses rank it as one of the top priorities when planning nursing care.

ASSESSING COMPLIANCE

When assessing a patient's ability to comply, you'll need to evaluate his physical ability to take drugs. Can he read drug labels and directions? Does he identify drugs by sight or touch? Can he open drug bottles easily? If he's disabled, by Parkinson's disease or arthritis, for example, or if he lacks manual dexterity for any reason, advise him to ask his pharmacist for snap or screw caps (rather than childproof closures) for his drug containers.

You can use the Drugs Regimen Unassisted Grading Scale (DRUGS) Tool to assess the patient's ability to self-administer his medications. This tool assesses the patient's ability to perform four tasks critical to self-administration. The patient is asked to:

- identify the appropriate medication
- open the container
- select the correct dose
- report the appropriate timing of doses.

Evaluate the patient's cognitive skills. Can he remember to take prescribed drugs on time and regularly? Can he remember where he stored his drugs? If not, refer him to appropriate community resources for supervision.

Assess your patient's lifestyle. Does he live with family or friends? If so, include them in your patient-teaching sessions if possible. Does he live alone or with a debilitated spouse? If so, he'll need continuing support from a visiting nurse or other caregiver.

Ask the patient whether the prescribed medication regimen interferes with his daily routine. Keep in mind that inadequate supervision may result in drug misuse. Make appropriate referrals and contact appropriate social agencies to ensure compliance and safety and to provide financial assistance if necessary.

Assess the patient's beliefs concerning drug use. For example, he may believe that chronic medication use is a sign of illness or weakness. As a result, he may take his medications erratically.

PREVENTING REACTIONS THAT IMPEDE COMPLIANCE

Discuss the patient's drug therapy with him. As he receives drugs, name them, explain their intended effect, and describe possible adverse reactions to watch out for and report.

Tell the patient that you're going to ask him questions to help identify or reduce the risk of harmful food or drug interactions (such as those caused by alcohol or caffeine) that may interfere with compliance. Ask him about all drugs, both prescription and nonprescription, that he's currently taking as well as those he's taken in the past. If possible, ask to see samples. Have him name each drug and tell you why, when, and how often he takes it. Remember, the patient may have drugs prescribed by more than one physician. Also ask whether he's taking any drugs originally prescribed for another person (a common occurrence).

If your facility has a specially designed computer program, use it to help prevent possible drug interactions. Enter all the data you've collected on drug dosage, frequency, and administration route into a master file of drugs commonly used by older patients, such as anticoagulants (warfarin), benzodiazepines (diazepam), beta blockers (propranolol), calcium channel blockers (verapamil), digitalis glycosides (digoxin), and diuretics (furosemide). From this information, the computer can compile a list of the patient's drugs, possible adverse reactions, potential interactions, and suggested interventions. Then review the findings with the patient. If he knows what to expect, he'll be more likely to comply with treatment. (If you don't have access to such technology, you can compile a similar list using a reputable drug reference.)

You can also encourage the patient to purchase drugs from only one pharmacy, preferably one that maintains a drug profile for each customer. Advise him to consult the pharmacist, who can anticipate drug interactions before they occur.

Inform the patient about specific food-drug interactions. Based on the information in your drug history, provide a list of foods to avoid.

BOOSTING THERAPEUTIC COMPLIANCE

To circumvent noncompliance caused by visual impairment, provide dosage instructions in large print, if necessary.

To alter eating habits that lead to noncompliance, emphasize which drugs the patient must take with food and which he must take on an empty stomach. Explain that taking some drugs on an empty stomach may cause nausea, whereas taking some drugs on a full stomach may interfere with absorption. Also find out whether the patient eats regularly or skips meals. If he skips meals, he may be skipping doses, too. As needed, help him coordinate his drug administration schedule with his eating habits.

To correct problems related to drug form and administration, help the patient find easier ways to take medicine. For example, if he can't swallow pills or capsules, switch to a liquid or powdered form of the drug if possible. Or suggest that he slide the tablet down with a soft food such as applesauce. Keep in mind which tablets you can crush and which you can't. For example, enteric-coated tablets, timed-release capsules, and sublingual or buccal tablets shouldn't be crushed because doing so may affect absorption and effectiveness. Some crushed drugs may taste bitter and may stain or irritate oral mucosa. (See *Drugs that shouldn't be crushed or chewed*, pages 134 and 135.)

If mobility or transportation deters compliance, help the patient locate a pharmacy that

Rx *Medication Alert*   Drugs that Shouldn't be Crushed or Chewed

Crushing or chewing certain drugs—including enteric-coated tablets, timed-release capsules, and sublingual or buccal tablets—can interfere with absorption, effectiveness, taste, or another property of the drug. Here's a list of those drugs.

Aciphex	Cartia XT	DynaCirc CR	Ferro-Sequels	K-Lyte
Actonel	Cefaclor Extended-	Duraphen II	Flagyl ER	K-Lyte CL
Accutane	Release	Duraphen II DM	Fleet Laxative	K-Lyte DS
Actiq	Ceftin	Duraphen Forte	Flomax	K-Tab
Adalat CC	Cefuroxime	Duratuss	Focalin XR	Lescol XL
Adderall XR	CellCept	Duratuss A	Fosamax	Levbid
AeroHist Plus	Charcoal Plus	Duratuss PE	Geocillin	Levsinex Timecaps
Afeditab CR	Chlor-Trimeton	Dynex	Gleevec	Lexxel
Allegra-D	12 Hour	Easprin	Glipizide	Lialda
Allfen Jr	Cipro XR	EC-Naprosyn	Glucophage XR	Lipram 4500
Alophen	Claritin-D 12 Hour	Ecotrin Adult Low	Glucotrol XL	Lipram PN 10, 16, 20
Alprazolam ER	Claritin-D 24 Hour	Strength	Glumetza	Lipram UL 12, 18, 20
Altoprev	Colace	Ecotrin Maximum	Guaifed	Liquibid-D 1200
Ambien CR	Colestid	Strength	Guaifed-PD	Liquibid-PD
Aptivus	Concerta	Ecotrin Regular	Guaifenesin/	Lithobid
Aquatab C	Commit	Strength	Pseudoephedrine	Lodrane 24
Aquatab D	Cotazym-S	Ed A-Hist	Guaifenex DM	LoHist 12 Hour
Arthrotec	Covera-HS	E.E.S. 400	Guaifenex GP	Maxifed DM
Asacol	Creon 5, 10, 20	Effer-K	Guaifenex PSE	Maxifed DMX
Ascriptin A/D	Crixivan	Effervescent	GuaiMAX-D	Maxiphen DM
Azulfidine EN-tabs	Cymbalta	Potassium	Halfprin 81	Medent-DM
Augmentin XR	Cytoxan	Effexor XR	Heartline	Mestinon Timespan
Avinza	Cytovene	Efidac/24	H 9600 SR	Metadate ER
Avodart	Dallergy	Pseudoephedrine	Hista-Vent DA	Metadate CD
Bayer Enteric-Coated	Dallergy-JR	Efidac/24	Hydrea	Methylin ER
Bayer Low Adult	Deconamine SR	E-Mycin	Imdur	Micro K Extendcaps
Bayer Regular	Depakene	Enablex	Inderal LA	Miraphen PSE
Strength	Depakote	Entex LA	Indocin SR	Modane
Bellahist-D LA	Depakote ER	Entex PSE	Innopran XL	Morphine sulfate
Biaxin XL	Detrol LA	Entocort EC	Invega	extended-release
Bidhist	Dilacor XR	Equetro	Ionamin	Motrin
Bidhist-D	Dilatrate-SR	Ergomar	Isochron	MS Contin
Biltricide	Dilt-CD	Eryc	Isoptin SR	Mucinex
Bisa-Lax	Dilt-XR	Ery-Tab	Isordil Sublingual	Mucinex DM
Biohist LA	Diltia XT	Erythrocin Stearate	Isosorbide Dinitrate	Muco-Fen-DM
Bisac-Evac	Ditropan XL	Erythromycin Base	Sublingual	Myfortic
Bisacodyl	Doxidan	Evista	Isosorbide SR	Naprelan
Boniva	Drisdol	ExeFen PD	K + 8	Nasatab LA
Bromfed PD	DriHist SR	Extendryl JR	K + 10	Nexium
Budeprion SR	Drixoral Cold/Allergy	Extendryl SR	Kadian	Niaspan
Calan SR	Drixoral Nondrowsy	Feldene	Kaletra	Nicotinic Acid
Carbatrol	Drixoral Allergy Sinus	Feen-a-mint	Kaon CL-10	Nifediac CC
Cardene SR	Droxia	Fentora	Keppra	Nifedical XL
Cardizem	Drysec	Feosol	Ketek	NitroQuick
Cardizem CD	Dulcolax	Feratab	Klor-Con	Nitrostat
Cardizem LA	DuraHist	Fergon	Klor-Con M	Norpace CR
Cardura XL	DuraHist D	Fero-Grad 500 mg	Klotrix	Ondrox

Rx Medication Alert
Drugs that Shouldn't be Crushed or Chewed (*continued*)

Opana ER	Prilosec OTC	Ralix	Somnote	Trental
Oracea	Procanbid	Ranexa	Sprycel	Tylenol Arthritis
Oramorph SR	Procardia XL	Razadyne ER	Stahist	Ultram ER
OxyContin	Profen II	Renagel	Strattera	Uniphyl
Palcaps (all)	Profen II DM	Rescon	Sudafed 12 hour	Urocit-K
Pancrease MT	Profen Forte	Rescon JR	Sudafed 24 hour	Uroxatral
Pancrecarb MS	Profen Forte DM	Rescon MX	Sular	Valcyte
Pancrelipase	Propecia	Respa-1st	Symax Duotab	Verapamil SR
Panocaps	Proquin XR	Respa-DM	Symax SR	Verelan
Panocaps MT	Proscar	Respahist	Taztia XT	Verelan PM
Paxil CR	Protonix	Respaire 120 SR	Tegretol-XR	VesiCare
Pentasa	Prozac Weekly	Respaire 60 SR	Temodar	Videx EC
PhenaVent D	Pseudo CM TR	Ritalin LA	Tessalon Perles	Voltaren XR
PhenaVent LA	Pseudovent	Ritalin SR	Theo-24	VoSpire ER
Pre-Hist-D	Pseudovent 400	R-Tanna	Tiazac	Wellbutrin SR, XL
Plendil	Pseudovent-PED	Rythmol SR	Topamax	Xanax XR
Prevacid	Pseudovent DM	Sinemet CR	Toprol XL	
Prevacid SoluTab	Pytest	SINUvent PE	Touro CC-LD	
Prevacid Suspension	QDALL	Slo-Niacin	Touro LA-LD	
Prilosec	QDALL AR	Solodyn	Tracleer	

refills and delivers prescriptions. If appropriate, consider using a mail-order pharmacy.

If forgetfulness interferes with compliance, devise a system for helping the patient remember to take his drugs properly. Suggest that the patient or a family member purchase or make a scheduling aid, such as a calendar, checklist, alarm wristwatch, or compartmented drug container. (See *Using compliance aids,* page 136.)

Some patients may try to save money by not having prescriptions filled or refilled or by taking fewer doses than ordered to make the drug last longer. If financial considerations are interfering with your patient's compliance, help him explore available resources. Suggest using less-expensive generic equivalents of name-brand drugs whenever possible. Also, explore ways that family members

can help, or refer the patient to the social services department and appropriate community agencies. Many states have programs to help low-income, elderly patients buy needed drugs.

Advise the patient to contact you or his physician before taking any nonprescription drugs to avoid adverse drug interactions. If necessary, regularly monitor serum levels of drugs, such as digoxin or potassium, to avoid toxicity. When the physician advises discontinuing a drug, instruct the patient to discard it in the toilet, if possible. This prevents others from using the drug and ensures that the patient won't continue taking it by mistake.

To avoid improper storage and possible drug deterioration, advise the patient to keep all prescribed drugs in their original

USING COMPLIANCE AIDS

To help your patient comply with oral or injectable drug therapy safety, you or a family member may premeasure doses for him, using compliance aids such as those shown below or ones you create yourself. Most pharmacies or community service agencies can supply similar aids.

1-day Pill Pack

A plastic box with four lidded medication compartments marked "breakfast," "lunch," "dinner," and "bedtime" helps the patient see whether he has taken all of the medications prescribed for 1 day. The lids may be embossed with Braille characters if needed. The patient, caregiver, or visiting nurse must remember to fill the device each day. Because it's small, the device doesn't hold many tablets or capsules.

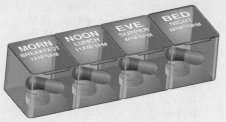

7-day Pill Reminder

The boxes shown here will help the patient remember whether he has taken all the tablets and capsules· prescribed for each day of the week. (The days of the week appear in both Braille characters and printed letters.) Like the 1-day pill container, this device is inappropriate for large numbers of tablets or capsules, or for tablets and capsules that must be taken at different times each day.

Some pill containers have extra-large compartments that can hold several pills and have a week's worth of separate morning and evening compartments.

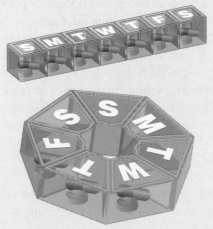

Homemade Dosing Aids

Show the patient and his caregivers how to make their own compliance aids by labeling clean, empty jars, extra prescription bottles (obtainable form the pharmacist), or envelopes with the drug name, the time of day, and the day of the week to take the medication. Recommend using a separate container for each time. Fill this container every morning with the correct doses of each medication.

Syringe-Filling Device

This device precisely measures insulin doses for a visually impaired diabetic patient. Designed for use with a disposable U-IOO syringe and an insulin bottle, the device is set by the caregiver to accommodate the syringe's width. The caregiver then positions the plunger at the point determined by the dose and tightens the stop. When the device is set, the patient can draw up the precise dose ordered for each injection.

As with any device, you'll need to take the drawbacks into account. This device can't be used if insulin needs to be mixed or if doses vary. The settings must be checked and adjusted whenever the syringe size or type changes. The screws must be checked regularly because they loosen with repeated use.

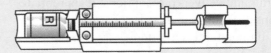

Syringe Scale Magnifier

This device helps a visually impaired diabetic patient read syringe markings, which allows him to fill his own syringe. The plastic magnifier snaps onto the syringe barrel. This device may be impractical for a patient with arthritis who can't easily attach the magnifier to the syringe.

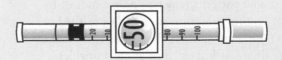

containers. Tell him to keep in mind that some drugs deteriorate when exposed to light; others decompose if they come in contact with other drugs, for example, in a pillbox. Before the patient stores drugs together, advise him to consult his pharmacist or physician. Suggest a storage area that's well-lighted (but protected from direct sunlight), not too warm or humid (not the bathroom medicine chest), and some distance from the patient's bedside (not on a bedside table). If he keeps drugs at his bedside, he may give himself an accidental overdose by taking them before he's fully awake and alert.

Knowledge: The Best Medicine

As the U.S. population continues to age, knowing how to manage medications for older patients becomes increasingly important. Recognizing and understanding the effects aging has on all aspects of medication management—from the way changes in physiology affects how drugs work in the body to the prevalence and risks of polypharmacy in older adults—gives you the advantage in caring for all your older patients.

Case Study

You're visiting an 88-year-old woman who lives with her adult daughter. During your visit, the daughter is at work, and the patient tells you she won't be home until later in the evening. The patient doesn't give a clear report of what food she ate during the day, but you notice crackers and tea on the table.

The patient's medical diagnoses include glaucoma, depression, heart failure, and arrhythmias. She appears anxious and irritable and complains that she can't sleep. She also reports nausea and says she hasn't felt like eating. She can't recall if she took all of her medications today.

Her vital signs include a temperature of 97.2° F (36.2° C), a pulse rate of 54 beats/minute, a respiratory rate of 20 breaths/minute, and blood pressure of 130/94 mm Hg. She weighs 110 lb (50 kg) and is 5´4˝ (1.6 m) tall.

Her prescribed medications include:

- digoxin (Lanoxin) 0.25 mg daily
- furosemide (Lasix) 60 mg daily

- phenytoin (Dilantin) 200 mg three times a day
- sertraline (Zoloft) 50 mg daily
- timolol (Timoptic) 0.25%, one drop in each eye twice a day.

You also notice a container of 5-mg tablets of diazepam (Valium) on the counter with a prescription date of more than a year ago. The patient tells you she also takes aspirin for joint pain and ginkgo biloba for memory.

Critical thinking questions

1. What can you do to help the patient and her daughter better manage the patient's medications?
2. What questions should you ask the patient and her daughter about the prescription and over-the-counter medications the patient is taking?
3. What other questions should you ask the patient and her daughter about the patient's medical history and medications?

6

Common Disorders:
A Systematic Approach

Older adults must cope with many challenges as they age, from normal body changes that occur with aging to a possible decline in their economic well-being as they leave the workforce and enter retirement. Many must even cope with a new living environment if they relocate to a retirement community, move in with a caregiver, or enter a long-term care facility. But one of the greatest challenges older adults face are the various diseases and disorders that can threaten their independence and overall well-being.

You can help your patients cope with the disorders that commonly occur in older adults by knowing which disorders pose the greatest risk and by understanding how they affect older patients in particular. This chapter can help you gain the understanding you need. It looks closely at each body system—from the cardiovascular, to the neurologic, to the sensory system—and covers what happens within that system as the body ages. Then, for each body system, the chapter details the particular disorders most likely to affect older adults. For each disorder, you'll find information on causes and incidence, pathophysiology, assessment findings, complications, treatment, and nursing considerations. Armed with detailed knowledge about the disorders most likely to affect your older patients and how the aging body responds to disease, you can help each of your older patients face the challenge of disease—and live as healthy a life as possible.

⧖ *Timeline Discoveries, Advances, and Cures*

Hundreds, if not thousands, of scientific, medical, and technological feats were achieved over the course of the past century, leading to breakthrough discoveries, advances, and cures—and ultimately a longer lifespan and higher quality of life for generations of Americans.

1913 Henry Ford creates assembly line

1913 American Society for the control of Cancer (later renamed American Cancer Society) founded

1913 Modern zipper invented

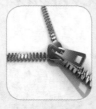

1916 First self-service grocery store opens

1918 Daylight Savings Time introduced

1920 Insulin discovered

1921 First robot built

1928 Penicillin discovered

1932 Air conditioning invented

1934 First multivitamins marketed

1935 Nylon invented

1937 First blood bank started in U.S.

1938 Annual *March of Dimes* campaign to eradicate birth defects begins

1945 Microwave oven invented

1944 First kidney dialysis machine built

1946 The Center for Disease Control and Prevention founded in Atlanta

1947 Chuck Yeager breaks the sound barrier

1900   10   20   30   40

Cardiovascular System

The cardiovascular system is more likely to wear out, break down, or otherwise malfunction than any other body system. Heart disease affects people of all ages and takes many forms, but it's especially prevalent among older adults.

As the body ages, changes occur that reduce functional status and compromise cardiovascular health. The walls of the aorta and ventricles become stiffer, decreasing the heart's ability to pump efficiently. Atherosclerotic lesions develop in the coronary and peripheral arteries, compromising the heart's blood supply. Also, the vasculature's ability to react to oxygen demand declines, which may increase the risk of ischemia. Delayed ventricular filling, vascular disease, stiffening of the myocardium, and decreased heart rate responses that prolong the relaxation phase contribute to impaired diastolic performance.

These changes don't occur all at once, and they may vary from person to person. Over all, however, they increase the likelihood that an older person will experience one or more common cardiovascular disorders. The risk of heart failure, for example, is highest in people over age 65—and with the baby boomers

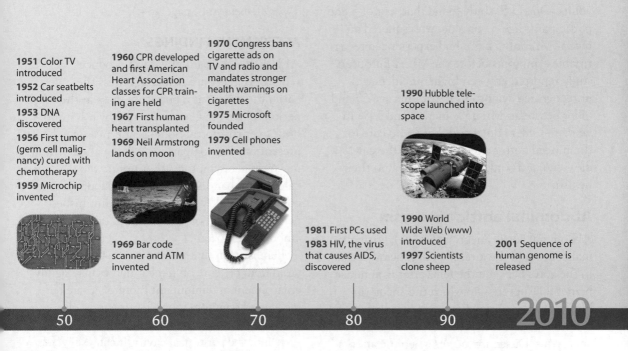

1951 Color TV introduced

1952 Car seatbelts introduced

1953 DNA discovered

1956 First tumor (germ cell malignancy) cured with chemotherapy

1959 Microchip invented

1960 CPR developed and first American Heart Association classes for CPR training are held

1967 First human heart transplanted

1969 Neil Armstrong lands on moon

1969 Bar code scanner and ATM invented

1970 Congress bans cigarette ads on TV and radio and mandates stronger health warnings on cigarettes

1975 Microsoft founded

1979 Cell phones invented

1981 First PCs used

1983 HIV, the virus that causes AIDS, discovered

1990 Hubble telescope launched into space

1990 World Wide Web (www) introduced

1997 Scientists clone sheep

2001 Sequence of human genome is released

50   60   70   80   90   2010

approaching age 65, the number of adults surviving into their older years is projected to double. With improved medical treatment and earlier identification of heart disease, adults diagnosed in their middle adult years are now surviving into their older years. Despite these improvements, less than 25% of women and 20% of men survive 6 years after being discharged from the hospital with heart failure, and a third die in the first year.

The incidence of hypertension also increases with age. Hypertension is a key risk factor for cardiovascular disorders, such as coronary artery disease (CAD) and stroke, as well as renal disorders. CAD, one of the primary causes of impaired function among older people, occurs in more than 30% of people age 65 and older and in more than 70% of those age 70 or older.

Acute myocardial infarction (MI) also has a higher incidence in older adults, with those age 65 and older having a 60% chance of experiencing an MI; a third of MI cases occur in those age 75 or older. For patients who don't closely follow current post-MI protocols after release from the hospital, the 30-day mortality rate is 26%; for those who do follow post-MI protocol, the incidence drops to 15%. But the older an adult grows, the less likely he is to report chest pain, increasing his post-MI mortality risk. Confusion from dementia also increases the likelihood that an older adult won't follow a post-MI protocol.

A lack of recognizable symptoms before an MI occurs contributes to the risk for older adults. One U.S. study found that, out of 5,888 participants age 65 or older who suffered a recent MI, only 22.3% had experienced recognizable symptoms before the MI. A European study reported an even higher incidence of unrecognized symptoms in patients age 55 and older before an MI: 33% in men and 54% in women. Older adults and those who care for them need better education about the cardiovascular disorders that can threaten their health.

Abdominal aortic aneurysm

Abdominal aortic aneurysm (AAA), an abnormal dilation in the arterial wall, generally occurs in the aorta between the renal arteries and iliac branches. Rupture—in which the aneurysm breaks open, resulting in profuse bleeding—is a common complication that occurs in larger aneurysms. Dissection occurs when the artery's lining tears and blood leaks into the walls.

CAUSES AND INCIDENCE

AAAs result from arteriosclerosis, hypertension, congenital weakening, cystic medial necrosis, trauma, syphilis, and other infections.

This disorder is four times more common in men than in women and is most prevalent in whites ages 40 to 70. Less than 20% of people with a ruptured AAA survive.

PATHOPHYSIOLOGY

AAAs develop slowly. First, a focal weakness in the muscular layer of the aorta (tunica media), caused by degenerative changes, allows the inner layer (tunica intima) and outer layer (tunica adventitia) to stretch outward. Blood pressure within the aorta progressively weakens the vessel walls and enlarges the aneurysm. Nearly all AAAs are fusiform, which causes the arterial walls to balloon on all sides. The resulting sac fills with necrotic debris and thrombi. (See *Locations of aortic aneurysms* and *Types of aneurysms*, page 144.)

ASSESSMENT FINDINGS

Although AAAs usually don't produce symptoms, most are evident (unless the patient is obese) as a pulsating mass in the periumbilical area, accompanied by a systolic bruit over the aorta. Some tenderness may be present on deep palpation. A large aneurysm may produce symptoms that mimic renal calculi, lumbar disk disease, and duodenal compression. AAAs rarely cause diminished peripheral pulses or claudication, unless embolization occurs.

Lumbar pain that radiates to the flank and groin from pressure on lumbar nerves may signify enlargement and imminent rupture. A rare but recognized symptom is unrelenting testicular pain with no other cause. If the aneurysm ruptures into the peritoneal cavity, it causes severe, persistent abdominal and back pain, mimicking renal or ureteral colic. Signs of hemorrhage—such as weakness, sweating, tachycardia, and hypotension—may be subtle because rupture into the retroperitoneal space produces a tamponade effect that prevents continued hemorrhage. Patients with such rupture may remain stable for hours before shock and death occur, although 20% die immediately.

COMPLICATIONS

- Rupture
- Obstruction of blood flow to other organs
- Embolization to a peripheral artery
- Diminished blood supply to vital organs, resulting in organ failure (with rupture)

- Hemorrhage
- Shock

TREATMENT

Usually, AAAs require resection of the aneurysm and replacement of the damaged aortic section with a Dacron graft. If the aneurysm is small and asymptomatic, surgery may be delayed and the aneurysm may be followed and allowed to expand to a certain size because of possible surgical complications; however, small aneurysms may also rupture. Because of this risk, surgical repair or replacement is recommended for symptomatic patients and for patients with aneurysms greater than 5 cm (2") in diameter. (See *Endovascular grafting for repair of an AAA*, page 145.)

Stenting is also a treatment option. It can be performed without an abdominal incision by introducing the catheters through arteries in the groin. However, not all patients with AAAs are candidates for this treatment.

Regular physical examination and ultrasound checks are necessary to detect enlargement, which may forewarn rupture. Large aneurysms or those that produce symptoms pose a significant risk of rupture and necessitate immediate repair. In patients with poor distal runoff, external grafting may be done.

Risk factor modification is fundamental in the medical management of abdominal aneurysm, including control of hypocholesterolemia and hypertension. Beta-adrenergic blockers are commonly prescribed to reduce the risk of aneurysm expansion and rupture.

NURSING CONSIDERATIONS

AAAs require meticulous preoperative and postoperative care, psychological support, and comprehensive patient teaching. Following diagnosis, if rupture isn't imminent, elective

LOCATIONS OF AORTIC ANEURYSMS

Aortic aneurysms are localized outpouching or abnormal dilation in a weakened arterial wall of the aorta. There are several types.

- Syphilitic aneurysms are the common variety in the ascending aorta, which is usually spared by the atherosclerotic process.
- Atherosclerotic aneurysms usually occur in the abdominal aorta or upper leg arteries.
- Mycotic aneurysms occur anywhere that bacteria can deposit on vessel walls.
- Dissecting-type aneurysms are most commonly seen in the descending or thoracic aorta.

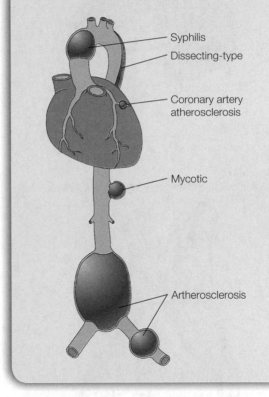

Syphilis
Dissecting-type
Coronary artery atherosclerosis
Mycotic
Artherosclerosis

surgery allows time for additional preoperative tests to evaluate the patient's clinical status.

You should also take the following steps:

- Monitor the patient's vital signs, and type and crossmatch blood.
- Use only gentle abdominal palpation.

TYPES OF ANEURYSMS

Dissecting

A hemorrhage separation in the aortic wall, usually within the medial layer

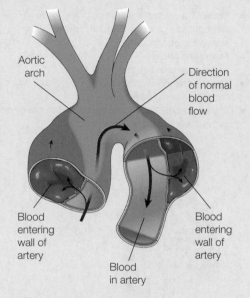

Aortic arch

Direction of normal blood flow

Blood entering wall of artery

Blood entering wall of artery

Blood in artery

Saccular

An outpouching of the arterial wall

Aortic arch aneurysm

Fusiform

A spindle-shaped enlargement encompassing the entire aortic circumference

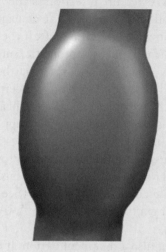

False

Occurs when the entire wall in injured, resulting in a break in all layers of the arterial wall; blood leaks out but is contained by the surrounding structures, creating a pulsatile hematoma

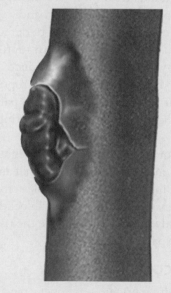

- As ordered, obtain renal function tests (blood urea nitrogen, creatinine, and electrolyte levels), blood samples (complete blood count with differential), electrocardiogram and cardiac evaluation, baseline pulmonary function tests, and arterial blood gas (ABG) analysis.
- Be alert for signs of rupture, which may be immediately fatal. Watch closely for signs of acute blood loss (decreasing blood pressure; increasing pulse and respiratory rate; cool, clammy skin; restlessness; and decreased sensorium).
- If rupture does occur, the first priority is to get the patient to surgery immediately. A pneumatic antishock garment may be used while transporting him to surgery. Surgery allows direct compression of the aorta to control hemorrhage. The patient may need large amounts of blood during the resuscitative period to replace blood loss. In such a patient, renal failure caused by ischemia is a major postoperative complication, possibly requiring hemodialysis.
- Before elective surgery, weigh the patient, insert an indwelling urinary catheter and an I.V. line, and assist with insertion of an arterial line and pulmonary artery catheter to monitor fluid and hemodynamic balance. Give prophylactic antibiotics as ordered.
- Explain the surgical procedure and the expected postoperative care in the intensive care unit (ICU) for patients undergoing complex abdominal surgery (I.V. lines, endotracheal [ET] and nasogastric [NG] intubation, and mechanical ventilation).
- After surgery, in the ICU, closely monitor vital signs, intake and hourly output, neurologic status (level of consciousness, pupil size, and sensation in arms and legs), and ABG values. Assess the depth, rate, and character of respirations and breath sounds at least every hour.

ENDOVASCULAR GRAFTING FOR REPAIR OF AN AAA

Endovascular grafting is a minimally invasive procedure for the repair of an abdominal aortic aneurysm (AAA). This procedure reinforces the walls of the aorta to prevent rupture and prevent expansion of the aneurysm.

Endovascular grafting is performed with fluoroscopic guidance: Using a guide wire, a delivery catheter with an attached compressed graft is inserted through a small incision into the femoral or iliac artery. The delivery catheter is advanced into the aorta, where it's positioned across the aneurysm. A balloon on the catheter expands the graft and affixes it to the vessel wall.

The procedure generally takes 2 to 3 hours to perform. Patients are instructed to walk the day after surgery and are generally discharged from the facility in 1 to 2 days.

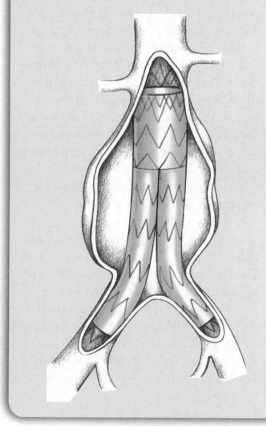

- Watch for signs of bleeding (increased pulse and respiratory rates and hypotension) and back pain, which may indicate the graft

SICK SINUS SYNDROME

Also called sinus nodal dysfunction, sick sinus syndrome results either from a dysfunction of the sinus node's automaticity or from abnormal conduction or blockages of impulses coming out of the nodal region.

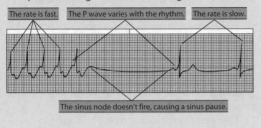

The rate is fast.   The P wave varies with the rhythm.   The rate is slow.

The sinus node doesn't fire, causing a sinus pause.

is tearing. Check abdominal dressings for excessive bleeding or drainage.

- Be alert for temperature elevations and other signs of infection. After NG intubation for intestinal decompression, irrigate the tube frequently to ensure patency. Record the amount and type of drainage.
- Suction the ET tube often. If the patient can breathe unassisted and has good breath sounds and adequate ABG values, tidal volume, and vital capacity 24 hours after surgery, he will be extubated and will require oxygen by mask.
- Weigh the patient daily to evaluate fluid balance.
- Help the patient walk as soon as he's able (generally the second day after surgery).
- Provide psychological support for the patient and his family. Help ease their fears about the ICU, the threat of impending rupture, and surgery by providing appropriate explanations and answering all questions.

Cardiac arrhythmias

Arrhythmias result from abnormal electrical conduction or automaticity that changes heart rate and rhythm. They vary in severity, from those that are mild, asymptomatic, and require no treatment (such as sinus arrhythmia, in which heart rate increases and decreases with respiration) to catastrophic ventricular fibrillation, which requires immediate resuscitation.

Any arrhythmia can occur in older adults as a result of medication or a disease process, but the most commonly occurring arrhythmias in older patients are sick sinus syndrome, heart block, and atrial fibrillation.

CAUSES AND INCIDENCE

Arrhythmias may be congenital or may result from myocardial ischemia or infarction, organic heart disease, drug toxicity, electrolyte imbalance, or degeneration of conductive tissue necessary to maintain normal heart rhythm (sick sinus syndrome). (See *Sick sinus syndrome.*)

Most serious arrhythmias happen in adults older than 60. This is because older adults are more likely to have heart disease and other health problems that can lead to arrhythmias. Older adults also tend to be more sensitive to the adverse effects of medications, some of which can cause arrhythmias. Some medicines used to treat arrhythmias can cause arrhythmias as an adverse effect.

PATHOPHYSIOLOGY

Arrhythmias may result from enhanced automaticity, reentry escape beats, or abnormal electrical conduction. (See *Recognizing bundle branch blocks* and *Common types of cardiac arrhythmias in the older adult*, pages 148 and 149.)

ASSESSMENT FINDINGS

Depending on the arrhythmia, the patient may exhibit signs and symptoms such as palpitations; a fast or racing heartbeat, a slow or irregular heartbeat; weakness; vertigo; light-headedness; diaphoresis; fainting; dyspnea; chest pain; anxiety; and syncope.

COMPLICATIONS

- Impaired cardiac output

TREATMENT

Effective treatment aims to return pacer function to the sinus node, increase or decrease the ventricular rate to normal, regain atrioventricular synchrony, and maintain normal sinus rhythm. Such treatment corrects abnormal rhythms through therapy with an antiarrhythmic agent; electrical conversion with precordial shock (defibrillation and cardioversion); physical maneuvers, such as carotid massage and Valsalva's maneuver; temporary or permanent placement of a pacemaker to maintain heart rate; or surgical removal or cryotherapy of an irritable ectopic focus to prevent recurring arrhythmias.

Arrhythmias may respond to treatment of the underlying disorder such as correction of hypoxia. However, arrhythmias associated with heart disease may require continuing and complex treatment.

NURSING CONSIDERATIONS

- Carefully assess the patient's cardiac, electrolyte, and overall clinical status to determine the effect on cardiac output and whether the arrhythmia is life-threatening.
- Assess an unmonitored patient for rhythm disturbances. If the patient's pulse rate is abnormally rapid, slow, or irregular, watch for signs of hypoperfusion, such as hypotension and diminished urine output.
- Document arrhythmias in a monitored patient, and watch for possible causes and effects.
- When life-threatening arrhythmias develop, quickly assess the patient's level of consciousness and pulse and respiratory

RECOGNIZING BUNDLE BRANCH BLOCKS

The normal width of a QRS complex is 0.006 to 0.10 second. However, prolonged ventricular depolarization widens the QRS complex. If the width increases to greater than 0.12 second, a bundle branch block is present.

After you identify a BBB, examine lead V_1, which lies to the right of the heart, and lead V_6, which lies to the left of the heart. You'll use these leads to determine whether the block is a right bundle branch block (RBBB) or a left bundle branch block (LBBB).

RBBB

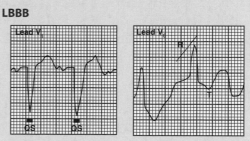

In RBBB, V_1 shows a small r wave (showing left ventricular depolarization), followed by a large R wave (confirming right ventricular depolarization). V_6 shows a widened S wave and an upright T wave.

LBBB

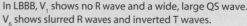

In LBBB, V_1 shows no R wave and a wide, large QS wave. V_6 shows slurred R waves and inverted T waves.

rates and initiate cardiopulmonary resuscitation, if indicated.

- Evaluate the patient for altered cardiac output resulting from arrhythmias. Administer medications as ordered, and prepare to assist with medical procedures (such as cardioversion), if indicated.

(*Text continues on page 150.*)

COMMON TYPES OF CARDIAC ARRHYTHMIAS IN THE OLDER ADULT

This chart reviews many common cardiac arrhythmias that occur in older adults and outlines their clinical features, causes, and usual treatments. Use a normal electrocardiogram, if available, to compare normal cardiac rhythm configurations with the rhythm strips shown here. Characteristics of normal sinus rhythm include:

- ventricular and atrial rates of 60 to 100 beats/minute
- regular and uniform QRS complexes and P waves
- PR interval of 0.12 to 0.20 second
- QRS duration of 0.06 second to 1.0 second
- identical atrial and ventricular rates, with constant PR intervals.

ARRHYTHMIA	FEATURES
Atrial fibrillation 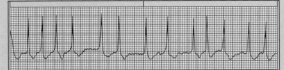	- Atrial rhythm grossly irregular; rate > 400 beats/minute - Ventricular rhythm grossly irregular - QRS complexes of uniform configuration and duration - PR interval indiscernible - No P waves, atrial activity appears as erratic, irregular, baseline fibrillatory waves
First-degree AV block 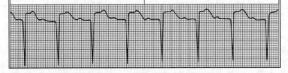	- Atrial and ventricular rhythms regular - PR interval > 0.20 second - P wave precedes QRS complex - QRS complex normal
Second-degree AV block *Mobitz I (Wenckebach)* 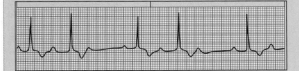	- Atrial rhythm regular - Ventricular rhythm irregular - Atrial rate exceeds ventricular rate - PR interval progressively, but only slightly, longer with each cycle until QRS complex disappears (dropped beat); PR interval shorter after dropped beat
Mobitz II 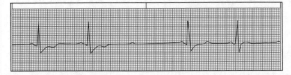	- Atrial rhythm regular - Ventricular rhythm regular or irregular, with varying degree of block - P-P interval constant - QRS complexes periodically absent
Third-degree AV block *(Complete heart block)* 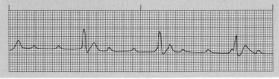	- Atrial rhythm regular - Ventricular rhythm regular and rate slower than atrial rate - No relation between P waves and QRS complexes - No constant PR interval - QRS complex normal (nodal pacemaker) or wide and bizarre (ventricular pacemaker)

CAUSES

- Heart failure, chronic obstructive pulmonary disease, thyrotoxicosis, constrictive pericarditis, ischemic heart disease, sepsis, pulmonary embolus, rheumatic heart disease, hypertension, mitral stenosis, atrial irritation, or complication of coronary bypass or valve replacement surgery
- Nifedipine and digoxin use

TREATMENT

- If patient's condition is unstable with a ventricular rate > 150 beats/minute, immediate cardioversion
- If patient's condition is stable, ACLS protocol and drug therapy, which may include a calcium channel blocker, a beta-adrenergic blocker, or an antiarrhythmic
- Possibly, anticoagulation therapy
- Class III antiarrhythmic dofetilide (Tikosyn) for conversion of atrial fibrillation and atrial flutter to normal sinus rhythm
- Radiofrequency catheter ablation to the bundle of His to interrupt all conduction between atria and ventricles (in resistant patients with recurring symptomatic atrial fibrillation)
- Maze procedure in which sutures are placed in strategic places in the atrial myocardium to prevent electrical circuits from developing perpetuating atrial fibrillation

---

- May be seen in healthy persons
- An inferior-wall MI or ischemia, hypothyroidism, hypokalemia, and hyperkalemia
- Digoxin toxicity; quinidine, procainamide, beta-adrenergic blocker, calcium channel blocker, or amiodarone use

- Correction of underlying cause
- Possibly atropine if severe symptomatic bradycardia develops
- Cautious use of digoxin, a calcium channel blocker, and a beta-adrenergic blocker

---

- An inferior-wall MI, cardiac surgery, acute rheumatic fever, and vagal stimulation
- Digoxin toxicity; propranolol, quinidine, or procainamide use

- Treatment of underlying cause
- Atropine or temporary pacemaker for symptomatic bradycardia
- Discontinuation of digoxin if appropriate

- Severe coronary artery disease, an anterior-wall MI, and acute myocarditis
- Digoxin toxicity

- Transcutaneous pacing until transvenous pacemaker placed
- Dopamine or epinephrine for symptomatic bradycardia
- Discontinuation of digoxin if appropriate

- An inferior- or anterior-wall MI, congenital abnormality, rheumatic fever, hypoxia, postoperative complication of mitral valve replacement, postprocedure complication of radiofrequency ablation in or near AV nodal tissue, Lev's disease (fibrosis and calcification that spreads from cardiac structures to the conductive tissue), and Lenègre's disease (conductive tissue fibrosis)
- Digoxin toxicity

- Transcutaneous pacing
- Dopamine or epinephrine for symptomatic bradycardia
- Temporary or permanent pacemaker

- Monitor the patient for predisposing factors, such as fluid and electrolyte imbalance, and signs of toxic reaction, especially if the patient is taking digoxin (Lanoxin). If you suspect a toxic reaction, report it to the physician immediately and withhold the next dose.
- To prevent arrhythmias postoperatively, provide adequate oxygen and reduce heart workload while carefully maintaining the patient's metabolic, neurologic, respiratory, and hemodynamic status.
- To avoid temporary pacemaker malfunction, install a fresh battery before each insertion. Carefully secure the external catheter wires and the pacemaker box. Assess the threshold daily. Watch closely for premature contractions, a sign of myocardial irritation.
- After pacemaker insertion, monitor the patient's pulse rate regularly and watch for signs of pacemaker failure and decreased cardiac output.

Coronary artery disease

Coronary artery disease (CAD) results from narrowing of the coronary arteries over time from atherosclerosis. The primary effect of CAD is the loss of oxygen and nutrients to myocardial tissue because of diminished coronary blood flow. As the population ages, the prevalence of CAD is increasing.

CAUSES AND INCIDENCE

CAD is commonly caused by atherosclerosis. Both modifiable and nonmodifiable risk factors affect the development of atherosclerosis and CAD.

Modifiable risk factors include:
- diabetes mellitus, especially in women
- elevated homocysteine levels
- inactivity
- increased low-density and decreased high-density lipoprotein levels

- obesity, which increases the risk of diabetes mellitus, hypertension, and high cholesterol
- smoking (the risk dramatically drops within 1 year of quitting)
- stress
- systolic blood pressure greater than 119 mm Hg or diastolic blood pressure greater than 79 mm Hg
- elevated hematocrit
- high resting heart rate
- hormonal contraceptive use
- increased levels of serum fibrinogen and uric acid
- reduced vital capacity
- thyrotoxicosis
- blood lead concentration higher than 8 mcg/dl in older women, which results in a three times higher risk.

Nonmodifiable factors include:
- age (risk increases after age 40)
- family history of CAD
- sex (incidence higher in men)
- race (incidence higher in whites).

Less common causes of reduced coronary artery blood flow include dissecting aneurysms, infectious vasculitis, syphilis, and congenital defects in the coronary vascular system.

The American Heart Association estimates that of the more than 71 million American adults with one or more types of cardiovascular disease—including CAD—more than 27 million are age 65 or older.

PATHOPHYSIOLOGY

Fatty fibrous plaques or calcium-plaque deposits, or a combination of both, narrow the lumens of coronary arteries, reducing the volume of blood that can flow through them and leading to myocardial ischemia. (See *Atherosclerotic plaque development*.)

As atherosclerosis develops, luminal narrowing is accompanied by vascular changes

ATHEROSCLEROTIC PLAQUE DEVELOPMENT

The coronary arteries are made up of three layers: intima (the innermost layer), media (the middle layer), and adventitia (the outermost layer).

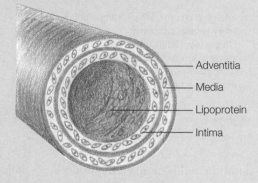

- Adventitia
- Media
- Lipoprotein
- Intima

Damaged by risk factors, a fatty streak begins to build up on the intimal layer.

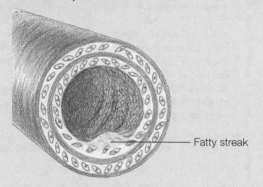

- Fatty streak

Fibrous plaque and lipids progressively narrow the lumen and impede blood flow to the myocardium.

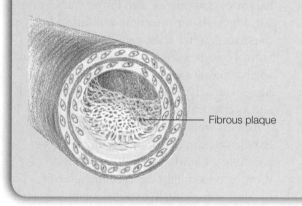

- Fibrous plaque

The plaque continues to grow and, in advanced stages, may become a complicated calcified lesion that may rupture.

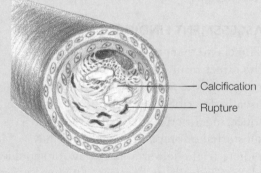

- Calcification
- Rupture

that impair the ability of the diseased vessel to dilate. This causes a precarious balance between myocardial oxygen supply and demand, threatening the myocardium beyond the lesion. When oxygen demand exceeds what the diseased vessel can supply, localized myocardial ischemia results.

Myocardial cells become ischemic within 10 seconds of a coronary artery occlusion. Transient ischemia causes reversible changes at the cellular and tissue levels, depressing myocardial function. Untreated, this can lead to tissue injury or necrosis. Within several

minutes, oxygen deprivation forces the myocardium to shift from aerobic to anaerobic metabolism, leading to an accumulation of lactic acid and a reduction of cellular pH.

The combination of hypoxia, reduced energy availability, and acidosis rapidly impairs left ventricular function. The strength of contractions in the affected myocardial region is reduced as the fibers shorten inadequately, resulting in less force and velocity. Moreover, wall function is abnormal in the ischemic area, resulting in the heart ejecting less blood with each contraction. Restoring blood flow

Culture — Atypical Signs of CAD

Not all patients experience angina in the same way. Some, particularly females, may not experience chest discomfort. Their symptoms may be primarily dyspnea and fatigue, which is called an anginal equivalent. This presentation is also seen in Blacks and Hispanic patients. Patients with diabetes may develop central neuropathies and therefore may not experience chest pain. Signs and sympathetic stimulation may be their primary anginal symptom.

In the older adult, CAD may be asymptomatic because of a decrease in sympathetic response. Dyspnea and fatigue are two key signals of ischemia in an active, older adult.

through the coronary arteries restores aerobic metabolism and contractility. However, if the blood flow isn't restored, myocardial infarction (MI) results.

ASSESSMENT FINDINGS

The classic symptom of CAD is angina, the direct result of inadequate flow of oxygen to the myocardium. The patient usually describes the sensation as a burning, squeezing, or crushing tightness in the substernal or precordial chest that may radiate to the left arm, neck, jaw, or shoulder blade. Typically, the patient clenches his fist over his chest or rubs his left arm when describing the pain. Nausea, vomiting, fainting, sweating, and cool extremities may accompany the tightness. (See *Atypical signs of CAD.*)

Angina commonly occurs after physical exertion but may also follow emotional excitement, exposure to cold, or a large meal. Angina may also develop during sleep, awakening the patient.

The patient's history suggests a pattern to the type and onset of pain. If the pain is predictable in frequency and duration and is relieved by rest or a nitrate, it's called stable angina. If it increases in frequency and duration and is more easily induced, it's called unstable angina.

If the angina results from unpredictable coronary artery spasm, it's called Prinzmetal's, or variant, angina. If impairment of vasodilator reserve causes angina-like chest pain in a patient with normal coronary arteries, it's called microvascular angina. Severe and prolonged angina generally suggests an MI, with potentially fatal arrhythmias and mechanical failure.

Inspection may reveal evidence of atherosclerotic disease, such as xanthelasma or xanthoma. Ophthalmoscopic inspection may show increased light reflexes and arteriovenous nicking, suggesting hypertension, an important risk factor of CAD.

Palpation can uncover thickened or absent peripheral arteries, signs of cardiac enlargement, and abnormal contraction of the cardiac impulse, such as left ventricular akinesia or dyskinesia.

Auscultation may detect bruits, an S_3 or S_4, or a late systolic murmur (if mitral insufficiency is present).

COMPLICATIONS

- Arrhythmias
- MI
- Ischemic cardiomyopathy

TREATMENT

The goal of treatment in a patient with angina is to reduce myocardial oxygen demand or increase the oxygen supply and reduce pain. The patient may need activity restrictions to prevent the onset of pain. Rather than eliminating activities, performing them more slowly can help avert pain. Stress reduction techniques are also essential, especially if known stressors precipitate pain.

Pharmacologic therapy consists primarily of a nitrate, such as nitroglycerin or isosorbide dinitrate, to reduce myocardial oxygen demand; a beta-adrenergic blocker to reduce the heart's workload and oxygen demands by reducing heart rate and peripheral resistance to blood flow; a calcium channel blocker to prevent coronary artery spasm; an antiplatelet drug to minimize platelet aggregation and the risk of coronary occlusion; a glycoprotein IIb to IIIa inhibitor such as abciximab (ReoPro) to reduce the risk of blood clots; an antilipemic to reduce serum cholesterol; and an antihypertensive to control hypertension. Obstructive lesions may necessitate atherectomy or coronary artery bypass graft (CABG) surgery, using vein grafts. A surgical technique available as an alternative to traditional CABG surgery is minimally invasive coronary artery bypass surgery, also known as keyhole surgery.

This procedure requires a shorter recovery period and has fewer postoperative complications. Instead of sawing open the patient's sternum and spreading the ribs apart, the surgeon makes several small incisions in the torso, through which he inserts small surgical instruments and fiber-optic cameras. This procedure was initially designed to correct blockages in just one or two easily reached arteries; it may be unsuitable for more complicated cases.

Percutaneous transluminal coronary angioplasty (PTCA) may be performed during cardiac catheterization to compress fatty deposits and relieve occlusion. In patients with calcification, PTCA may reduce the obstruction by fracturing the plaque. For older patients and those who otherwise can't tolerate cardiac surgery, it's a viable alternative to grafting. However, patients with a left main coronary artery occlusion, lesions in extremely tortuous vessels, or occlusions older than 3 months aren't candidates for PTCA.

PTCA may be performed along with coronary stenting, or stents may be placed alone. Stents provide a framework to hold an artery open by securing flaps of tunica media against an artery wall. Intravascular coronary stenting is done to reduce the incidence of restenosis. Prosthetic intravascular cylindrical stents made of stainless steel coil are positioned at the site of the occlusion. To be eligible for this procedure, the patient must be able to tolerate anticoagulant therapy and the vessel to be stented must be at least ⅛" (0.3 cm) in diameter.

Coronary brachytherapy, which involves delivering beta or gamma radiation into the coronary arteries, may be used in patients who have undergone stent implantation in a coronary artery but then developed such problems as diffuse in-stent restenosis. Brachytherapy is a promising technique, but its use is restricted to the treatment of stent-related problems because of complications and the unknown long-term effects of the radiation. However, in some facilities, brachytherapy is being studied as a first-line treatment for CAD.

Laser angioplasty corrects occlusion by vaporizing fatty deposits with the excimer or hot-tip laser device. Percutaneous myocardial revascularization (PMR) is a procedure that uses a laser to create channels in the heart muscle to improve perfusion to the myocardium. A carbon dioxide laser is used to create transmural channels from the epicardial layer to the myocardium, extending into the left ventricle. This technique is also known as transmyocardial revascularization and appears to be up to 90% effective in treating severe symptoms.

Rotational ablation (or rotational atherectomy) removes atheromatous plaque with a high-speed, rotating burr covered with diamond crystals. Enhanced external counterpulsation (EECP) provides pain relief for patients who suffer from recurrent stable angina when standard treatments fail. It's a noninvasive technique that increases oxygen-rich blood flow to the heart and reduces the heart's workload. EECP can reduce anginal pain, improve tolerance, and stimulate collateral circulation.

NURSING CONSIDERATIONS

- During anginal episodes, monitor the patient's blood pressure and heart rate. Take a 12-lead electrocardiogram before administering nitroglycerin or other nitrates. Record the duration of pain, the amount of medication required to relieve it, and accompanying symptoms.
- Ask the patient to grade the severity of pain on a scale of 0 to 10. This allows him to give his individual assessment of pain as well as of the effectiveness of pain-relieving medications.
- Keep nitroglycerin available for immediate use. Instruct the patient to call at once whenever he feels chest, arm, or neck pain and before taking nitroglycerin.
- During catheterization, monitor the patient for dye reactions. If signs and symptoms such as falling blood pressure, bradycardia, diaphoresis, and light-headedness appear, increase parenteral fluids as ordered, administer nasal oxygen, place the patient in Trendelenburg's position, and administer I.V. atropine if necessary.
- After catheterization, review the expected course of treatment with the patient and

family members. Monitor the catheter site for bleeding. Also, check for distal pulses. To counter the diuretic effect of the dye, increase I.V. fluids and make sure the patient drinks plenty of fluids. Assess potassium levels, and add potassium to the I.V. fluid if necessary.
- After PTCA and intravascular stenting, maintain heparinization, observe the patient for bleeding systemically at the site, and keep the affected leg immobile. If the patient undergoes PMR, he must also remain immobile because the stents are left in the patient until his clotting time is less than 180 seconds. Precordial blood must be taken every 8 hours for 24 hours for cardiac enzyme levels. Monitor complete blood count and electrolyte levels.
- After rotational ablation, monitor the patient for chest pain, hypotension, coronary artery spasm, and bleeding from the catheter site. Provide heparin and antibiotic therapy for 24 to 48 hours as ordered.
- After bypass surgery, provide care for the I.V. set, pulmonary artery catheter, and endotracheal tube. Monitor the patient's blood pressure, intake and output, breath sounds, chest tube drainage, and cardiac rhythm, watching for signs of ischemia and arrhythmias. The patient may need I.V. epinephrine, nitroprusside, dopamine, albumin, potassium, or blood products. He may also need temporary epicardial pacing, especially if the surgery included replacement of the aortic valve.
- The patient may need an intra-aortic balloon pump inserted until his condition stabilizes. Watch for and treat chest pain, perform vigorous chest physiotherapy, and guide the patient in pulmonary self-care.

Femoral and popliteal aneurysms

Because femoral and popliteal aneurysms occur in the two major peripheral arteries, they're also known as peripheral arterial aneurysms. They may be fusiform (spindle shaped) or saccular (pouchlike), with fusiform types occurring three times more often. They may be singular or multiple segmental lesions, in many instances affecting both legs, and may accompany other arterial aneurysms located in the abdominal aorta or iliac arteries.

CAUSES AND INCIDENCE

Femoral and popliteal aneurysms usually result from progressive atherosclerotic changes in the arterial walls (medial layer). Rarely, they result from congenital weakness in the arterial wall. They may also result from trauma (blunt or penetrating), bacterial infection, or peripheral vascular reconstructive surgery (which causes "suture line" aneurysms, also called false aneurysms, in which a blood clot forms a second lumen).

This condition is most common in men older than age 50. Elective surgery before complications arise greatly improves the prognosis.

PATHOPHYSIOLOGY

Atherosclerotic plaque formation or loss of elastin and collagen in the vessel wall causes localized outpouching or dilation of a weakened arterial wall.

ASSESSMENT FINDINGS

The patient may report pain in the popliteal space when a popliteal aneurysm is large enough to compress the medial popliteal nerve. Inspection may reveal edema and venous distention if the vein is compressed.

Femoral and popliteal aneurysms can produce signs and symptoms of severe ischemia in the leg or foot resulting from acute thrombosis within the aneurysmal sac, embolization of mural thrombus fragments and, rarely, rupture.

A patient with acute aneurysmal thrombosis may report severe pain. Inspection may reveal distal petechial hemorrhages from aneurysmal emboli. The affected leg or foot may show loss of color. Palpation of the affected leg or foot may indicate coldness and a loss of pulse. Gangrene may develop.

Bilateral palpation that reveals a pulsating mass above or below the inguinal ligament in femoral aneurysm and behind the knee in popliteal aneurysm usually confirms the diagnosis. When thrombosis has occurred, palpation detects a firm, nonpulsating mass.

COMPLICATIONS

- Amputation of thrombosis
- Emboli
- Gangrene

TREATMENT

Femoral and popliteal aneurysms require surgical bypass and reconstruction of the artery, usually with an autogenous saphenous vein graft replacement. Arterial occlusion that causes severe ischemia and gangrene may require leg amputation.

NURSING CONSIDERATIONS

Before corrective surgery:

- Assess and record the patient's circulatory status, noting the location and quality of peripheral pulses in the affected leg.
- Administer a prophylactic antibiotic or anticoagulant as ordered.

After corrective surgery:

- Carefully monitor the patient for early signs and symptoms of thrombosis or graft occlusion (such as loss of pulse, decreased skin temperature and sensation, and severe pain) and infection (such as fever).
- Palpate distal pulses at least every hour for the first 24 hours and then as often as ordered. Correlate these findings with the

preoperative circulatory assessment. Mark the sites on the patient's skin where pulses are palpable to facilitate repeated checks.

- Help the patient walk soon after surgery to prevent venous stasis and, possibly, thrombus formation.
- If the patient is receiving an anticoagulant, suggest measures to prevent accidental bleeding, such as using an electric razor. Tell the patient to report any signs of bleeding immediately (for example, bleeding gums, tarry stools, and easy bruising). Explain the importance of follow-up blood studies to monitor anticoagulant therapy. Warn the patient to avoid trauma, tobacco, and aspirin.

Heart failure

Heart failure is a syndrome rather than a disease and occurs when the heart can't pump enough blood to meet the body's metabolic needs. Heart failure results in intravascular and interstitial volume overload and poor tissue perfusion. A patient with heart failure experiences reduced exercise tolerance, a reduced quality of life, and a shortened life span.

Although the most common cause of heart failure is coronary artery disease, it also occurs in adults with congenital and acquired heart defects. The incidence of heart failure increases with age. Although advances in diagnostic and therapeutic techniques have greatly improved the outlook for patients with heart failure, the prognosis still depends on the underlying cause and its response to treatment.

CAUSES AND INCIDENCE

Causes of heart failure may be classified into four general categories. (See *Causes of heart failure.*)

CAUSES OF HEART FAILURE	
CAUSE	**EXAMPLES**
Abnormal cardiac muscle function	• Cardiomyopathy • Myocardial infarction
Abnormal left ventricular filling	• Atrial fibrillation • Atrial myxoma • Constrictive pericarditis • Impaired ventricular relaxation —Hypertension —Myocardial hibernation —Myocardial stunning • Mitral valve stenosis • Tricuspid valve stenosis
Abnormal left ventricular pressure	• Aortic or pulmonic valve stenosis • Chronic obstructive pulmonary disease • Hypertension • Pulmonary hypertension
Abnormal left ventricular volume	• High-output states —Arteriovenous fistula —Chronic anemia —Infusion of a large amount of fluids in a short period —Septicemia —Thyrotoxicosis • Valvular insufficiency

Of those affected with heart failure, 75% have preexisting hypertension. The risk doubles for those with blood pressure readings greater than 160/90 mm Hg. Heart failure also becomes more common with advancing age, affecting 1 out of every 100 people over age 65. By age 40, both men and women have a 1 in 5 lifetime risk for developing heart failure.

PATHOPHYSIOLOGY

Heart failure may be classified according to the side of the heart affected (left- or right-sided heart failure) or by the cardiac cycle involved (systolic or diastolic dysfunction). However, it becomes harder to distinguish between left- and right-sided heart failure in older adults because of the normal effects of aging on the heart as well as heart damage from chronic illness.

Left-sided heart failure

Left-sided heart failure occurs as a result of ineffective left ventricular contractile function. As the pumping ability of the left ventricle fails, cardiac output fails. The heart no longer effectively pumps blood out into the body, and the blood backs up into the left atrium and then into the lungs, causing pulmonary congestion, dyspnea, and activity intolerance. If the congestion persists, pulmonary edema and right-sided heart failure may result. Common causes include left ventricular infarction, hypertension, and aortic and mitral valve stenosis.

Right-sided heart failure

Right-sided heart failure results from ineffective right ventricular contractile function. Consequently, blood isn't pumped effectively through the right ventricle to the lungs, causing blood to back up into the right atrium and the peripheral circulation. The patient gains weight and develops peripheral edema and engorgement of the kidneys and other organs. Right-sided heart failure may result from an acute right ventricular infarction, pulmonary hypertension, or a pulmonary embolus. However, the most common cause is profound backward blood flow due to left-sided heart failure.

Systolic dysfunction

Systolic dysfunction occurs when the left ventricle can't pump enough blood out to the systemic circulation during systole and the ejection fraction falls. Consequently, blood backs up into the pulmonary circulation and pressure increases in the pulmonary venous system. Cardiac output fails, and weakness, fatigue, and shortness of breath may occur. Causes of systolic dysfunction include a myocardial infarction (MI) and dilated cardiomyopathy.

Diastolic dysfunction

Diastolic dysfunction occurs when the ability of the left ventricle to relax and fill during diastole is reduced and the stroke volume falls. As a result, the ventricles need higher volumes of blood to maintain cardiac output and pulmonary congestion and peripheral edema develop. Diastolic dysfunction may occur as a result of left ventricular hypertrophy, hypertension, or restrictive cardiomyopathy. This type of heart failure is less common than systolic dysfunction, and its treatment isn't as clear.

All causes of heart failure eventually lead to reduced cardiac output, which triggers compensatory mechanisms, such as increased sympathetic activity, activation of the renin-angiotensin-aldosterone system, ventricular dilation, and hypertrophy. These mechanisms improve cardiac output at the expense of increased ventricular work.

Increased sympathetic activity—a response to decreased cardiac output and blood pressure—enhances peripheral vascular resistance, contractility, heart rate, and venous return. Signs of increased sympathetic activity, such as cool extremities and clamminess, may indicate impending heart failure.

Increased sympathetic activity also restricts blood flow to the kidneys, causing them to secrete rennin. This then converts angiotensinogen to angiotensin I, which then becomes angiotensin II—a potent vasoconstrictor. Angiotensin causes the adrenal cortex to release aldosterone, leading to sodium and water retention and an increase in circulating blood volume. This renal mechanism is initially helpful; however, if it persists unchecked, it can aggravate heart failure as the heart struggles to pump against the increased volume.

In ventricular dilation, an increase in end-diastolic ventricular volume (preload) causes increased stroke work and stroke volume during contraction, stretching cardiac muscle fibers so that the ventricle can accept the increased intravascular volume. Eventually, the muscle becomes stretched beyond optimum limits and contractility declines.

In ventricular hypertrophy, an increase in ventricular muscle mass allows the heart to pump against increased resistance to the outflow of blood, improving cardiac output. However, this increased muscle mass also increases myocardial oxygen requirements. An increase in the ventricular diastolic pressure necessary to fill the enlarged ventricle may compromise diastolic coronary blood flow, limiting the oxygen supply to the ventricle and causing ischemia and impaired muscle contractility.

In heart failure, counterregulatory substances—prostaglandins and atrial natriuretic factor—are produced in an attempt to reduce the negative effects of volume overload and vasoconstriction caused by the compensatory mechanisms.

The kidneys release the prostaglandins prostacyclin and prostaglandin E2, which are potent vasodilators. These vasodilators also act to reduce volume overload produced by the renin-angiotensin-aldosterone system by inhibiting sodium and water reabsorption by the kidneys.

Atrial natriuretic factor is a hormone secreted mainly by the atria in response to stimulation of the stretch receptors in the atria from excess fluid volume. Fluid volume overload also causes the ventricles to secrete B-type natriuretic factor. These natriuretic factors work to counteract the negative effects of sympathetic nervous system stimulation and the renin-angiotensin-aldosterone system by producing vasodilation and diuresis.

ASSESSMENT FINDINGS

Left-sided heart failure primarily produces pulmonary signs and symptoms; right-sided heart failure, primarily systemic signs and symptoms. However, heart failure often affects both sides of the heart.

Signs and symptoms of left-sided heart failure include dyspnea, orthopnea, crackles, possibly wheezing, hypoxia, respiratory acidosis, cough, cyanosis or pallor, palpitations, arrhythmias, elevated blood pressure, and pulsus alternans. Signs and symptoms of right-sided heart failure include dependent edema, hepatomegaly, jugular vein distention, splenomegaly, ascites, slow weight gain, arrhythmias, positive hepatojugular reflex, abdominal distention, weakness, fatigue, dizziness, and syncope.

COMPLICATIONS

- Pulmonary edema
- Multiple organ failure
- MI

TREATMENT

Treatment for heart failure may include:

- treatment of the underlying cause, if known
- an angiotensin-converting enzyme inhibitor for left ventricle dysfunction to reduce production of angiotensin II, resulting in preload and afterload reduction; older patients may require lower doses because of impaired renal clearance and require monitoring for severe hypotension, signaling a toxic effect
- digoxin (Lanoxin) for heart failure caused by left ventricular systolic dysfunction to increase myocardial contractility, improve cardiac output, reduce the volume of the ventricle, and decrease ventricular stretch
- diuretics to reduce fluid volume overload and venous return
- beta-adrenergic blockers for New York Heart Association (NYHA) class II or III heart failure caused by left ventricular systolic dysfunction to prevent remodeling
- inotropic therapy with dobutamine or milrinone for acute treatment of heart failure exacerbation
- long-term or long-term intermittent inotropic therapy to augment ventricular contractility and to avoid exacerbations of heart failure in patients with NYHA class IV heart failure
- nesiritide (Natrecor), a human B-type natriuretic peptide, to augment diuresis and to decrease afterload in short-term management of heart failure exacerbation
- diuretics, nitrates, morphine, and oxygen to treat pulmonary edema
- lifestyle modifications (to reduce symptoms of heart failure), such as weight loss if necessary, limited sodium (3 g/day) and alcohol intake, reduced fat intake, smoking cessation, stress reduction, and development of an exercise program (heart failure no longer contraindicates exercise and cardiac rehabilitation)
- a biventricular pacemaker to control ventricular dyssynchrony
- coronary artery bypass surgery or angioplasty for heart failure due to coronary artery disease
- valve surgery to reshape and support the mitral valve and improve cardiac functioning
- left ventricular remodeling surgery to return the ventricle to a more normal shape and allow the heart to pump blood more efficiently
- a left ventricular assist device, also known as the "bridge to transplantation," to improve the pumping ability of the heart until transplantation can be performed
- heart transplantation in the patient who's receiving aggressive medical treatment but still experiencing limitations or repeated hospitalizations.

NURSING CONSIDERATIONS

During the acute phase of heart failure, take the following steps:

- Place the patient in Fowler's position and give him supplemental oxygen to help him breathe more easily.
- Weigh the patient daily and check for peripheral edema. Carefully monitor I.V. intake and urine output, vital signs, and mental status. Auscultate the patient's heart for abnormal sounds (S_3 gallop) and his lungs for crackles or rhonchi. Report changes at once.
- Frequently monitor the patient's blood urea nitrogen, creatinine, and serum potassium, sodium, chloride, and magnesium levels.
- Make sure the patient has continuous cardiac monitoring during acute and advanced stages to identify and treat arrhythmias promptly.
- To reduce the risk of deep vein thrombosis from vascular congestion, help the patient with range-of-motion exercises. Enforce

bed rest and apply antiembolism stockings. Check regularly for calf pain and tenderness.

- Allow adequate rest periods.

To prepare the patient for discharge, take the following steps:

- Advise the patient to avoid foods high in sodium, such as canned or commercially prepared foods and dairy products, to curb fluid overload.
- Encourage participation in an outpatient cardiac rehabilitation program.
- Explain to the patient that he may need to replace the potassium he loses through diuretic therapy by taking a prescribed potassium supplement and eating high-potassium foods, such as bananas and apricots.
- Stress the need for regular checkups.
- Stress the importance of taking digoxin exactly as prescribed. Tell the patient to watch for and immediately report signs of toxicity, such as anorexia, vomiting, and yellow vision.
- Tell the patient to notify his practitioner promptly if his pulse is unusually irregular or drops to less than 60 beats/minute; if he experiences dizziness, blurred vision, shortness of breath, a persistent dry cough, palpitations, increased fatigue, paroxysmal nocturnal dyspnea, swollen ankles, or decreased urine output; or if he notices rapid weight gain (3 to 5 lb [1.4 to 2.3 kg] in 1 week).

Hypertension

Hypertension, an intermittent or sustained elevation in diastolic or systolic blood pressure, occurs as two major types: primary (also called essential or idiopathic) hypertension, the most common, and secondary hypertension, which results from renal disease or another identifiable cause. Malignant hypertension is a severe, fulminant form of hypertension common to

both types. Hypertension is a major cause of stroke, cardiac disease, and renal failure. The prognosis is good if this disorder is detected early and treatment begins before complications develop. Severely elevated blood pressure (hypertensive crisis) may be fatal.

CAUSES AND INCIDENCE

Hypertension affects 29% of adults age 18 and older in the United States. Another 28%, or 59 million, are considered to be prehypertensive. If untreated, hypertension carries a high mortality. Risk factors for hypertension include family history, race (most common in African-Americans), stress, obesity, a diet high in saturated fats or sodium, tobacco use, a sedentary lifestyle, and aging.

Secondary hypertension may result from renal vascular disease; pheochromocytoma; primary hyperaldosteronism; Cushing's syndrome; thyroid, pituitary, or parathyroid dysfunction; coarctation of the aorta; neurologic disorders; and use of drugs, such as cocaine, epoetin alfa (erythropoietin), and cyclosporine.

Cardiac output and peripheral vascular resistance determine blood pressure. Increased blood volume, cardiac rate, and stroke volume as well as arteriolar vasoconstriction can raise blood pressure. The link to sustained hypertension, however, is unclear.

Hypertension may also result from the failure of intrinsic regulatory mechanisms:

- Renal hypoperfusion causes the release of renin, which angiotensin (a liver enzyme) converts to angiotensin I. Angiotensin I, in turn, is converted to angiotensin II, a powerful vasoconstrictor, and the resulting vasoconstriction increases afterload. Angiotensin II also stimulates adrenal secretion of aldosterone, which increases sodium reabsorption. Hypertonic-stimulated release of antidiuretic hormone from the pituitary gland follows, increasing water reabsorption, plasma volume, cardiac output, and blood pressure.

- Autoregulation changes an artery's diameter to maintain perfusion, despite fluctuations in systemic blood pressure. The intrinsic mechanisms responsible include stress relaxation (vessels gradually dilate when blood pressure rises to reduce peripheral resistance) and capillary fluid shift (plasma moves between vessels and extravascular spaces to maintain intravascular volume).

- When blood pressure drops, baroreceptors in the aortic arch and carotid sinuses decrease their inhibition of the medulla's vasomotor center, which increases sympathetic stimulation of the heart by norepinephrine. This, in turn, increases cardiac output by strengthening the contractile force, increasing the heart rate, and augmenting peripheral resistance by vasoconstriction. Stress can also stimulate the sympathetic nervous system to increase cardiac output and peripheral vascular resistance.

PATHOPHYSIOLOGY

Arterial blood pressure is a product of total peripheral resistance and cardiac output. Cardiac output is increased by conditions that increase heart rate, stroke volume, or both. Peripheral resistance is increased by factors that increase blood viscosity or reduce the lumen size of vessels, especially the arterioles.

Several theories help to explain the development of hypertension, including:

- changes in the arteriolar bed, causing increased peripheral vascular resistance

- abnormally increased tone in the sympathetic nervous system that originates in the vasomotor system centers, causing increased peripheral vascular resistance

- increased blood volume resulting from renal or hormonal dysfunction

- an increase in arteriolar thickening caused by genetic factors, leading to increased peripheral vascular resistance

- abnormal renin release, resulting in the formation of angiotensin II, which constricts the arteriole and increases blood volume. (See *Understanding blood pressure regulation*, page 162.)

Prolonged hypertension increases the heart's workload as resistance to left ventricular ejection increases. To increase contractile force, the left ventricle hypertrophies, raising the heart's oxygen demands and workload. Cardiac dilation and failure may occur when hypertrophy can no longer maintain sufficient cardiac output. Because hypertension promotes coronary atherosclerosis, the heart may be further compromised by a reduced blood flow to the myocardium, resulting in angina or a myocardial infarction (MI). Hypertension also causes vascular damage, which can lead to accelerated atherosclerosis and target-organ damage, including retinal injury, renal failure, stroke, and aortic aneurysm and dissection.

The pathophysiology of secondary hypertension depends on the underlying disease:

- The most common cause of secondary hypertension is chronic renal disease. Insult to the kidneys from chronic glomerulonephritis or renal artery stenosis interferes with sodium excretion, the renin-angiotensin-aldosterone system, or renal perfusion, causing blood pressure to increase.

- In Cushing's syndrome, increased cortisol levels raise blood pressure by increasing renal sodium retention, angiotensin II levels, and vascular response to norepinephrine.

- In primary aldosteronism, increased intravascular volume, altered sodium

UNDERSTANDING BLOOD PRESSURE REGULATION

Hypertension may result from a disturbance in one of these intrinsic mechanisms.

Renin-Angiotensin-Aldosterone System

The renin-angiotensin-aldosterone system acts to increase blood pressure through these mechanisms:

- sodium depletion, reduced blood pressure, and dehydration stimulate renin release
- renin reacts with angiotensin, a liver enzyme, and converts it to angiotensin I, which increases preload and afterload
- angiotensin I converts to angiotensin II in the lungs; angiotensin II is a potent vasoconstrictor that targets the arterioles
- angiotensin II works to increase preload and afterload by stimulating the adrenal cortex to secrete aldosterone; this increases blood volume by conserving sodium and water.

Autoregulation

Several intrinsic mechanisms work to change an artery's diameter to maintain tissue and organ perfusion despite fluctuations in systemic blood pressure.

These mechanisms include stress relaxation and capillary fluid shifts:

- in stress relaxation, blood vessels gradually dilate when blood pressure increases to reduce peripheral resistance
- in capillary fluid shift, plasma moves between vessels and extravascular spaces to maintain intravascular volume.

Sympathetic Nervous System

When blood pressure drops, baroreceptors in the aortic arch and carotid sinuses decrease their inhibition of the medulla's vasomotor center. The consequent increases in sympathetic stimulation of the heart by norepinephrine increases cardiac output by strengthening the contractile force, raising the heart rate, and augmenting peripheral resistance by vasoconstriction. Stress can also stimulate the sympathetic nervous system to increase cardiac output and peripheral vascular resistance.

Antidiuretic Hormone

The release of antidiuretic hormone can regulate hypotension by increasing reabsorption of water by the kidney. With reabsorption, blood plasma volume increases, thus raising blood pressure.

---

concentrations in vessel walls, and high aldosterone levels cause vasoconstriction and increased resistance.

- Pheochromocytoma, a chromaffin cell tumor of the adrenal medulla, secretes epinephrine and norepinephrine, which increase blood pressure; the epinephrine increases cardiac contractility and rate, and the norepinephrine increases peripheral vascular resistance.

ASSESSMENT FINDINGS

Although hypertension isn't typically symptomatic, it may cause:

- elevated blood pressure readings on at least two consecutive occasions after initial screening, the result of pathophysiologic changes in blood vessels (See *Classifying blood pressure readings.*)

- occipital headache (may worsen on rising in the morning as a result of increased intracranial pressure) resulting from vascular changes; nausea and vomiting may also occur
- epistaxis possibly due to vascular involvement
- bruits (which may be heard over the abdominal aorta or carotid, renal, or femoral arteries) caused by stenosis or aneurysm
- dizziness, confusion, and fatigue from decreased tissue perfusion, the result of vasoconstriction
- blurry vision as a result of retinal damage
- nocturia caused by an increase in blood flow to the kidneys and an increase in glomerular filtration
- edema caused by increased capillary pressure.

CLASSIFYING BLOOD PRESSURE READINGS

In 2003, the National Institutes of Health issued The Seventh Report of the Joint National Committee on Prevention, Detection, Evaluation, and Treatment of High Blood Pressure (The JNC 7 Report). Updates since The JNC 6 report include a new category, prehypertension, and the combining of stages 2 and 3 hypertension. categories now are normal, prehypertension, and stages I and 2 hypertension.

The revised categories are based on the average of two or more readings taken on separate visits after an initial screening. They apply to adults ages 18 and older. (If the systolic and diastolic pressures fall into different categories, use the higher of the two pressures to classify the reading. For example, a reading of 160/92 mm Hg should be classified as stage 2.)

Normal blood pressure with respect to cardiovascular risk is a systolic reading below 120 mm Hg and a diastolic reading below SO mm Hg. Patients with prehypertension are at increased risk for developing hypertension and should follow health promoting lifestyle modifications to prevent cardiovascular disease.

In addition to classifying stages of hypertension based on average blood pressure readings, physicians should also take note of target organ disease and additional risk factors, such as a patient with diabetes, left ventricular hypertrophy, and chronic renal disease. This additional information is important to obtain a true picture of the patient's cardiovascular health.

Category	Systolic	Diastolic
Normal	< 120 mm Hg and	< 80 mmHg
Prehypertension	120 to 139 mm Hg or	80 to 89 mm Hg
Hypertension		
Stage 1	140 to 159 mm Hg or	90 to 99 mm Hg
Stage 2	160 mmHg or	I00 mm Hg

If secondary hypertension exists, other signs and symptoms may be related to the cause. For example, Cushing's syndrome may cause truncal obesity and purple striae, whereas patients with pheochromocytoma may develop headache, nausea, vomiting, palpitations, pallor, and profuse perspiration.

COMPLICATIONS

- Stroke
- Coronary artery disease
- Angina
- MI
- Heart failure
- Arrhythmias
- Sudden death
- Cerebral infarction
- Hypertensive encephalopathy
- Hypertensive retinopathy
- Renal failure

TREATMENT

The National Institutes of Health recommends the following approach for treating primary hypertension:

- First, help the patient start needed lifestyle modifications, including weight reduction, moderation of alcohol intake, regular physical exercise, reduction of sodium intake, and smoking cessation.
- If the patient fails to achieve the desired blood pressure or make significant progress, continue lifestyle modifications and begin drug therapy.
- For stage 1 hypertension (systolic blood pressure of 140 to 159 mm Hg, or diastolic

blood pressure of 90 to 99 mm Hg) in the absence of compelling indications (heart failure, post-MI, high coronary disease risk, diabetes, chronic kidney disease, or recurrent stroke prevention), give most patients thiazide-type diuretics. Consider using an angiotensin-converting enzyme (ACE) inhibitor, a beta-adrenergic blocker, a calcium channel blocker (CCB), an angiotensin-receptor blocker (ARB), or a combination.

- For stage 2 hypertension (systolic blood pressure greater than or equal to 160 mm Hg or diastolic blood pressure greater than or equal to 100 mm Hg) in the absence of compelling indications, give most patients a two-drug combination (usually a thiazide-type diuretic and an ACE inhibitor, ARB, CCB, or beta-adrenergic blocker).
- If the patient has one or more compelling indications, base drug treatment on the benefits from outcome studies or existing clinical guidelines.
- Treatment may include the following, depending on indication:
  - heart failure—diuretic, beta-adrenergic blocker, ACE inhibitor, ARB, or aldosterone antagonist
  - high coronary disease risk—diuretic, beta-adrenergic blocker, ACE inhibitor, or CCB
  - diabetes — diuretic, beta-adrenergic blocker, ACE inhibitor, or CCB
  - chronic kidney disease—ACE inhibitor or ARB
  - post-MI failure—ACE inhibitor, beta-adrenergic blocker, or aldosterone antagonist
  - recurrent stroke prevention—diuretic or ACE inhibitor.
- Give other antihypertensive drugs as needed.
- If the patient fails to achieve the desired blood pressure, continue lifestyle

modifications and optimize drug dosages or add drugs until the goal blood pressure is achieved. Also, consider consultation with a hypertension specialist.

Treatment of secondary hypertension focuses on correcting the underlying cause and controlling hypertensive effects.

Typically, hypertensive emergencies—whether from primary or secondary hypertension— require parenteral administration of a vasodilator or an adrenergic inhibitor or oral administration of a selected drug, such as nifedipine (Procardia), captopril (Capoten), clonidine (Catapres), or labetalol (Trandate), to rapidly reduce blood pressure. The initial goal is to reduce mean arterial blood pressure by no more than 25% (within minutes to hours), then to 160/110 mm Hg within 2 hours while avoiding an excessive fall in blood pressure that could precipitate renal, cerebral, or myocardial ischemia.

Examples of hypertensive emergencies include hypertensive encephalopathy, intracranial hemorrhage, acute left-sided heart failure with pulmonary edema, and dissecting aortic aneurysm. Hypertensive emergencies can also occur with eclampsia or severe gestational hypertension, unstable angina, and acute MI.

Hypertension without accompanying signs and symptoms or target-organ disease seldom requires emergency drug therapy.

NURSING CONSIDERATIONS

- Because many older adults have a wide auscultatory gap—the hiatus between the first Korotkoff sound and the next sound—failure to pump the blood pressure cuff up high enough can lead to missing the first beat and underestimating systolic blood pressure. To avoid missing the first Korotkoff sound, palpate the radial artery and inflate the cuff to a point about 20 mm Hg beyond which the pulse beat disappears.

- To encourage adherence to antihypertensive therapy, suggest that the patient establish a daily routine for taking his medication. Warn that uncontrolled hypertension may cause stroke and heart attack. Tell him to report adverse drug effects. Also, advise him to avoid high-sodium antacids and over-the-counter cold and sinus medications, which contain harmful vasoconstrictors.
- Encourage a change in dietary habits. Help the obese patient plan a weight-reduction diet; tell him to avoid high-sodium foods (pickles, potato chips, canned soups, and cold cuts) and table salt.
- Help the patient examine and modify his lifestyle (for example, by reducing stress and exercising regularly).
- If a patient is hospitalized with hypertension, find out if he was taking his prescribed medication. If he wasn't, ask why. If he can't afford the medication, refer him to appropriate social service agencies. Tell the patient and his family to keep a record of drugs used in the past, noting especially which ones were or weren't effective. Suggest recording this information on a card so that the patient can show it to his practitioner.
- When a routine blood pressure screening reveals elevated pressure, first make sure the cuff size is appropriate for the patient's upper arm circumference. Take the pressure in both arms in lying, sitting, and standing positions. Ask the patient if he smoked, drank a beverage containing caffeine, or was emotionally upset before the test. Advise him to return for blood pressure testing at frequent and regular intervals.
- To help identify hypertension and prevent untreated hypertension, participate in public education programs dealing with hypertension and ways to reduce risk factors. Encourage public participation in blood pressure screening programs. Routinely screen all patients, especially those at risk (African-Americans and people with family histories of hypertension, stroke, or heart attack).

Myocardial infarction

Myocardial infarction (MI), commonly known as a heart attack and part of a broader category of disease known as acute coronary syndrome, results from prolonged myocardial ischemia due to reduced blood flow through one of the coronary arteries. In cardiovascular disease—the leading cause of death in the United States and western Europe—death usually results from the cardiac damage or complications of MI. Mortality is high when treatment is delayed, and almost one-half of sudden deaths due to MI occur before hospitalization, within 1 hour of the onset of symptoms. The prognosis improves if vigorous treatment begins immediately.

CAUSES AND INCIDENCE
Predisposing risk factors include:
- diabetes mellitus
- drug use, especially cocaine
- elevated serum triglyceride, total cholesterol, and low-density lipoprotein levels
- hypertension
- obesity or excessive intake of saturated fats, carbohydrates, or salt
- positive family history
- sedentary lifestyle
- smoking
- stress or a type A personality.

The site of the MI depends on the vessels involved. Occlusion of the circumflex branch of the left coronary artery causes a lateral wall infarction; occlusion of the anterior descending branch of the left coronary artery, an anterior wall infarction. True posterior or inferior wall infarctions generally result from occlusion of the right coronary artery or one of its branches. Right ventricular infarctions can also result from right coronary artery occlusion, can accompany inferior infarctions, and may cause right-sided heart failure. In Q-wave (transmural) MI, tissue damage extends through all myocardial layers; in non-Q-wave (subendocardial) MI, tissue damage occurs only in the innermost and possibly the middle layers.

Incidence is high: About 1 million patients visit the hospital each year with an MI and another 200,000 to 300,000 people die from MI-related complications without seeking medical care. Men and postmenopausal women are more susceptible to MI than premenopausal women, although incidence is rising among women, especially among those who smoke or take hormonal contraceptives. Those 65 and older also have an increased risk of MI, and have a particularly high rate of silent MI.

PATHOPHYSIOLOGY

An acute coronary syndrome most commonly results when plaque ruptures inside a coronary artery and a resulting thrombus occludes blood flow. The effect is an imbalance in myocardial oxygen supply and demand.

The degree and duration of blockage indicate the type of ischemia or infarct that occurs:

- If the patient has unstable angina, a thrombus partially occludes a coronary vessel. This thrombus is full of platelets. The partially occluded vessel may have distal microthrombi that cause necrosis in some myocytes. The patient typically experiences symptoms.
- ST-segment myocardia infarction results when reduced blood flow through of the coronary arteries causes myocardial ischemia, injury, and necrosis. The damage extends through myocardial layers.
- If smaller vessels infarct, the patient is at higher risk for MI, which may progress to

a non-ST-segment myocardial infarction. Usually, only the innermost layer of the heart is damaged.

ASSESSMENT FINDINGS

The cardinal symptom of MI is persistent, crushing substernal pain that may radiate to the left arm, jaw, neck, or shoulder blades. Such pain is usually described as heavy, squeezing, or crushing and may persist for 12 hours or more. However, in some MI patients—particularly older people or those with diabetes—pain may not occur at all; in others, it may be mild and confused with indigestion. In patients with coronary artery disease, angina of increasing frequency, severity, or duration (especially if not provoked by exertion, a heavy meal, or cold and wind) may signal impending infarction.

Other clinical effects include a feeling of impending doom, fatigue, nausea, vomiting, and shortness of breath. Some patients may have no symptoms. The patient may experience catecholamine responses, such as coolness in extremities, perspiration, anxiety, and restlessness. Fever is unusual at the onset of an MI, but a low-grade temperature elevation may develop during the next few days. Blood pressure varies; hypotension or hypertension may be present.

COMPLICATIONS

- Recurrent or persistent chest pain
- Arrhythmias
- Left-sided heart failure
- Thromboembolism
- Papillary muscle dysfunction or rupture
- Rupture of the ventricular septum
- Dressler's syndrome

TREATMENT

Treatment aims to relieve chest pain, stabilize heart rhythm, reduce cardiac workload, revascularize the coronary artery, and preserve myocardial tissue. Arrhythmias, the predominant problem during the first 48 hours after the infarction, may require antiarrhythmics, possibly a pacemaker and, rarely, cardioversion. Arrhythmias are best detected using a 12-lead ECG.

To preserve myocardial tissue in ST-elevation MI, fibrinolytic therapy should be started I.V. within 30 minutes of arrival in the emergency department, if not contraindicated. Fibrinolytic therapy includes a choice of streptokinase, alteplase, urokinase, tenecteplase, or reteplase.

Primary percutaneous transluminal coronary angioplasty is a Class I recommendation as an alternative to thrombolytic therapy only if performed in a timely manner by physicians skilled in the procedure and supported by experienced personnel in high-volume centers.

Other treatments consist of:

- lidocaine, vasopressin, or amiodarone for ventricular arrhythmias, or other drugs, such as procainamide, quinidine, or disopyramide (Norpace)
- antiplatelet therapy with glycoprotein IIb-IIIa inhibitors, such as ticlopidine (Ticlid) and clopidogrel (Plavix) for non-ST-elevation MI
- atropine I.V. or a temporary pacemaker for heart block or bradycardia
- nitroglycerin (sublingual, topical, transdermal, or I.V.); calcium channel blockers, such as nifedipine (Procardia), verapamil (Calan), or diltiazem (Cardizem) sublingual, oral, or I.V.; or isosorbide dinitrate sublingual, oral, or I.V. to relieve pain by redistributing blood to ischemic areas of the myocardium, increasing cardiac output and reducing myocardial workload
- heparin I.V. (usually follows thrombolytic therapy)
- morphine I.V. for pain and sedation

- bed rest with a bedside commode to decrease cardiac workload
- oxygen administration at a modest flow rate for 2 to 3 hours (the patient should receive a lower concentration if he has chronic obstructive pulmonary disease)
- angiotensin-converting enzyme inhibitors for a patient with a large anterior wall MI as well as for a patient with an MI and a left ventricular ejection fraction of less than 40%
- drugs to increase myocardial contractility or blood pressure
- beta-adrenergic blockers, such as propranolol (Inderal) or atenolol (Tenormin), after acute MI to help prevent reinfarction by reducing the heart's workload
- aspirin to inhibit platelet aggregation (should be initiated immediately and continued for years)
- pulmonary artery catheterization to detect left- or right-sided heart failure and to monitor the patient's response to treatment.

NURSING CONSIDERATIONS

Care for patients who have suffered an MI is directed toward detecting complications, preventing further myocardial damage, and promoting comfort, rest, and emotional well-being. Most MI patients receive treatment in the intensive care unit (ICU), where they're under constant observation for complications.

When caring for a patient who has suffered from an MI, take the following steps:

- On admission to the ICU, monitor and record the patient's ECG, blood pressure, temperature, and heart and breath sounds.
- Assess and record the severity and duration of pain, and administer analgesics. Avoid I.M. injections; absorption from the muscle is unpredictable and bleeding is likely if the patient is receiving thrombolytic therapy.

- Check the patient's blood pressure after giving nitroglycerin, especially after the first dose.
- Frequently monitor the ECG to detect rate changes or arrhythmias. Place rhythm strips in the patient's chart periodically for evaluation.
- During episodes of chest pain, obtain a 12-lead ECG (before and after nitroglycerin therapy as well), blood pressure readings, and pulmonary artery catheter measurements and monitor them for changes.
- Watch for signs and symptoms of fluid retention (crackles, cough, tachypnea, and edema), which may indicate impending heart failure. Carefully monitor the patient's daily weight, intake and output, respirations, serum enzyme levels, and blood pressure. Auscultate for adventitious breath sounds periodically (patients on bed rest frequently have atelectatic crackles, which disappear after coughing), for S_3 or S_4 gallops, and for new-onset heart murmurs.
- Organize patient care and activities to maximize periods of uninterrupted rest.
- Initiate a cardiac rehabilitation program. This usually includes education for the patient and his family about heart disease and exercise, along with emotional support.
- Ask the dietary department to provide a clear liquid diet until nausea subsides. A low-cholesterol, low-sodium, low-fat, high-fiber diet may be prescribed.
- Provide a stool softener to prevent straining during defecation, which causes vagal stimulation and may slow the heart rate. Allow use of a bedside commode and provide as much privacy as possible.
- Assist with range-of-motion exercises. If the patient is completely immobilized by a severe MI, turn him often. Antiembolism stockings help prevent venostasis and thrombophlebitis.

- Provide emotional support and help reduce stress and anxiety; administer tranquilizers as needed. Explain procedures and answer questions. Explaining the ICU environment and routine can ease anxiety. Involve the patient's family in his care as much as possible.

To prepare the patient for discharge, take the following steps:

- Thoroughly explain dosages and therapy to promote compliance with the prescribed medication regimen and other treatment measures. Warn about drug adverse effects, and advise the patient to watch for and report signs of toxicity (anorexia, nausea, vomiting, and yellow vision, for example, if the patient is receiving digoxin).
- Review dietary restrictions with the patient. If he must follow a low-sodium or low-fat and low-cholesterol diet, provide a list of foods that he should avoid. Ask the dietitian to speak to the patient and his family.
- Counsel the patient to resume sexual activity progressively.
- Advise the patient to report typical or atypical chest pain. Postinfarction syndrome may develop, producing chest pain that must be differentiated from recurrent MI, pulmonary infarct, or heart failure.
- If the patient has a Holter monitor in place, explain its purpose and use.
- Stress the need to stop smoking.
- Encourage participation in a cardiac rehabilitation program.
- Review follow-up procedures, such as office visits and treadmill testing, with the patient.

Peripheral arterial occlusive disease

Peripheral arterial occlusive disease (PAOD) is the obstruction or narrowing of the lumen of the aorta or its major branches, causing an interruption of blood flow, most commonly to the legs and feet. PAOD may affect the carotid, vertebral, innominate, subclavian, mesenteric, and celiac arteries. Occlusions may be acute or chronic and commonly cause severe ischemia, skin ulceration, and gangrene.

The prognosis depends on the occlusion's location; the development of collateral circulation to counteract reduced blood flow and, in acute disease, the time elapsed between occlusion and its removal.

CAUSES AND INCIDENCE

PAOD is common complication of atherosclerosis. The occlusive mechanism may be endogenous, due to emboli formation or thrombosis, or exogenous, due to trauma or fracture. Predisposing factors include smoking; aging; such conditions as hypertension, hyperlipidemia, and diabetes; and a family history of vascular disorders, myocardial infarction, or stroke.

Although PAOD doesn't affect any one race in particular, men older than age 50 have an increased risk for intermittent claudication, a common sign of peripheral artery disease.

The incidence of PAOD increases with age. It's also associated with higher mortality rates from cardiac disease.

PATHOPHYSIOLOGY

Narrowing of blood vessels leads to interrupted blood flow, usually to the legs and feet. During times of increased activity or exercise, blood flow to surrounding muscles can't meet the metabolic demand.

ASSESSMENT FINDINGS

The signs and symptoms of PAOD depend on the site of the occlusion. (See *Types of peripheral arterial occlusive disease*, page 170.)

COMPLICATIONS

- Severe ischemia
- Skin ulceration
- Gangrene
- Limb loss

TREATMENT

Treatment depends on whether the obstruction is acute or chronic as well as the cause, location, and size of the occlusion. For mild chronic disease, supportive measures include elimination of smoking, hypertension control, and walking exercises. For carotid artery occlusion, antiplatelet therapy may begin with ticlopidine or clopidogrel and aspirin. For intermittent claudication of chronic occlusive disease, pentoxifylline and cilostazol may improve blood flow through the capillaries, particularly for patients who are poor candidates for surgery.

Acute peripheral arterial occlusion usually requires surgery to restore circulation to the affected area. Specific procedures include:

- atherectomy, which uses a drill or slicing mechanism to excise plaque
- balloon angioplasty, which compresses the obstruction by inflating a balloon in the affected area
- bypass grafting, which diverts blood flow past the thrombosed section through an anastomosed autogenous or Dacron graft
- combined therapy, which uses a combination of any of the above treatments
- embolectomy, which uses a balloon-tipped Fogarty catheter to remove thrombotic material from the artery; this procedure is used mainly for mesenteric, femoral, or popliteal artery occlusion
- laser angioplasty, which uses excision and hot-tip lasers to vaporize the obstruction
- patch arterioplasty, which involves the removal of the thrombosed arterial segment

TYPES OF PERIPHERAL ARTERIAL OCCLUSIVE DISEASE

SITE OF OCCLUSION	ASSESSMENT FINDINGS
Carotid Arterial System ● Internal carotids	● Absent or decreased pulsation with an ausculatory bruit over the affected vessels ● Neurologic dysfunction: transient ischemic attacks (TIAs) due to reduced cerebral circulation producing unilateral sensory or motor dysfunction (transient monocular blindness, and hemiparesis), possible aphasia or dysarthria, confusion, decreased mentation, and headache (These are recurrent features that usually last 5 to 10 minutes but may persist up to 24 hours and may herald a stroke.)
Vertebrobasilar System ● Vertebral arteries ● Basilar arteries	● Neurologic dysfunction: TIAs of the brain stem and cerebellum producing biocular vision disturbances, vertigo, dysarthria, and "drop attacks" (falling down without loss of consciousness); less common than carotid TIA
Innominate ● Brachiocephalic artery	● Indications of ischemia (claudication) or the right arm ● Neurologic dysfunction: signs and symptoms of vertebrobasilar occlusion ● Possible bruit over the right side of the chest
Subclavian Artery	● Clinical effects of vertebrobasilar occlusion and exercise induced arm claudication ● Subclavian steal syndrome (characterized by the backflow of blood from the brain through the vertebral artery on the same side as the occlusion, into the subclavian artery distal to the occlusion) ● Rarely gangrene (usually limited to the digits)
Mesenteric Artery ● Superior (most commonly affected) ● Celiac axis ● Inferior	● Bowel ischemia, infarct necrosis, and gangrene ● Diarrhea ● Leukocytosis ● Nausea and vomiting with eating ● Shock due to massive intraluminal fluid and plasma loss ● Sudden, acute abdominal pain
Aortic Bifurcation (saddle block occlusion, a medical emergency associated with cardiac embolization)	● Sensory and motor deficits (muscle weakness, numbness, paresthesias, and paralysis) in both legs ● Signs of ischemia (sudden pain and cold, pale legs with decreased or absent peripheral pulses) in both legs
Iliac Artery (Leriche's syndrome)	● Absent or reduced femoral or distal pulses ● Impotence ● Intermittent claudication of the lower back, buttocks, and thighs, relieved by rest ● Possible bruit over femoral arterial ● Generally bilateral
Femoral And Popliteal Artery	● Gangrene ● Intermittent claudication of the calves on exertion ● Ischemic pain in feet ● Leg pallor and coolness; blanching of the feet on elevation ● No palpable pulses in the ankles and feet ● Pretrophic pain (heralds necrosis and ulceration)

and replacement with an autogenous vein or Dacron graft
- stent insertion, in which the surgeon inserts a mesh of wires that stretch and mold to the arterial wall to prevent reocclusion; this new adjunct follows laser angioplasty or atherectomy
- thromboendarterectomy, in which the surgeon opens the occluded artery and directly removes the obstructing thrombus and the medial layer of the arterial wall; it's usually performed after angiography and commonly used with autogenous vein or Dacron bypass surgery (femoral-popliteal or aortofemoral)
- thrombolytic therapy, which involves the lysis of any clot around or in the plaque with urokinase, streptokinase, or alteplase.

Amputation becomes necessary with failure of arterial reconstructive surgery or with the development of gangrene, persistent infection, or intractable pain. Other therapy includes heparin to prevent emboli (for embolic occlusion) and bowel resection after restoration of blood flow (for mesenteric artery occlusion).

NURSING CONSIDERATIONS

Throughout treatment, provide comprehensive patient teaching, including proper foot care. Explain all diagnostic tests and procedures, and advise the patient to stop smoking and to follow the prescribed medical regimen.

Preoperatively, during an acute episode, take the following steps:
- Assess the patient's circulatory status by checking for the most distal pulses and by inspecting his skin color and temperature.
- Provide pain relief as needed.
- Administer heparin by continuous I.V. drip as ordered. Use an infusion monitor or pump to ensure the proper flow rate.

- Wrap the patient's affected foot in soft cotton batting, and reposition it frequently to prevent pressure on any one area. Strictly avoid elevating or applying heat to the affected leg.
- Watch for signs of fluid and electrolyte imbalance, and monitor intake and output for signs of renal failure (urine output less than 30 ml/hour).
- If the patient has carotid, innominate, vertebral, or subclavian artery occlusion, monitor him for signs of stroke, such as numbness in an arm or leg and intermittent blindness.

After the procedure, take the following steps:
- Monitor the patient's vital signs. Continuously assess his circulatory function by inspecting skin color and temperature and by checking for distal pulses. In charting, compare earlier assessments and observations. Watch closely for signs of hemorrhage (tachycardia and hypotension), and check dressings for excessive bleeding.
- In carotid, innominate, vertebral, or subclavian artery occlusion, assess neurologic status frequently for changes in level of consciousness as well as muscle strength and pupil size.
- In mesenteric artery occlusion, connect the nasogastric tube to low intermittent suction. Monitor intake and output (low urine output may indicate damage to renal arteries during surgery). Check bowel sounds for return of peristalsis. Increasing abdominal distention and tenderness may indicate extension of bowel ischemia with resulting gangrene, necessitating further excision, or it may indicate peritonitis.
- In saddle block occlusion, check distal pulses for adequate circulation. Watch for signs of renal failure and mesenteric artery occlusion (severe abdominal pain), and for

cardiac arrhythmias, which may precipitate embolus formation.

- In iliac artery occlusion, monitor urine output for signs of renal failure from decreased perfusion to the kidneys as a result of surgery. Provide meticulous catheter care.
- In both femoral and popliteal artery occlusions, assist with early ambulation; discourage prolonged sitting.
- After amputation, check the patient's stump carefully for drainage and record its color and amount as well as the time. Elevate the stump as ordered, and administer adequate analgesic medication. Because phantom limb pain is common, explain this phenomenon to the patient.
- When preparing the patient for discharge, instruct him to watch for signs of recurrence (pain, pallor, numbness, paralysis, and absence of pulse) that can result from graft occlusion or occlusion at another site. Warn him against wearing constrictive clothing.

Valvular heart disease

In valvular heart disease, three types of mechanical disruption can occur: stenosis, or narrowing, of the valve opening; incomplete closure of the valve; and prolapse of the valve. A combination of these three in the same valve may also occur. They can result from such disorders as endocarditis (most common), congenital defects, and inflammation, and they can lead to heart failure.

In older adults, the most common valvular disorders are aortic stenosis and mitral valve regurgitation. However, any valve can be affected.

CAUSES AND INCIDENCE

The etiology of acquired valvular heart disease can be ischemic (postmyocardial infarction), inflammatory (connective tissue disease), degenerative (age-related stiffness and wear and tear) or infectious (rheumatic fever). Aortic stenosis may result from rheumatic fever

or atherosclerosis. It can also stem from an infective process on the heart valve such as in endocarditis.

In older adults, mitral insufficiency may occur because the mitral annulus has become calcified. Although it isn't known why this occurs, it may be linked to a degenerative process. Mitral insufficiency is sometimes associated with congenital anomalies, such as transposition of the great vessels and rheumatic fever.

PATHOPHYSIOLOGY

In aortic stenosis, increased left ventricular pressure tries to overcome the resistance of the narrowed valvular opening. The added workload increases the body's demand for oxygen while diminished cardiac output causes poor coronary artery perfusion, ischemia of the left ventricle, and left-sided heart failure.

In mitral insufficiency—also referred to as mitral regurgitation—a damaged mitral valve allows blood flow from the left ventricle to flow back into the left atrium during systole. As a result, the atrium enlarges to accommodate the backflow. The left ventricle also dilates to accommodate the increased volume of blood from the atrium and to compensate for diminishing cardiac output. Ventricular hypertrophy and increased end-diastolic pressure result in increased pulmonary artery pressure, eventually leading to both left- and right-sided heart failure.

ASSESSMENT FINDINGS

Specific findings depend on the affected valve.

Aortic stenosis

Even with severe aortic stenosis (narrowing to about one-third of the normal opening), the patient may be asymptomatic. Eventually, the patient complains of exertional dyspnea, fatigue, exertional syncope, angina, and palpitations. If left-sided heart failure develops, the patient may complain of orthopnea and paroxysmal nocturnal dyspnea.

Inspection may reveal peripheral edema if the patient has left-sided heart failure. Palpation may detect diminished carotid pulses and alternating pulse. If the patient has left-sided heart failure, the apex of the heart may be displaced inferiorly and laterally. If the patient has pulmonary hypertension, you may be able to palpate a systolic thrill at the base of the heart, at the jugular notch, and along the carotid arteries. Occasionally, it may be palpable only during expiration and when the patient leans forward.

Auscultation may uncover an early systolic ejection murmur in children and adolescents who have noncalcified valves. The murmur begins shortly after S_1 and increases in intensity to reach a peak toward the middle of the ejection period. It diminishes just before the aortic valve closes. (See *Identifying the murmur of aortic stenosis*.)

The murmur is low-pitched, rough, and rasping and is loudest at the base at the second intercostal space. In patients with stenosis, the murmur is at least grade 3 or 4. It disappears when the valve calcifies. A split S_2 develops as aortic stenosis becomes more severe. An S_4 reflects left ventricular hypertrophy and may be heard at the apex in patients with severe aortic stenosis.

Mitral insufficiency

Depending on the severity of the disorder, the patient with mitral insufficiency may be asymptomatic, or he may complain of orthopnea, exertional dyspnea, fatigue, weakness, weight loss, chest pain, and palpitations.

Inspection may reveal jugular vein distention. You may also note peripheral edema.

On auscultation, you may detect a soft S_1 buried in the systolic murmur. A grade 3 to 6

IDENTIFYING THE MURMUR OF AORTIC STENOSIS

A low-pitched, harsh crescendo-decrescendo murmur that radiates from the aortic valve area to the carotid artery characterizes aortic stenosis.

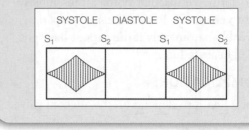

or louder holosystolic murmur, most characteristic of mitral insufficiency, is best heard at the apex. You may also hear a split S_2 and a low-pitched S_3, after which you may detect a short, rumbling diastolic murmur. In a patient in normal sinus rhythm who has experienced a recent onset of severe mitral insufficiency, you may hear a fourth heart sound. (See *Identifying the murmur of mitral insufficiency*.)

Auscultation of the lungs may reveal crackles if the patient has pulmonary edema.

Chest palpation may disclose a regular pulse rate with a sharp upstroke. You can probably palpate a systolic thrill at the apex. In a patient

IDENTIFYING THE MURMUR OF MITRAL INSUFFICIENCY

A high-pitched, rumbling pansystolic murmur that radiates from the mitral area to the left axillary line characterizes mitral insufficiency.

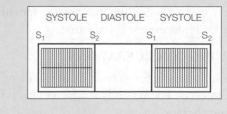

with marked pulmonary hypertension, you may be able to palpate a right ventricular tap and the shock of the pulmonic valve closing. When the left atrium is markedly enlarged, you may be able to palpate it along the sternal border late during ventricular systole; it resembles a right ventricular lift. Abdominal palpation may reveal hepatomegaly if the patient has right-sided heart failure.

COMPLICATIONS

Complications depend on the affected valve.

Aortic stenosis

- Left-sided heart failure (usually after age 70)
- Sudden death

Mitral insufficiency

- Left- and right-sided heart failure
- Pulmonary edema
- Cardiovascular collapse

TREATMENT

Treatment depends on the nature and severity of associated symptoms. For example, heart failure requires digoxin, diuretics, a sodium-restricted diet and, in acute cases, oxygen. Other measures may include anticoagulant therapy or antiplatelet medications to prevent thrombus formation around diseased or replaced valves, prophylactic antibiotics before and after surgery or dental care, and valvulo-plasty. An intra-aortic balloon pump may be used temporarily to reduce backflow by enhancing forward blood flow into the aorta.

If the patient has severe signs and symptoms that can't be managed medically, open-heart surgery using cardiopulmonary bypass for valve repair or replacement is indicated.

NURSING CONSIDERATIONS

- Watch closely for signs of heart failure or pulmonary edema and for adverse effects of drug therapy.

- Teach the patient about diet restrictions, medications, and the importance of consistent follow-up care.
- If the patient has undergone surgery, watch for hypotension, arrhythmias, and thrombus formation. Monitor his vital signs, arterial blood gas values, intake and output, daily weight, blood chemistries, chest X-rays, and pulmonary artery catheter readings.

Varicose veins

Varicose veins are dilated, tortuous veins, engorged with blood resulting from improper venous valve function. Primary varicose veins originate in superficial veins (the saphenous veins and branches). Secondary varicose veins occur in deep and perforating veins.

As a person ages, veins dilate and stretch, increasing susceptibility to varicose veins and chronic venous insufficiency. Because older adults typically have more friable skin that can easily break down, ulcers that result from chronic venous insufficiency may take longer to heal.

CAUSES AND INCIDENCE

Conditions that can predispose a person to primary varicose veins include:

- anything that produces venous stasis or increased intra-abdominal pressure, such as obesity or constipation
- congenital weakness of the valves or venous walls
- a family history of varicose veins
- an occupation that requires standing for extended periods.

Conditions that can predispose a person to secondary varicose veins include:

- arteriovenous fistulas
- deep vein thrombosis
- occlusion

- trauma to the venous system
- venous malformation.

Primary varicose veins tend to run in families and to affect both legs; they're twice as common in women as in men. They account for about 90% of varicose veins. Between 10% and 20% of Americans have primary varicose veins. Secondary varicose veins typically occur in one leg. Both types of varicose veins occur more commonly in middle adulthood, and the incidence increases with age.

PATHOPHYSIOLOGY

Veins are thin-walled, distensible vessels with valves that keep blood flowing in one direction. Any condition that weakens, destroys, or distends these valves allows blood backflow to the previous valve. If a valve can't hold the pooling blood, it can become incompetent, allowing even more blood to flow backward.

As the volume of venous blood builds, pressure in the vein increases and the vein becomes distended. As the veins stretch, their walls weaken and they lose their elasticity. The veins enlarge, becoming lumpy and tortuous. Hydrostatic pressure increases, forcing plasma out of the veins and into the surrounding tissues, which causes edema.

People who stand for prolonged periods may also develop venous pooling because the muscles in the legs don't contract and force the blood back up to the heart. If the valves in the veins are too weak to hold the pooling blood, they begin to leak, allowing blood to flow backward.

ASSESSMENT FINDINGS

A person with varicose veins may be asymptomatic or may complain of mild to severe leg symptoms, including a heavy feeling that worsens in the evening and in warm weather; cramps at night; diffuse, dull aching after prolonged standing or walking; and fatigue. Exercise may relieve symptoms because venous return improves.

Inspection of the affected leg reveals dilated, tortuous, purplish, ropelike veins, particularly in the calves, from venous pooling. Deep vein incompetence causes orthostatic edema and stasis of the calves and ankles. Palpation may reveal nodules along affected veins and valve incompetence.

COMPLICATIONS

- Blood clots secondary to venous stasis
- Venous stasis ulcers
- Chronic venous insufficiency

TREATMENT

Treatment for varicose veins may include:

- treatment of the underlying cause, such as an abdominal tumor or obesity, if possible
- antiembolism stockings or elastic bandages to counteract swelling by supporting the veins and improving circulation
- regular exercise to promote muscular contraction to force blood through the veins and reduce venous pooling
- injection of a sclerosing agent into small or medium-sized varicosities
- surgical stripping and ligation (for severe varicose veins)
- phlebectomy (removal of the varicose vein through a small incisions in the skin, which may be performed in an outpatient setting).

NURSING CONSIDERATIONS

- Teach the patient to avoid wearing constrictive clothing that interferes with venous return.
- Encourage the obese patient to lose weight to reduce increased intra- abdominal pressure.
- Teach the patient to elevate the legs above the heart whenever possible to promote venous return.

- Instruct the patient to avoid prolonged standing or sitting because these actions enhance venous pooling.
- After stripping and ligation or after injection of a sclerosing agent, administer an analgesic as ordered to relieve pain.
- Frequently check circulation in the patient's toes, noting color and temperature, and observe elastic bandages for bleeding. When ordered, rewrap bandages at least once per shift, wrapping from toe to thigh, with the leg elevated.
- Watch for signs and symptoms of complications, such as sensory loss in the leg (which could indicate saphenous nerve damage), calf pain (which could indicate thrombophlebitis), and fever (a sign of infection).

Respiratory System

Like the cardiovascular system, the respiratory system undergoes significant changes as adults age. Aging slowly degrades the respiratory system's structure and function, putting older adults at greater risk for respiratory disorders and diseases.

Specific anatomic changes that typically occur with aging include an increased anteroposterior chest diameter—the result of altered calcium metabolism and costal cartilage calcification—which reduces chest wall mobility. Osteoporosis and vertebral collapse result in kyphosis, adding to the problem. Respiratory muscles also degenerate or atrophy with aging, decreasing pulmonary function.

Ventilatory capacity diminishes with age for several reasons. First, the lung's diffusing capacity declines, and decreased inspiratory and expiratory muscle strength diminishes vital capacity. The lung tissue itself also degenerates, causing a decrease in the lungs' elastic recoil. This results in elevated residual

volume that, in some older adults, can even cause signs and symptoms consistent with emphysema. Finally, the closing of some airways produces poor ventilation of the basal areas, resulting in a decreased surface area for gas exchange and reduced partial pressure of oxygen.

In the typical older adult, normal partial pressure of arterial oxygen drops to 70 to 85 mm Hg, and oxygen saturation decreases by 5%. The lungs become more rigid, and the number and size of alveoli decline. A 40% reduction in respiratory fluids heightens the risk of pulmonary infection and mucus plugs. Maximum breathing capacity, forced vital capacity, vital capacity, and inspiratory reserve volume all diminish with age, leaving the older adult with a lowered tolerance for oxygen debt. Add in outside factors—including environmental hazards such as poor air quality for some older adults who live in polluted areas, a lifetime of poor habits such as lack of exercise or smoking for others—and it becomes all too clear why older adults are at such high risk for respiratory disorders.

For such patients, you'll need to perform respiratory assessments frequently. You're likely to be the first person to encounter older adults in the health care setting, where you can detect early changes in pulmonary function and get your patients the prompt treatment they need. But make sure you're on alert: Missing or misinterpreting the sometimes-misleading signs and symptoms of respiratory disease in these patients can place them at risk for late diagnosis and a more complicated illness.

Chronic obstructive pulmonary disease

Chronic obstructive pulmonary disease (COPD) is chronic airway obstruction that results from either emphysema or chronic bronchitis, or from a combination of these disorders. In most cases, bronchitis and emphysema occur together. COPD doesn't always produce signs and symptoms and causes only minimal disability in many patients. However, it tends to worsen with age, especially if older patients have other aggravating conditions.

CAUSES AND INCIDENCE

Predisposing factors for COPD include cigarette smoking, recurrent or chronic respiratory infections, air pollution, occupational exposure to chemicals, and allergies. Smoking is by far the most important of these factors; it impairs ciliary action and macrophage function, inflames airways, increases mucus production, destroys alveolar septae, and causes peribronchiolar fibrosis. Early inflammatory changes may reverse if the patient stops smoking before lung destruction is extensive. Familial and hereditary factors (such as deficiency of $alpha_1$-antitrypsin) may also predispose a person to COPD.

The most common chronic lung disease, COPD (also known as chronic obstructive lung disease) affects an estimated 17 million Americans, and its incidence is rising. It affects more men than women, probably because until recently men were more likely to smoke heavily. COPD occurs mostly in people older than age 40.

PATHOPHYSIOLOGY

Emphysema and bronchitis each has its own pathophysiology.

Emphysema

In emphysema, the release of proteolytic enzymes from lung cells results in recurrent inflammation, which causes irreversible enlargement of the air spaces distal to the terminal bronchioles. Enlargement of air spaces destroys the alveolar walls, which results in a

breakdown of elasticity and loss of fibrous and muscle tissue, making the lungs less compliant.

A change in airway size compromises the lungs' ability to circulate sufficient air. Inflammation damages and eventually destroys the alveolar walls, creating large air spaces. (See *Looking at abnormal alveoli*.) The alveolar septa

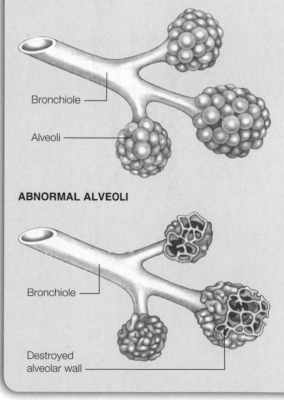

LOOKING AT ABNORMAL ALVEOLI

In the patient with emphysema, recurrent pulmonary inflammation damages and eventually destroys the alveolar walls, creating large air spaces. The damaged alveoli can't recoil normally after expanding; therefore, bronchioles collapse on expiration, trapping the air in the lungs and causing overdistention. As the alveolar walls are destroyed, the lungs become enlarged, and the total lung capacity and residual volume then increase. Shown here are changes that occur during emphysema.

NORMAL ALVEOLI

Bronchiole

Alveoli

ABNORMAL ALVEOLI

Bronchiole

Destroyed alveolar wall

are initially destroyed, leaving the alveoli unable to recoil normally after expanding and resulting in bronchiolar collapse on expiration. The amount of air that can be expired passively diminishes, trapping air in the lungs and leading to overdistention. (See *Air trapping in emphysema.*) Septal destruction may affect only respiratory bronchioles and alveolar ducts, leaving alveolar sacs intact (called centriacinar emphysema), or it may involve the entire acinus (called panacinar emphysema), with more random damage that involves the lower lobes of the lungs. (See *Two types of emphysema,* page 179.)

Chronic bronchitis

Chronic bronchitis occurs when the patient inhales irritants for a prolonged period. The irritants inflame the tracheobronchial tree, leading to increased mucus production and a narrowed or blocked airway. As the inflammation continues, changes in the cells lining the respiratory tract result in resistance of the small airways and severe ventilation-perfusion

---

AIR TRAPPING IN EMPHYSEMA

After alveolar walls are damaged or destroyed, they can't support and keep the airways open. The alveolar walls then lose their capability of elastic recoil. Collapse then occurs on expiration, as shown here.

Normal expiration
Note normal recoil and the open bronchiole.

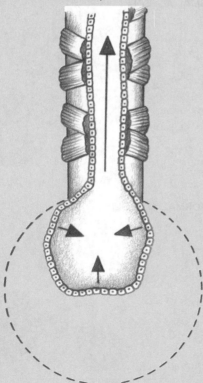

Impaired expiration
Note decreased elastic recoil and narrowed bronchiole.

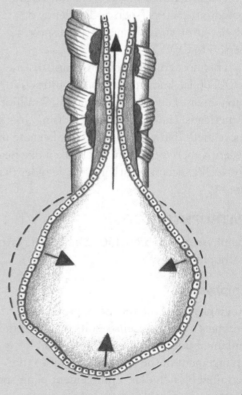

($\dot{V}/\dot{Q}$) imbalance, which decreases arterial oxygenation.

Chronic bronchitis results in hypertrophy and hyperplasia of the mucus glands, increased goblet cells, ciliary damage, squamous metaplasia of the columnar epithelium, and chronic leukocytic and lymphocytic infiltration of the bronchial walls. (See *Changes in chronic bronchitis.*) Hypersecretion of the goblet cells blocks free movement of the cilia, which normally sweep dust, irritants, and mucus away from the airways. The mucus and debris accumulating in the patient's airways leave him more susceptible to respiratory tract infections.

The disorder also causes widespread inflammation, airway narrowing, and the buildup of mucus within the airways. As a result, airways become obstructed and can close, trapping gas in the distal porion of the lungs. This results in hypoventilation, which leads to a $\dot{V}/\dot{Q}$ mismatch and hypoxemia.

ASSESSMENT FINDINGS

Findings may vary for the two disorders.

Emphysema

The patient's history may reveal a long-time smoking habit. Other findings may include:

- shortness of breath
- chronic cough
- anorexia with resultant weight loss and a general feeling of malaise
- barrel chest
- pursed-lip breathing
- peripheral cyanosis
- clubbed fingers and toes
- tachypnea
- decreased tactile fremitus
- decreased chest expansion
- decreased breath sounds
- crackles and wheezing during inspiration

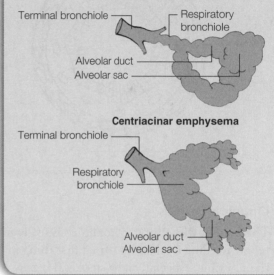

TWO TYPES OF EMPHYSEMA

Two types of emphysema are most common among older adults. Panacinar (panlobular) emphysema destroys alveoli and alveolar ducts. It's typically associated with aging and alpha$_1$-antitrypsin deficiency. Centriacinar (centrilobular) emphysema, which is associated with chronic bronchitis and smoking, destroys the respiratory bronchioles.

Panacinar emphysema

Terminal bronchiole — Respiratory bronchiole

Alveolar duct
Alveolar sac

Centriacinar emphysema

Terminal bronchiole

Respiratory bronchiole

Alveolar duct
Alveolar sac

- prolonged expiratory phase with grunting respirations
- distant heart sounds.

Age-related respiratory changes can worsen the signs and symptoms of emphysema. The decreased peak airflow, gas exchange, and vital capacity that can result from aging can aggravate the older patient's shortness of breath. Smoking—which actually speeds up the aging process in the lungs—can make signs and symptoms even worse. Defense mechanisms in the lungs and immune system also decrease with aging, increasing the risk of pneumonia after bacterial or viral infection.

CHANGES IN CHRONIC BRONCHITIS

In chronic bronchitis, irritants inflame the tracheobronchial tree over time, leading to increased mucus production and a narrowed or blocked airway. As the inflammation continues, goblet and epithelial cells hypertrophy. Because the natural defense mechanisms are blocked, the airways accumulate debris in the respiratory tract. The illustrations here show these changes.

Cross section of normal bronchial tube

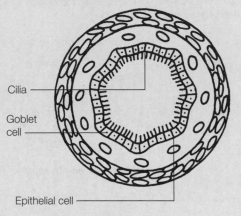

Narrowed bronchial tube in chronic bronchitis

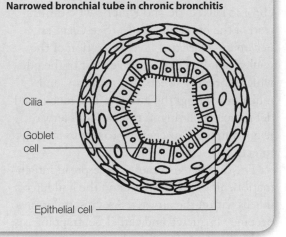

Chronic bronchitis

The patient with chronic bronchitis is likely to report needing to clear his throat first thing in the morning, especially if he smokes. He may also complain of a chronic cough that produces yellowish sputum, shortness of breath, and frequent respiratory infections.

COMPLICATIONS

- Disability from weakness that results from inadequate oxygenation
- Cor pulmonale
- Severe respiratory failure
- Death

TREATMENT

Treatment is designed to relieve symptoms and prevent complications. Because most patients with COPD receive outpatient treatment, they need comprehensive teaching to help them comply with therapy and understand the nature of this chronic, progressive disease. If programs in pulmonary rehabilitation are available, encourage the patient to enroll.

Urge the patient to stop smoking. Provide smoking cessation counseling or refer him to a program. Tell him to avoid other respiratory irritants, such as secondhand smoke, aerosol spray products, and outdoor air pollution. He may find an air conditioner with an air filter in his home helpful; a humidifier may make it easier for him to move bronchial secretions.

Treatment also typically includes a beta-agonist bronchodilator (albuterol [AccuNeb] or salmeterol [Serevent]), an anticholinergic bronchodilator (ipratropium [Atrovent]), and a corticosteroid (beclomethasone [Qvar] or triamcinolone [Azmacort]). The patient will most likely take these with a metered-dose inhaler. If the patient develops a respiratory infection, he may need antibiotics.

Lung volume reduction surgery is a new procedure for carefully selected patients with primarily emphysema. The surgeon removes nonfunctional parts of the lung (diseased tissue that provides little ventilation or perfusion), allowing functional lung tissue to expand and the diaphragm to return to its normally elevated position.

NURSING CONSIDERATIONS

- Teach the patient and his family how to recognize early signs of infection, and warn the patient to avoid contact with people with respiratory infections. To help prevent infection, encourage good oral hygiene (coughing into a tissue, or sneezing or coughing into the crook of the elbow) and hand washing. Recommend pneumococcal and annual influenza vaccinations.
- To promote ventilation and reduce air trapping, teach the patient to breathe slowly, prolonging expirations to two to three times the duration of inspiration, and to exhale through pursed lips.
- To help mobilize secretions, teach the patient how to cough effectively. If the patient with copious secretions has difficulty mobilizing secretions, teach his family how to perform postural drainage and chest physiotherapy. If secretions are thick, urge the patient to drink 12 to 15 glasses of fluid each day. Recommend using a home humidifier, particularly in the winter.
- Administer low concentrations of oxygen as ordered. Obtain an arterial blood gas analysis to determine the patient's oxygen needs and to avoid carbon dioxide narcosis.
- If the patient will continue oxygen therapy at home, teach him how to use the equipment correctly. A patient with COPD rarely requires more than 2 to 3 L/minute of oxygen to maintain adequate oxygenation; higher flow rates will further increase the partial pressure of arterial oxygen, but the patient whose ventilatory drive is largely based on hypoxemia commonly develops markedly increased partial pressure of arterial carbon dioxide. In such cases, chemoreceptors in the brain are relatively insensitive to the increase in carbon dioxide. Teach the patient and his family that excessive oxygen therapy may eliminate the hypoxic respiratory drive, causing confusion and drowsiness, signs of carbon dioxide narcosis or impending death.
- Emphasize the importance of a balanced diet. Because the patient may tire easily when eating, suggest that he eat frequent, small meals and consider using oxygen, administered by nasal cannula, during meals.
- If the patient has a metered-dose inhaler, teach him how to use it correctly.
- If the patient is on antibiotics for a respiratory infection, stress the importance of finishing the prescribed course of treatment.
- Help the patient and his family adjusts their lifestyles to accommodate the limitations imposed by this debilitating chronic disease. Instruct the patient to allow for daily rest periods and to exercise daily as his physician directs. If he has a motorized scooter, recommend that he limit its use to shopping trips or other activities that require extra effort.
- As COPD progresses, encourage the patient to discuss his fears.
- To help prevent COPD, advise all patients, especially those with a family history of COPD or those in its early stages, not to smoke.
- Assist in the early detection of COPD by urging your patients to have periodic physical examinations, including spirometry and medical evaluation of a chronic cough, and to seek treatment for recurring respiratory infections promptly.

Influenza

Influenza (also called grippe or flu), an acute, highly contagious infection of the respiratory tract, results from three different types of *Myxovirus influenzae*. It occurs sporadically or in epidemics (usually during the colder months), which tend to peak 2 to 3 weeks after initial cases and subside within a month.

One of the remarkable features of the influenza virus is its capacity for antigenic variation into several distinct strains, allowing it to infect new populations that have little or no immunologic resistance. An antigenic variation can occur as antigenic drift (minor changes that occur yearly or every few years) or antigenic shift (major changes that lead to pandemics).

Older people and those with chronic diseases are more likely to experience serious effects from influenza. In these groups, influenza may even lead to death.

CAUSES AND INCIDENCE

Transmission of influenza occurs through inhalation of respiratory droplets from an infected person or by indirect contact with a contaminated object, such as a drinking glass or other item contaminated with respiratory secretions.

Influenza viruses are classified into three groups. Type A, the most prevalent, strikes every year, with new serotypes causing epidemics every 3 years. Type B also strikes annually but causes epidemics only every 4 to 6 years. Type C is endemic and causes only sporadic cases.

PATHOPHYSIOLOGY

The influenza virus invades the epithelium of the respiratory tract, causing inflammation and desquamation. (See *How influenza viruses multiply.*)

ASSESSMENT FINDINGS

After an incubation period of 24 to 48 hours, flu symptoms begin to appear and can include the sudden onset of chills, fever of 101° to 104° F (38.3° to 40° C), headache, malaise, myalgia (particularly in the back and limbs), and a nonproductive cough. Occasionally, the patient may complain of laryngitis, hoarseness, conjunctivitis, rhinitis, and rhinorrhea. Signs and symptoms usually subside in 3 to 5 days, but cough and weakness may persist.

In some patients—especially older patients—lack of energy and easy fatigability may persist for several weeks. Fever that persists longer than 5 days signals the onset of complications. Pneumonia, the most common complication, occurs as primary influenza virus pneumonia or secondary to bacterial infection. The signs and symptoms of the older patient's comorbidities may worsen, despite resolution of the influenza, calling for close monitoring.

COMPLICATIONS

- Pneumonia
- Myositis
- Exacerbation of chronic obstructive pulmonary disease
- Myocarditis (rare)
- Pericarditis (rare)
- Transverse myelitis (rare)
- Encephalitis (rare)

TREATMENT

Treatment of uncomplicated influenza includes bed rest, adequate fluid intake, aspirin or acetaminophen to relieve fever and muscle pain, and dextromethorphan or another antitussive to relieve nonproductive coughing. Prophylactic antibiotics aren't recommended because they have no effect on the influenza virus.

HOW INFLUENZA VIRUSES MULTIPLY

An influenza virus, classified as type A, B, or C, contains the genetic material ribonucleic acid (RNA), which is covered and protected by protein. RNA is arranged in the genes that carry the instruction for viral replication. This genetic material has an extraordinary ability to mutate, causing the generation of new serologically distinct strains of influenza virus. Being a virus, the pathogen can't reproduce or carry out chemical reactions on its own. It needs a host cell.

After attaching to the host cell, the viral RNA enters the host cell and causes the host components to replicate its genetic material and protein, which are then assembled into the new virus particles. These newly produced viruses can burst forth to invade other healthy cells.

The viral invasion destroys the host cells, impairing respiratory defenses, especially the mucociliary transport system, and predisposing the patient to secondary bacterial infection.

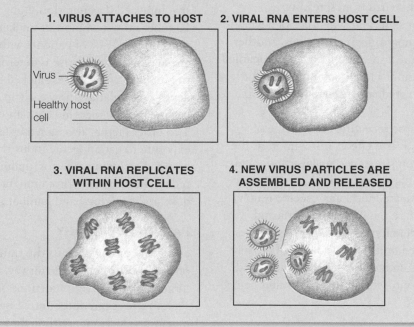

1. VIRUS ATTACHES TO HOST

Virus

Healthy host cell

2. VIRAL RNA ENTERS HOST CELL

3. VIRAL RNA REPLICATES WITHIN HOST CELL

4. NEW VIRUS PARTICLES ARE ASSEMBLED AND RELEASED

In influenza complicated by pneumonia, supportive care (fluid and electrolyte supplements, oxygen, and assisted ventilation) and treatment of bacterial superinfection with appropriate antibiotics are necessary. No specific therapy exists for cardiac, central nervous system, or other complications.

Antiviral drugs, such as oseltamivir (Tamiflu), zanamivir (Relenza), amantadine (Symmetrel), and rimantadine (Flumadine), inhibit neuraminidase, decreasing the release of viruses from infected cells and limiting viral spread. These drugs reduce the severity of signs and symptoms as well as the length of illness by an average of 1.5 days. The patient must receive the antiviral within 48 hours of the onset of signs and symptoms. To help prevent influenza types A and B, people should receive the influenza virus vaccine (Fluzone) or intranasal vaccine (FluMist).

NURSING CONSIDERATIONS

Unless complications occur, influenza doesn't require hospitalization; patient care focuses on relief of symptoms.

- Advise the patient to increase his fluid intake. Warm baths or heating pads may relieve myalgia. Give him nonopioid analgesics and antipyretics as ordered.
- Screen visitors to protect the patient from bacterial infection and the visitors from influenza. Use droplet precautions.
- Teach the patient proper disposal of tissues and proper hand-washing technique to prevent the virus from spreading.
- Watch for signs and symptoms of developing pneumonia, such as crackles, another temperature rise, or coughing accompanied by purulent or bloody sputum. Help the patient to gradually resume his normal activities.
- Inform those receiving the vaccine of possible adverse effects (discomfort at the vaccination site, fever, malaise and, rarely, Guillain-Barré syndrome).
- Live-attenuated influenza vaccine is now available as a nasal spray. Criteria and contraindications for use vary from the inactivated, injectable vaccine. Make sure recipients understand that they may shed influenza virus for up to 21 days after being immunized.

Lung cancer

Even though it's largely preventable, lung cancer is the most common cause of cancer death in both men and women. Lung cancer usually develops within the wall or epithelium of the bronchial tree. Its most common types are epidermoid (squamous cell) carcinoma, small-cell (oat cell) carcinoma, adenocarcinoma, and large-cell (anaplastic) carcinoma. Although the prognosis is usually poor, it varies with the extent of metastasis at the time of diagnosis and the cell type growth rate. Only about 13% of patients with lung cancer survive 5 years after diagnosis.

CAUSES AND INCIDENCE

Most experts agree that lung cancer is attributable to inhalation of carcinogenic pollutants by a susceptible host. Any smoker older than age 40, especially if he began to smoke before age 15, has smoked a whole pack or more per day for 20 years, or works with or near asbestos, is susceptible.

Pollutants in tobacco smoke cause progressive lung cell degeneration. Lung cancer is 10 times more common in smokers than in nonsmokers; 90% of patients with lung cancer are smokers. Cancer risk is determined by the number of cigarettes smoked daily, the depth of inhalation, how early in life smoking began, and the nicotine content of cigarettes. Two other factors also increase susceptibility: exposure to carcinogenic industrial and air pollutants (including asbestos, uranium, arsenic, nickel, iron oxides, chromium, radioactive dust, and coal dust) and familial susceptibility.

PATHOPHYSIOLOGY

Lung cancer begins with the transformation of one epithelial cell of the airway. The bronchi in general and certain portions of the bronchi, such as the segmental bifurcations and sites of mucus production, are thought to be more vulnerable to injury from carcinogens.

As a lung tumor grows, it can partially or completely obstruct the airway, resulting in lobar collapse distal to the tumor. A lung tumor can also hemorrhage, causing hemoptysis. Early metastasis may occur to other thoracic structures, such as the hilar lymph nodes or the mediastinum. Distant metastasis can occur to the brain, liver, bone, and adrenal glands. (See *Tumor infiltrations in lung cancer*.)

ASSESSMENT FINDINGS

Because early-stage lung cancer usually produces no symptoms, this disease is usually in an

TUMOR INFILTRATION IN LUNG CANCER

The illustrations below show a lung tumor projecting into the bronchi and metastasis to the hilar and carinal lymph nodes.

Right lung — Anterior view

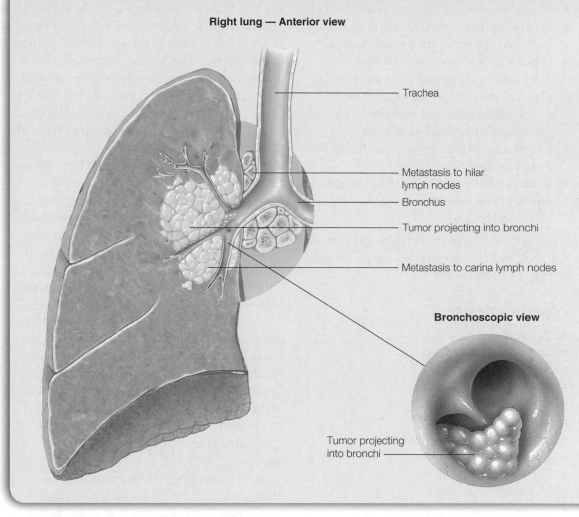

Trachea

Metastasis to hilar lymph nodes

Bronchus

Tumor projecting into bronchi

Metastasis to carina lymph nodes

Bronchoscopic view

Tumor projecting into bronchi

advanced state at diagnosis, with late-stage signs and symptoms commonly leading to diagnosis. Epidermoid and small-cell carcinomas cause a smoker's cough, hoarseness, wheezing, dyspnea, hemoptysis, and chest pain. Adenocarcinoma and large-cell carcinoma result in fever, weakness, weight loss, anorexia, and shoulder pain.

Metastatic signs and symptoms vary greatly, depending on the effect of tumors on intrathoracic and distant structures:

- Bronchial obstruction causes hemoptysis, atelectasis, pneumonitis, and dyspnea.
- Cervical thoracic sympathetic nerve involvement causes miosis, ptosis, exophthalmos, and reduced sweating.

- Chest wall invasion results in piercing chest pain, increasing dyspnea, and severe shoulder pain that radiates down the arm.
- Esophageal compression causes dysphagia.
- Local lymphatic spread results in coughing, hemoptysis, stridor, and pleural effusion.
- Pericardial involvement results in pericardial effusion, tamponade, and arrhythmias.
- Phrenic nerve involvement can cause dyspnea, shoulder pain, and unilateral paralyzed diaphragm with paradoxical motion.
- Recurrent nerve invasion causes hoarseness and vocal cord paralysis.
- Vena caval obstruction results in venous distention and edema of the face, neck, chest, and back.

Distant metastasis may involve any part of the body, most commonly the central nervous system, liver, and bone.

COMPLICATIONS

- Anorexia
- Esophageal compression
- Tracheal obstruction
- Cachexia
- Clubbing of fingers and toes
- Dyspnea
- Hypertrophic osteoarthropathy
- Dysphagia
- Phrenic nerve paralysis
- Hypoxemia
- Pleural effusion

TREATMENT

More recent treatment options, which consist of combinations of surgery, radiation, and chemotherapy, may improve the prognosis and prolong survival. Nevertheless, because treatment usually begins at an advanced stage, it's largely palliative.

Surgery is the preferred treatment for stage I, stage II, or selected stage III squamous cell cancer; adenocarcinoma; and large-cell carcinoma, unless the tumor is nonresectable or other conditions rule out surgery. Surgery may include partial removal of a lung (wedge resection, segmental resection, lobectomy, or radical lobectomy) or total removal (pneumonectomy or radical pneumonectomy). A less invasive form of surgery that's used for small (1½" or less) tumors is video-assisted thoracic surgery (VATS). VATS requires small incisions and causes less pain than other types of surgery.

Preoperative radiation therapy may reduce tumor bulk to allow for surgical resection. Preradiation chemotherapy helps improve response rates. Radiation therapy is ordinarily recommended for stage I and stage II lesions, if surgery is contraindicated, and for stage III lesions when the disease is confined to the involved hemithorax and the ipsilateral supraclavicular lymph nodes.

Generally, radiation therapy is delayed for a month after surgery to allow the wound to heal. Radiation is then directed to the part of the chest most likely to develop metastasis. High-dose radiation therapy or radiation implants may also be used.

In laser therapy, laser energy is directed through a bronchoscope to destroy local tumors.

Chemotherapy combinations of paclitaxel, gemcitabine, docetaxel, irinotecan, and vinorelbine are more active and better tolerated when combined with cisplatin or carboplatin. Many of these drugs are also used alone to treat small-cell and non–small-cell lung cancers. Bevacizumab (Avastin) works by stopping tumors from developing new blood vessels, which deprives tumors of the oxygen and nutrients they need to grow. Erlotinib (Tarceva) works by blocking chemicals that signal the cancer cells to grow and divide.

NURSING CONSIDERATIONS

Comprehensive supportive care and patient teaching can minimize complications and speed recovery from surgery, radiation, and chemotherapy.

Before surgery, take the following steps:

- Supplement and reinforce the information given to the patient by the health care team about the disease and the surgical procedure.
- Explain expected postoperative procedures, such as insertion of an indwelling catheter, use of an endotracheal tube or chest tube (or both), dressing changes, and I.V. therapy.
- Teach the patient how to perform coughing, deep diaphragmatic breathing, and range-of-motion (ROM) exercises.
- Reassure the patient that he'll receive analgesics and proper positioning to control postoperative pain.
- Inform the patient that he may take nothing by mouth beginning on midnight of the night before surgery, that he'll shower with a soaplike antibacterial agent the night or morning before surgery, and that he'll receive preoperative medications, such as a sedative and an anticholinergic to dry secretions.

After thoracic surgery, take the following steps:

- Maintain a patent airway, and monitor the patient's chest tubes to reestablish normal intrathoracic pressure and prevent postoperative and pulmonary complications.
- Check the patient's vital signs every 15 minutes during the 1st hour after surgery, every 30 minutes during the next 4 hours, and then every 2 hours. Watch for and report abnormal respiration and other changes.
- Suction the patient as needed, and encourage him to begin deep breathing and coughing as soon as possible. Check secretions often. Initially, sputum will be thick

and dark with blood, but it should become thinner and grayish yellow within a day.

- Monitor and record closed chest drainage. Keep chest tubes patent and draining effectively. Fluctuation in the water-seal chamber on inspiration and expiration indicates that the chest tube is patent. Watch for air leaks, and report them immediately. Position the patient on the surgical side to promote drainage and lung reexpansion.
- Watch for and report foul-smelling discharge and excessive drainage on dressings. Usually, the dressing is removed after 24 hours, unless the wound appears infected.
- Monitor intake and output, and maintain adequate hydration.
- Watch for and treat infection, shock, hemorrhage, atelectasis, dyspnea, mediastinal shift, and pulmonary embolus, as ordered.
- To prevent pulmonary embolus, apply antiembolism stockings and encourage ROM exercises.

If the patient is receiving chemotherapy and radiation, take the following steps:

- Explain possible adverse effects of radiation and chemotherapy. Watch for, treat and, when possible, try to prevent them.
- Ask the dietary department to provide soft, nonirritating foods that are high in protein, and encourage the patient to eat high-calorie between-meal snacks.
- Give antiemetics and antidiarrheals as needed.
- Schedule patient care activities in a way that helps the patient conserve his energy.
- During radiation therapy, administer skin care to minimize skin breakdown. If the patient receives radiation therapy in an outpatient setting, warn him to avoid tight clothing, exposure to the sun, and harsh ointments on his chest. Teach him exercises to help prevent shoulder stiffness.

- If the patient and family decide to discontinue treatment and participate in palliative treatment only, offer them your support. Help them cope with end-of-life issues, and recognize that you will have your own responses to these issues.

Obstructive sleep apnea

Sleep apnea is a disruption in breathing during sleep. An episode generally lasts at least 10 seconds and typically occurs more than five times in 1 hour. Sleep apnea is more likely to occur as a persons ages.

CAUSES AND INCIDENCE

Although sleep apnea can have a central or a neurologic origin, it's more commonly the result of a type of respiratory obstruction, such as the soft palate or tongue obstructing the upper airway. Factors that contribute to the disorder include obesity, family history, large neck circumference, and abnormal anatomy (recessed chin, abnormal upper airway, large tonsils or adenoids, nasal obstruction, or craniofacial anomalies).

Sleep apnea has been linked to such conditions as hypertension, atrial fibrillation, hypothyroidism, atherosclerosis, and diabetes. Central nervous system (CNS) depressants, such as muscle relaxants, sedatives, analgesics, and alcohol, can worsen or cause sleep apnea by further relaxing the airway muscles and reducing respiratory drive. Smoking can aggravate the condition by causing swelling, inflammation, and narrowing of the upper airway. The supine position may also trigger apnea because gravity increases the likelihood that the tongue will occlude the airway, or that muscles and tissues will collapse.

Sleep apnea is more common in men and in those over age 40. Menopausal and postmenopausal women also have a higher incidence.

PATHOPHYSIOLOGY

Skeletal muscles relax during sleep. This relaxation displaces the tongue and other anatomic structures of the head and neck, which obstruct the upper airway, even though the chest wall continues to move. Absence of breathing causes an increase in arterial carbon dioxide levels and lowers the pH level. These changes stimulate the nervous system, and the sleeping person responds after 10 or more seconds of apnea. This arousal episode serves to correct the obstruction, and breathing resumes. The cycle repeats itself as often as every 5 minutes during sleep, affecting the patient's ability to get a restful night of sleep. (See *Understanding obstructive sleep apnea*.)

ASSESSMENT FINDINGS

The patient's partner may complain that the patient snores, tosses and turns, and has fitful sleep. The partner may report hearing periods of no breathing and then the restart of the snoring.

The patient may complain of excessive daytime sleepiness, intellectual impairment, poor judgment, memory loss, morning headache, daytime fatigue, gastroesophageal reflux, impotence and a decreased libido, and weight gain.

COMPLICATIONS

- Hypertension
- Heart failure
- Stroke

TREATMENT

For mild to moderate sleep apnea, treatment aims to keep the keep the airway clear without surgical intervention:

- Continuous positive airway pressure (CPAP) is the first line treatment for moderate to severe sleep apnea. Improvements

UNDERSTANDING OBSTRUCTIVE SLEEP APNEA

When breathing is unobstructed, air flows normally. During an apneic event, the airway becomes blocked and air ceases to flow.

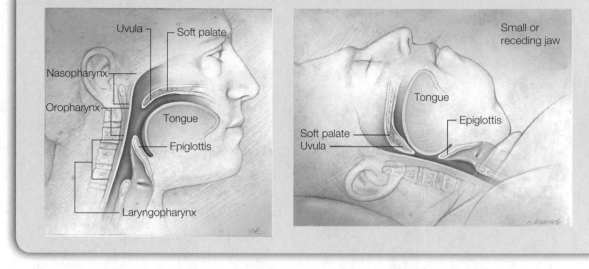

continue to make the equipment more comfortable and less physically restrictive, allowing for more restful sleep.

- Weight loss or a change in sleeping position may resolve mild cases of sleep apnea. Elevating the head of the bed 30 degrees allows the tongue to lie flat, helping to maintain a patent airway. The side-lying position also prevents the tongue from falling to the back of the throat.
- Avoiding alcohol and other CNS depressants for at least 6 hours before going to bed can help prevent relaxation of the pharyngeal muscles.
- Devices that prevent obstruction by the tongue or nonsurgical neck structures can help in mild cases.

For more severe cases, surgery can correct abnormalities of the soft tissue or bone structure that obstruct the patient's airway:

- Uvulopalatopharyngoplasty, a laser-assisted procedure, removes part of the uvula and excess soft tissue on the palate and posterior pharyngeal wall.
- Nasal surgery removes polyps or corrects such abnormalities as a deviated septum to improve airway patency.
- Maxillomandibular advancement enlarges the entire upper airway by expanding the bones that surround the airway.
- Genioglossus advancement places tension on the tongue to prevent it from displacing backward during sleep.
- Hyoid advancement repositions the hyoid bone to expand the airway.

NURSING CONSIDERATIONS

- Teach the patient and his family about the disorder and its possible causes. Explain the risks to the patient's health, including possible cardiac risks.
- Perform an assessment and collect a health history to determine contributing factors.

PNEUMONIA IN TWO LOCATIONS

These two illustrations show consolidation associated with lobar pneumonia (shown on the left) and bronchopneumonia (shown on the right).

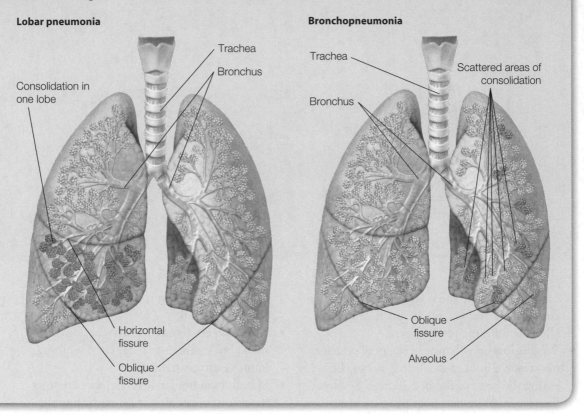

Lobar pneumonia

Trachea

Bronchus

Consolidation in one lobe

Horizontal fissure

Oblique fissure

Bronchopneumonia

Trachea

Scattered areas of consolidation

Bronchus

Oblique fissure

Alveolus

- Using the health history, assess the patient's sleep patterns, including the degree of fatigue during the day and interference in the ability to function because of interrupted sleep.
- Encourage the patient who smokes to join a smoking-cessation program.
- Encourage the obese patient to join a weight-loss program.
- Teach the patient how to use CPAP, and give him information about the device.
- Make sure the nasal or full-face mask on the CPAP fits properly to ensure optimal functioning.

- If the patient requires surgery, provide preoperative and postoperative teaching for the patient and his partner.
- Administer medication as ordered, and explain possible adverse reactions and what to do if they occur.

Pneumonia

Pneumonia is an acute infection of the lung parenchyma that commonly impairs gas exchange. The prognosis is generally good for people who have normal lungs and adequate host defenses before the onset of pneumonia; however, pneumonia is the sixth leading cause of death in the United States.

CAUSES AND INCIDENCE

Pneumonia can be classified in several ways:

- Microbiologic etiology: Pneumonia can result from viral, bacterial, fungal, protozoan, mycobacterial, mycoplasmal, or rickettsial infection.
- Location: Bronchopneumonia involves distal airways and alveoli; lobular pneumonia, part of a lobe; and lobar pneumonia, an entire lobe. (See *Pneumonia in two locations*, page 190.)
- Type: Primary pneumonia results from inhalation or aspiration of a pathogen; it includes pneumococcal and viral pneumonia. Secondary pneumonia may follow initial lung damage from a noxious chemical or other insult (superinfection), or it may result from hematogenous spread of bacteria from a distant focus. (See *Types of pneumonia*, pages 192 and 193.)

Predisposing factors for bacterial and viral pneumonia include chronic illness and debilitation, cancer (particularly lung cancer), abdominal and thoracic surgery, atelectasis; the common cold and other viral respiratory infections such as acquired immunodeficiency syndrome, chronic respiratory disease (including chronic obstructive pulmonary disease, asthma, bronchiectasis, and cystic fibrosis), influenza, smoking, malnutrition, alcoholism, sickle cell disease, tracheostomy, exposure to noxious gases, aspiration, and immunosuppressive therapy.

Predisposing factors for aspiration pneumonia include advanced age, debilitation, artificial airway use, nasogastric (NG) tube feedings, impaired gag reflex, poor oral hygiene, and decreased level of consciousness.

In older and debilitated patients, bacterial pneumonia may follow bronchitis, sinusitis, influenza, or even a common cold.

PATHOPHYSIOLOGY

In bacterial pneumonia, which can occur in any part of the lungs, an infection initially triggers alveolar inflammation and edema. Capillaries become engorged with blood, causing stasis. As the alveolocapillary membrane breaks down, alveoli fill with blood and exudate, resulting in atelectasis. In severe bacterial infections, the lungs assume a heavy, liverlike appearance, as in acute respiratory distress syndrome (ARDS).

Viral infection, which typically causes diffuse pneumonia, first attacks bronchiolar epithelial cells, causing interstitial inflammation and desquamation. It then spreads to the alveoli, which fill with blood and fluid. In advanced infection, a hyaline membrane may form. As with bacterial infection, severe viral infection may clinically resemble ARDS.

In aspiration pneumonia, aspiration of gastric juices or hydrocarbons triggers similar inflammatory changes and also inactivates surfactant over a large area. Decreased surfactant leads to alveolar collapse. Acidic gastric juices may directly damage the airways and alveoli. Particles with the aspirated gastric juices may obstruct the airways and reduce airflow, which, in turn, leads to secondary bacterial pneumonia.

ASSESSMENT FINDINGS

The main signs and symptoms of pneumonia are coughing, sputum production, pleuritic chest pain, shaking chills, shortness of breath, rapid shallow breathing, and fever. Physical findings vary widely, ranging from diffuse, fine crackles to signs of localized or extensive consolidation and pleural effusion. There may also be associated signs and

TYPES OF PNEUMONIA

TYPE	CHARACTERISTICS	TREATMENT
Viral Pneumonias		
Influenza	• Poor prognosis even with treatment • 50% mortality rate from cardiovascular collapse • Signs and symptoms: cough (initially nonproductive; later, purulent sputum), marked cyanosis, dyspnea, high fever, chills, substernal pain and discomfort, moist crackles, frontal headache, myalgia	• Supportive treatment for respiratory failure includes endotracheal intubation and ventilator assistance; for fever, hypothermia blanket or antipyretics; for influenza A, amantadine or rimantadine.
Adenovirus	• Insidious onset (generally affects young adults) • Good prognosis; usually clears without residual effects • Signs and symptoms: sore throat, fever, cough, chills, malaise, small amounts of mucoid sputum, retrosternal chest pain, anorexia, rhinitis, adenopathy, scattered crackles, rhonchi	• Treatment goal is to relieve symptoms.
Chickenpox (varicella)	• Present in about 30% of adults with varicella • Signs and symptoms: characteristic rash, cough, dyspnea, cyanosis, tachypnea, pleuritic chest pain, hemoptysis and rhonchi 1 to 6 days after onset of rash	• Supportive treatment includes adequate hydration and, in critically ill patients, oxygen therapy. • Patients who are immunocompromised also receive I.V. acyclovir.
Cytomegalovirus	• Difficult to distinguish from other nonbacterial pneumonias. In adults with healthy lung tissue, resembles mononucleosis and is generally benign; in immunocompromised hosts, varies from clinically inapparent to fatal infection • Signs and symptoms: fever, cough, shaking chills, dyspnea, cyanosis, weakness, diffuse crackles	• Supportive treatment includes adequate hydration and nutrition, oxygen therapy, and bed rest. • Disease is more severe in patients who are immunocompromised, warranting ganciclovir or foscarnet.
Protozoal Pneumonia		
Pneumocystis jiroveci	• Occurs in immunocompromised patients • Signs and symptoms: dyspnea, nonproductive cough, anorexia, weight loss, fatigue, low-grade fever	• Antimicrobial therapy consists of cotrimoxazole or pentamidine therapy. • Supportive treatment includes oxygen therapy, improved nutrition, and mechanical ventilation.
Bacterial Pneumonias		
Streptococcus	• Caused by *Streptococcus pneumoniae* • Signs and symptoms: sudden onset of a single, shaking chill and sustained temperature of 102° to 104 ° F (38.9° to 40° C); commonly preceded by upper respiratory tract infection	• Antimicrobial therapy consists of penicillin G or, if the patient is allergic to penicillin, erythromycin; therapy is begun after obtaining culture specimen, but without waiting for results and continues for 7 to 10 days.

TYPES OF PNEUMONIA (*Continued*)

TYPE	CHARACTERISTICS	TREATMENT
Bacterial Pneumonias		
Klebsiella	• More likely in patients with chronic alcoholism, pulmonary disease, and diabetes • Signs and symptoms: fever and recurrent chills; cough producing rusty, bloody, viscous sputum (currant jelly); cyanosis of lips and nail beds from hypoxemia; shallow, grunting respirations	• Antimicrobial therapy consists of an aminoglycoside and, in serious infections, a cephalosporin.
Staphylococcus	• More likely in patients with viral illness, such as influenza or measles, and in those with cystic fibrosis • Signs and symptoms: temperature of 102° to 104° F, recurrent shaking chills, bloody sputum, dyspnea, tachypnea, hypoxemia	• Antimicrobial therapy consists of nafcillin or oxacillin for 14 days if staphylococci are producing Penicillinase. • A chest tube may be used to drain empyema.
Aspiration Pneumonia	• Results from vomiting and aspiration of gastric or oropharyngeal contents into trachea and lungs from ineffective swallowing muscles • Noncardiogenic pulmonary edema possible with damage to respiratory epithelium from contact with gastric acid • Subacute pneumonia possible with cavity formation • Lung abscess possible if foreign body present • Signs and symptoms: crackles, dyspnea, cyanosis, hypotension, tachycardia	

symptoms of headache, sweating, loss of appetite, and excess fatigue. An older patient may not have the more commons signs of cough and fever; instead, confusion may be the presenting sign.

COMPLICATIONS
• Septic shock
• Hypoxemia
• Respiratory failure
• Empyema
• Lung abscess
• Bacteremia
• Endocarditis
• Pericarditis
• Meningitis

TREATMENT
Antimicrobial therapy varies with the causative agent, and therapy requires reevaluation early in the course of treatment. Supportive measures include humidified oxygen therapy for hypoxemia, mechanical ventilation for respiratory failure, a high-calorie diet and adequate fluid intake, bed rest, and analgesics to relieve pleuritic chest pain. Patients with severe pneumonia on mechanical ventilation may require positive

end-expiratory pressure to promote adequate oxygenation.

NURSING CONSIDERATIONS

Correct supportive care can increase patient comfort, avoid complications, and speed recovery:

- Maintain a patent airway and adequate oxygenation. Monitor pulse oximetry and obtain arterial blood gas levels, especially if the patient is hypoxemic. If the partial pressure of arterial oxygen drops below 55 mm Hg, administer supplemental oxygen. If the patient has an underlying chronic lung disease, give oxygen cautiously.
- Teach the patient how to cough and perform deep-breathing exercises to clear secretions; encourage him to do so often. In severe pneumonia that requires endotracheal intubation or tracheostomy (with or without mechanical ventilation), provide thorough respiratory care. Suction often, using sterile technique, to remove secretions.
- Obtain sputum specimens as needed, by suction if the patient can't produce specimens independently. Collect specimens in a sterile container and deliver them promptly to the microbiology laboratory.
- Administer antibiotics as ordered and pain medication as needed; record the patient's response to medications. Fever and dehydration may necessitate I.V. fluids and electrolyte replacement.
- Maintain adequate nutrition to offset a hypermetabolic state secondary to infection. Ask the dietary department to provide a high-calorie, high-protein diet consisting of soft, easy-to-eat foods. Encourage the patient to eat. As necessary, supplement oral feedings with NG tube feedings or parenteral nutrition.
- Monitor fluid intake and output. Consider limiting milk products because they may increase sputum production.

- Provide a quiet, calm environment for the patient, with frequent rest periods.
- Give emotional support by explaining all procedures (especially intubation and suctioning) to the patient and his family. Encourage family visits. Provide diversionary activities appropriate to the patient's age.
- To control the spread of infection, dispose of secretions properly. Tell the patient to sneeze and cough into a disposable tissue; tape a lined bag to the side of the bed for used tissues.
- Administer pneumococcal vaccine (Pneumovax) to patients age 65 and older according to guidelines from the Centers for Disease Control and Prevention.

Pulmonary embolism

The most common pulmonary complication in hospitalized patients, pulmonary embolism is an obstruction of the pulmonary arterial bed by a dislodged thrombus, heart valve vegetation, or foreign substance. Although pulmonary infarction that results from embolism may be so mild as to be asymptomatic, massive embolism (more than 50% obstruction of pulmonary arterial circulation) and the accompanying infarction can be rapidly fatal. (See *Looking at pulmonary emboli*, page 195.)

CAUSES AND INCIDENCE

Pulmonary embolism generally results from dislodged thrombi originating in the leg veins. More than half of such thrombi arise in the deep veins of the legs. Other less common sources of thrombi include the pelvic, renal, and hepatic veins; right side of the heart; and upper extremities.

Predisposing factors for pulmonary embolism include long-term immobility, chronic pulmonary disease, heart failure or atrial fibrillation, thrombophlebitis, polycythemia vera, thrombocytosis, autoimmune hemolytic

LOOKING AT PULMONARY EMBOLI

The illustration below shows multiple emboli in small branches of the left lateral pulmonary artery and a single embolus in a branch of the right pulmonary artery. An area of infarction is also visible.

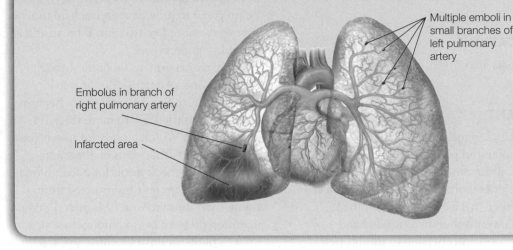

Multiple emboli in small branches of left pulmonary artery

Embolus in branch of right pulmonary artery

Infarcted area

anemia, sickle cell disease, varicose veins, recent surgery, lower-extremity fractures or surgery, burns, obesity, vascular injury, and cancer. Dehydration can also be a complicating factor. Pulmonary embolism is more likely to occur as a person ages.

PATHOPHYSIOLOGY

Thrombus formation results directly from vascular wall damage, venostasis, or hypercoagulability of the blood. Trauma, clot dissolution, sudden muscle spasm, intravascular pressure changes, or a change in peripheral blood flow can cause the thrombus to loosen or fragment. Then the thrombus—now called an embolus—floats to the heart's right side and enters the lungs through the pulmonary artery. There, the embolus may dissolve, continue to fragment, or grow.

If the embolus occludes the pulmonary artery, it prevents alveoli from producing enough surfactant to maintain alveolar integrity. As a result, alveoli collapse and atelectasis

develops. If the embolus enlarges, it may clog most or all of the pulmonary vessels and cause death.

Rarely, the emboli contain air, fat, bacteria, amniotic fluid, talc (from drugs intended for oral administration that are injected I.V. by addicts), or tumor cells.

ASSESSMENT FINDINGS

Total occlusion of the main pulmonary artery is rapidly fatal; smaller or fragmented emboli produce signs and symptoms that vary with the size, number, and location of the emboli. Usually, the first symptom of pulmonary embolism is dyspnea, which may be accompanied by anginal or pleuritic chest pain. Other clinical features include tachycardia, productive cough (sputum may be blood-tinged), low-grade fever, and pleural effusion. Less common signs include massive hemoptysis, chest splinting, leg edema and, with a large embolus, cyanosis, syncope, and distended jugular veins.

In addition, pulmonary embolism may cause pleural friction rub and signs and symptoms of circulatory collapse (weak, rapid pulse and hypotension) and hypoxia (restlessness and anxiety).

COMPLICATIONS

- Pulmonary infarction
- Death

TREATMENT

Treatment is designed to maintain adequate cardiovascular and pulmonary function during resolution of the obstruction and to prevent recurrence of embolic episodes. Because most emboli resolve in 10 to 14 days, treatment consists of oxygen therapy as needed and anticoagulation with heparin to inhibit new thrombus formation, followed by oral warfarin. Heparin therapy is monitored by daily coagulation studies (partial thromboplastin time [PTT]).

Patients with massive pulmonary embolism and shock may need fibrinolytic therapy with thrombolytic agents (streptokinase, urokinase, or tissue plasminogen activator) to enhance fibrinolysis of the pulmonary emboli and remaining thrombi. Emboli that cause hypotension may require the use of vasopressors. Treatment of septic emboli requires antibiotics—not anticoagulants—and evaluation for the infection's source, particularly endocarditis.

Surgery is performed on patients who can't take anticoagulants, who have recurrent emboli during anticoagulant therapy, or who have been treated with thrombolytic agents or pulmonary thromboendarterectomy. This procedure (which shouldn't be performed without angiographic evidence of pulmonary embolism) consists of vena caval ligation, plication, or insertion of an inferior vena cava device to filter blood returning to the heart and lungs.

NURSING CONSIDERATIONS

- Give oxygen by nasal cannula or mask. Check arterial blood gas levels if the patient develops fresh emboli or worsening dyspnea. Be prepared to provide endotracheal intubation with assisted ventilation if breathing is severely compromised.
- Administer heparin, as ordered, through I.V. push or continuous drip. Monitor coagulation studies daily; effective heparin therapy raises the PTT to more than 1½ times normal. Watch closely for nosebleeds, petechiae, and other signs of abnormal bleeding, and check stools for occult blood. Make sure the patient is protected from trauma and injury; avoid I.M. injections and maintain pressure over venipuncture sites for 5 minutes, or until bleeding stops, to reduce hematoma.
- After the patient is stable, encourage him to move about often, and assist with isometric and range-of-motion exercises. Check the patient's pedal pulses, temperature, and the color of his feet to detect venostasis. *Never* massage the patient's legs.
- Offer diversional activities to promote rest and relieve restlessness.
- Help the patient walk as soon as possible after surgery to prevent venostasis.
- Maintain adequate nutrition and fluid balance to promote healing.
- Don't attempt to elicit the Homan's sign.
- Report frequent pleuritic chest pain so that analgesics can be prescribed. Also, incentive spirometry can assist in deep breathing. Provide tissues and a bag for easy disposal of expectorations.
- Warn the patient not to cross his legs; this promotes thrombus formation.
- To relieve anxiety, explain procedures and treatments. Encourage the patient's family to participate in his care.

- Most patients need treatment with an oral anticoagulant (warfarin) for 3 to 6 months after a pulmonary embolism. Advise such a patient to watch for signs of bleeding (bloody stools, blood in urine, and large ecchymoses), to take the prescribed medication exactly as ordered, not to change dosages without consulting the physician, and to avoid taking additional medication (including aspirin and vitamins). Stress the importance of follow-up laboratory tests (International Normalized Ratio) to monitor anticoagulant therapy.

Tuberculosis

An acute or chronic infection caused by *Mycobacterium tuberculosis*, tuberculosis (TB) is characterized by pulmonary infiltrates, formation of granulomas with caseation, fibrosis, and cavitation. People who live in crowded, poorly ventilated conditions and those who are immunocompromised are most likely to become infected. The close living quarters found in long-term care facilities can potentially pose a risk to older patients, calling for careful screening of residents—including new admissions—for signs of TB.

In patients with strains that are sensitive to the usual antitubercular agents, the prognosis is excellent with correct treatment. However, in those with strains that are resistant to two or more of the major antitubercular agents, mortality is 50%.

CAUSES AND INCIDENCE

After exposure to M. *tuberculosis*, roughly 5% of infected people develop active TB within 1 year; in the remainder, microorganisms cause a latent infection. The host's immune system usually controls the tubercle bacillus by enclosing it in a tiny nodule (tubercle). The bacillus may lie dormant within the tubercle for years and later reactivate and spread.

In older patients, dormant bacilli from previous infection pose a particular threat. Older patients typically have a less robust immune system and are more likely to have chronic illnesses than younger patients, putting them at greater risk if the bacilli reactivate.

The incidence of TB has been increasing in the United States secondary to homelessness, drug abuse, and human immunodeficiency virus infection. Globally, TB is the leading infectious cause of morbidity and mortality, generating 8 to 10 million new cases each year.

PATHOPHYSIOLOGY

Although the primary infection site is the lungs, mycobacteria commonly exist in other parts of the body. Several factors increase the risk of infection reactivation, including gastrectomy, uncontrolled diabetes mellitus, Hodgkin's lymphoma, leukemia, silicosis, acquired immunodeficiency syndrome, treatment with corticosteroids or immunosuppressants, and advanced age.

Transmission is by droplet nuclei produced when an infected person coughs or sneezes. People with cavitary lesions are particularly infectious because their sputum usually contains 1 to 100 million bacilli per milliliter. If an inhaled tubercle bacillus settles in an alveolus, infection occurs, with alveolocapillary dilation and endothelial cell swelling. Alveolitis results, with replication of tubercle bacilli and influx of polymorphonuclear leukocytes. These organisms spread through the lymph system to the circulatory system and then through the body.

Cell-mediated immunity to the mycobacteria, which develops 3 to 6 weeks later, usually contains the infection and arrests the disease.

THE APPEARANCE OF TUBERCULOSIS ON LUNG TISSUE

The chest X-ray of a patient with tuberculosis is likely to show nodular lesions, patchy infiltrates (mainly in upper lobes), cavity formation, scar tissue, and calcium deposits.

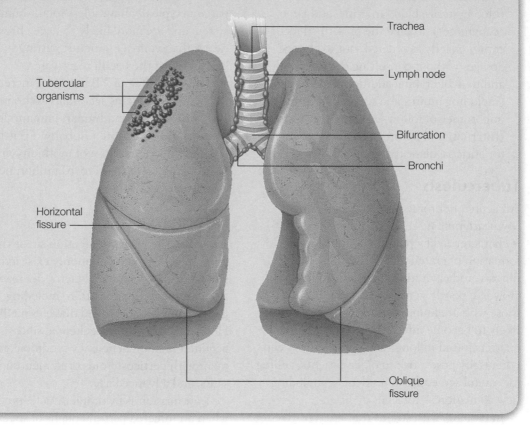

Trachea

Lymph node

Tubercular organisms

Bifurcation

Bronchi

Horizontal fissure

Oblique fissure

If the infection reactivates, the body's response characteristically leads to caseation—the conversion of necrotic tissue to a cheeselike material. The caseum may localize, undergo fibrosis, or excavate and form cavities, the walls of which are studded with multiplying tubercle bacilli. If this happens, infected caseous debris may spread throughout the lungs by the tracheobronchial tree. Sites of extrapulmonary TB include the pleurae, meninges, joints, lymph nodes, peritoneum, genitourinary tract, and bowel. However, extrapulmonary TB rarely occurs in the United States because

of our close monitoring of milk pasteurization and use of antibiotics. (See *The appearance of tuberculosis on lung tissue.*)

ASSESSMENT FINDINGS

After an incubation period of 4 to 8 weeks, TB is usually asymptomatic in primary infection but may produce nonspecific signs and symptoms, such as fatigue, weakness, anorexia, weight loss, night sweats, and low-grade fever.

Fever and night sweats, the typical hallmarks of TB, may not be present in older patients, who instead may exhibit a change in activity or weight loss. Assess older patients carefully.

In reactivation, signs and symptoms may include a cough that produces mucopurulent sputum, occasional hemoptysis, and chest pain. Assessment may include a chest X-ray, sputum collection for acid-fast bacillus (AFB) culture, and possibly lung biopsy. AFB culture results can take up to 8 weeks.

COMPLICATIONS

- Respiratory failure
- Bronchopleural fistulas
- Pneumothorax
- Hemorrhage
- Pleural effusion
- Pneumonia

TREATMENT

The four first-line agents that form the core of treatment for TB are isoniazid (INH), rifampin (RIF), ethambutol (EMB), and pyrazinamide, although rifapentine is also considered a first-line drug for TB. Latent TB is usually treated with daily INH for 9 months; a person with latent TB whose contacts are resistant to INH can receive treatment with RIF daily for 4 months.

For most adults with active TB, recommended treatment includes taking all four first-line drugs daily for 2 months, followed by 4 months of INH and RIF; specific drug therapy depends on the patient's condition and organism susceptibility. If drug therapy is interrupted, the patient may need to start therapy again from the beginning or receive additional treatment. Second-line agents—including cycloserine, ethionamide, p-Aminosalicylic acid, streptomycin, and capreomycin—are reserved for special circumstances or drug-resistant strains.

Some patients may require directly observed therapy (DOT), in which an assigned caregiver directly observes the administration of the drug. The goal of DOT is to monitor the treatment regimen and reduce the development of resistant organisms.

NURSING CONSIDERATIONS

For patients with TB, take the following steps:

- Initiate AFB isolation precautions immediately for all patients suspected or confirmed to have TB. AFB isolation precautions include a private room with negative pressure in relation to surrounding areas and a minimum of six air exchanges per hour (air should be exhausted directly outside the building).
- Continue AFB isolation until there's clinical evidence of reduced infectiousness (substantially decreased cough and fewer organisms on sequential sputum smears).
- Teach the infectious patient to cough and sneeze into tissues and to dispose of all secretions properly. Place a covered trash can nearby, or tape a lined bag to the side of the bed to dispose of used tissues.
- Instruct the patient to wear a mask when outside his room that meets current Centers for Disease Control and Prevention standards to prevent the spread of microorganisms.
- Make sure visitors and staff members wear particulate respirators that fit closely around the face when they're in the patient's room.
- Remind the patient to get plenty of rest. Stress the importance of eating balanced meals to promote recovery. If the patient is anorexic, urge him to eat small meals frequently. Record weight weekly.
- Be alert for adverse effects of medications. Because INH sometimes leads to hepatitis or peripheral neuritis, monitor aspartate aminotransferase and alanine aminotransferase levels. To prevent or treat peripheral neuritis, give pyridoxine (vitamin B_6)

as ordered. If the patient receives EMB, watch for optic neuritis; if it develops, discontinue the drug. If he receives RIF, watch for hepatitis and purpura. Observe the patient for other complications such as hemoptysis.

Teach the patient on medication the following as appropriate:

- Warn the patient who wears contact lenses that RIF can cause discoloration.
- If the patient is taking INH, monitor his skin and sclera for yellowing.
- If the patient is taking EMB, tell him to report any changes in his color vision or visual acuity immediately.
- Before discharge, advise the patient to watch for adverse effects from the medication and report them immediately. Emphasize the importance of regular follow-up examinations. Teach the patient and his family the signs and symptoms of recurring TB. Stress the need to follow long-term treatment faithfully.
- Emphasize to the patient the importance of taking the medications daily as prescribed. He may enroll in a supervised administration program to avoid the development of drug-resistant organisms.

For older patients, take the following steps:

- Help your older patient maintain good respiratory status. Watch for and report any changes in respiratory status from one visit to the next. For a hospitalized patient, watch for signs that the patient's condition is deteriorating, such as worsening shortness of breath or increased sputum production.
- If your older patient who smokes, recommend the American Cancer Society's smoking-cessation programs, which is free to the public, or a similar program. If the patient is regularly exposed to other airway irritants, explore ways to improve the situation to decrease or eliminate exposure.

Neurologic System

The neurologic system coordinates and regulates all body systems, governing every mental and physical function from birth to death. Because of this, a neurologic change can affect every body system.

With age, the number of neurons in the brain and spinal cord decreases, and the brain's overall weight drops by about 5% to 17%. Synthesis and metabolism of neurotransmitters diminish, slowing nerve impulse transmission and delaying reaction time. In addition, kinetic sensing declines, leading to impaired balance and further slowing of reaction time. The sleep cycle is altered, resulting in frequent awakenings and reduction in deep sleep and rapid eye movement sleep. Sensory organs also lose efficiency as the body ages.

Common neurologic problems among older patients include Alzheimer's disease, stroke and transient ischemic attack, aphasia, delirium, dysphagia, Parkinson's disease, and sensory deprivation.

You'll need to perform neurologic assessments frequently because older adults are prone to neurologic disorders, which can develop rather quickly. Promptly recognizing and intervening for such disorders can help older adults reach their highest level of functioning and independence. However, don't automatically assume that all neurologic changes in an older adult are age-related: first look for a pathologic explanation for the symptoms. If pathology is ruled out, plan interventions to help the patient maximize his abilities and functioning.

TYPES OF ALZHEIMER'S DISEASE

Alzheimer's disease may occur as one of two types: familial or sporadic.

Familial Alzheimer's Disease

According to the Alzheimer's Association, familial Alzheimer's disease results from a mutation in one of three genes: PS1, PS2, or APP. Individuals having one of these mutated genes have a 50% chance of passing the affected gene on to their offspring. In turn, individuals who have the mutated gene usually develop Alzheimer's disease. Scientists don't fully understand how these mutations cause the disease; however, they do know that each of these genes influences beta-amyloid production.

Sporadic Alzheimer's Disease

Sporadic Alzheimer's disease doesn't result from a mutation in one particular gene. Instead, slight gene variations may influence whether someone is more or less susceptible to the disease.

The most researched gene in sporadic Alzheimer's disease is APOE. This gene is responsible for the production of a protein that transports cholesterol and other fats throughout the body. The protein may also be involved in the structure and function of the outer wall of brain cells.

APOE has three common forms: APOE-epsilon 2, APOE-epsilon 3, and APOE-epsilon 4. An individual inherits one form of this gene from each parent. Of the three forms, APOE-epsilon 4 is the form of the gene associated with sporadic Alzheimer's disease. Studies have shown that 35% to 50% of individuals with Alzheimer's disease have at least one copy of this form of the gene. Therefore, scientists have concluded that individuals who carry at least one copy of APOE-epsilon 4 have a higher risk for developing Alzheimer's disease. Individuals who have two copies (one from each parent) have an even higher risk for developing the disease. In addition, when they develop the disease, they typically show symptoms at a younger age.

Alzheimer's disease

Alzheimer's disease (AD), also called primary degenerative dementia, is a progressive degenerative disorder of the cerebral cortex (especially the frontal lobe) that accounts for more than half of all cases of dementia. It results in memory loss (primarily short-term memory lost at first), confusion, impaired judgment, personality changes, disorientation, and loss of language skills. Because this is a primary progressive dementia, the prognosis for a patient with this disease is poor.

CAUSES AND INCIDENCE

The cause of AD is unknown; however, several factors have been implicated in the development of this disease. These include neurochemical factors, such as deficiencies in the neurotransmitter acetylcholine, somatostatin, substance P, and norepinephrine; viral factors, such as slow-growing central nervous system viruses; environmental factors, such as repeated head trauma or exposure to aluminum or manganese; and genetic immunologic factors. (See *Types of Alzheimer's disease*.)

Genetic studies show that an autosomal-dominant form of AD is associated with early onset and early death, accounting for about 100,000 deaths a year. A family history of AD and the presence of Down syndrome are two established risk factors.

AD isn't exclusive to older people; it typically starts soon after a person reaches age 60, and early-onset AD can occur as early as age 40. The number of people with AD doubles every 5 years after age 65, with at least 40% of people older than age 80 having the disease.

PATHOPHYSIOLOGY

The brain tissue of patients with AD has three hallmark features: neurofibrillary tangles, neuritic plaques, and granulovacuolar degeneration. (See *Tissue changes in Alzheimer's disease*, page 202.)

TISSUE CHANGES IN ALZHEIMER'S DISEASE

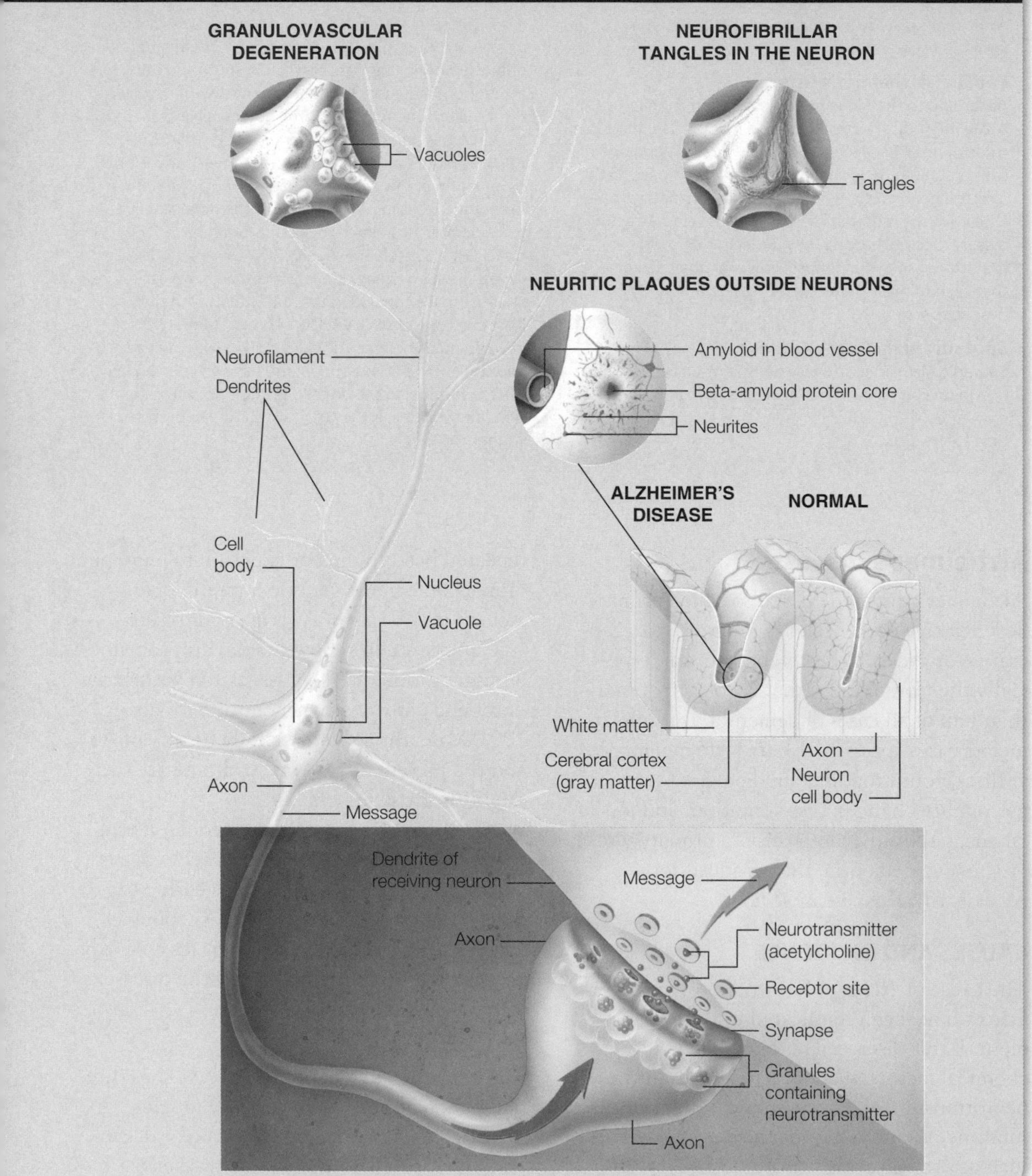

GRANULOVASCULAR DEGENERATION

Vacuoles

NEUROFIBRILLAR TANGLES IN THE NEURON

Tangles

NEURITIC PLAQUES OUTSIDE NEURONS

Amyloid in blood vessel

Beta-amyloid protein core

Neurites

Neurofilament

Dendrites

Cell body

Nucleus

Vacuole

Axon

Message

ALZHEIMER'S DISEASE

NORMAL

White matter

Cerebral cortex (gray matter)

Axon
Neuron cell body

Dendrite of receiving neuron

Message

Axon

Neurotransmitter (acetylcholine)

Receptor site

Synapse

Granules containing neurotransmitter

Axon

Additional structural changes include cortical atrophy, ventricular dilation, deposits of amyloid around the cortical blood vessels, and reduced brain volume. There's a selective loss of cholinergic neurons in the pathways to the frontal lobes and hippocampus. Postmortem examination of the brain reveals diffuse atrophy and a brain weight of less than 1,000 g compared with a normal brain weight of about 1,380 g. Functional changes don't necessarily reflect the extent of brain degeneration because patients typically compensate to a great degree for decreased brain function.

ASSESSMENT FINDINGS

Onset is insidious. Initially, the patient undergoes almost imperceptible changes, such as:

- forgetfulness
- recent memory loss
- difficulty learning and remembering new information
- deterioration in personal hygiene and appearance
- inability to concentrate
- a decrease in the ability to link multiple steps together to solve a problem (an early sign).

Gradually, tasks that require abstract thinking and activities that require judgment become more difficult. Progressive difficulty in communication and severe deterioration in memory, language, visuospatial skills, and motor function result in a loss of coordination and an inability to write or speak. Personality changes (such as restlessness and irritability) and nocturnal awakenings are common.

The patient may also exhibit:

- loss of eye contact
- a fearful look
- wringing of the hands and other signs of anxiety
- positive snout reflex.

Eventually, the patient becomes disoriented, and emotional lability and physical and intellectual disability progress. The patient becomes susceptible to malnutrition, infection, and accidents. Usually, death results from infection. (See *Stages of Alzheimer's disease*, page 204.)

COMPLICATIONS

- Injury
- Pneumonia and other infections
- Constipation
- Malnutrition
- Depression
- Dehydration

TREATMENT

Therapy attempts to slow disease progression, manage behavioral problems, modify the home environment for safety and function, and elicit family support. Underlying disorders that contribute to the patient's confusion, such as hypoxia, are also identified and treated.

Donepezil (Aricept), rivastigmine (Exelon), galantamine (Razadyne), and tacrine (Cognex) may be prescribed to slow loss of cognitive function and memory. Memantine (Namenda) combined with other AD drugs can slow the progression of symptoms of moderate to severe AD. Gabapentin (Neurontin) helps control behavioral problems. Valproic acid (Depakene) can treat mood disorders, which occur in 30% of patients with AD.

NURSING CONSIDERATIONS

- Establish an effective communication system with the patient and his family to help them adjust to the patient's altered cognitive abilities.
- Offer emotional support to the patient and family members. Explain that behavior problems may be worsened by excess

STAGES OF ALZHEIMER'S DISEASE

Alzheimer's disease progresses in three stages. The symptoms of each stage are outlined here.

STAGE	FUNCTIONS/TESTS	SYMPTOMS
Mild or early stage		
	Language	Anomia, empty speech
	Memory	Defective
	Visuospatial skills	Impaired
	Calculation	Impaired
	Personality	Indifferent, occasionally sad, irritable, or depressed
	Klüver-Bucy syndrome	Absent
	Motor system	Normal
	EEG	Normal
	Computed tomography (CT) scan/magnetic resonance imaging (MRI)	Normal
Moderate or middle stage		
	Language	Fluent aphasia
	Memory	Severely impaired
	Visuospatial skills	Severely impaired
	Personality	Indifferent or irritable; suspicious or angry
	Motor system	Restlessness, pacing
	EEG	Slowing of background rhythms
	CT scan/MRI	Atrophy
Severe or late stage		
	Intellectual function	Severely impaired
	Language	Palilalia, echolalia, or mutism
	Motor system	Limb rigidity
	Sphincter control	Incontinence
	EEG	Diffuse slowing
	CT scan/MRI	Diffuse atrophy

stimulation or changes in established routines. Teach them about the disease, and refer them to social service and community resources for legal and financial advice and support. Provide guidance to control negative behavioral manifestations. (See *The progression of Alzheimer's disease*.)

- Anxiety may cause the patient to become agitated or fearful. Intervene by helping him focus on another activity.
- Provide the patient with a safe environment. Encourage him to exercise, as ordered, to help maintain mobility.
- Monitor swallowing ability and assist with meals; assess for signs of aspiration.
- Assist with toileting habits as needed to prevent incontinence and constipation.
- Explain to the family that in the latter stages of the disease, the patient will require care for all his needs. Offer the family help with end-of-life issues as appropriate.

Parkinson's disease

Named for the English doctor who first accurately described the disease in 1817, Parkinson's disease characteristically produces progressive muscle rigidity, akinesia, involuntary tremors, and dementia. Also called parkinsonism, paralysis agitans, or shaking palsy, Parkinson's disease is one of the most common crippling diseases in the

THE PROGRESSION OF ALZHEIMER'S DISEASE

Counsel family members to expect progressive deterioration in the patient with Alzheimer's disease. To help them plan future patient care, discuss the stages of this neurodegenerative disease.

Bear in mind that family members may refuse to believe that the disease is advancing. Be sensitive to their concerns and, if necessary, review the information again when they're more receptive.

Forgetfulness

The patient becomes forgetful, especially of recent events. He frequently loses everyday objects such as keys. Aware of his loss of function, he may compensate by relinquishing tasks that might reveal his forgetfulness. Because his behavior isn't disruptive and may be attributed to stress, fatigue, or normal aging, he usually doesn't consult a physician at this stage.

Confusion

The patient has increasing difficulty with activities that require planning, decision making, and judgment, such as managing personal finances, driving a car, and performing his job. He retains skills such as personal grooming. Social withdrawal occurs when the patient feels overwhelmed by a changing environment and his inability to cope with multiple stimuli. Travel is difficult and tiring. As he becomes aware of his progressive loss of function, he may become severely depressed.

Safety becomes a concern when the patient forgets to turn off appliances or recognize unsafe situations (such as boiling water). At this point, the family may need to consider day care or a supervised residential facility.

Decline in Activities of Daily Living

The patient at this stage loses his ability to perform such daily activities as eating or washing without direct supervision. Weight loss may occur. He withdraws from the family and increasingly depends on the primary caregiver. Communication becomes difficult as his understanding of written and spoken language declines. Agitation, wandering, pacing, and nighttime awakening are linked to his inability to cope with a multisensory environment. He may mistake his mirror image for a real person (pseudohallucination). Caregivers must be constantly vigilant, which may lead to physical and emotional exhaustion. They may also become angry and feel a sense of loss.

Total Deterioration

In the final stage of Alzheimer's disease, the patient no longer recognizes himself, his body parts, or other family members. He becomes bedridden, and his activity consists of small, purposeless movements. Verbal communication stops, although he may scream spontaneously. Complications of immobility may include pressure ulcers, urinary tract infections, pneumonia, and contractures.

United States. Eventually, the progressive debilitating effects culminate in death, commonly as a result of aspiration pneumonia or some other infection.

CAUSES AND INCIDENCE

The exact cause of Parkinson's disease is unknown. Possible contributing factors include advanced age, genetics, environment (the incidence is higher in rural households that use well water and are exposed to herbicides and pesticides), and industrial chemicals (such as manganese, iron, and steel alloys).

Parkinson's disease strikes 2 in every 1,000 people, most often developing in those older than age 60. Incidence is higher in those who have suffered repeated brain injury.

PATHOPHYSIOLOGY

Parkinson's disease is a degenerative process involving the dopaminergic neurons in the substantia nigra (the area of the basal ganglia that produces and stores the neurotransmitter dopamine). This area plays an important role in the extrapyramidal system, which controls posture and coordination of voluntary motor movements.

Normally, stimulation of the basal ganglia results in refined motor movement because acetylcholine (excitatory) and dopamine (inhibitory) release is balanced. Degeneration of the dopaminergic neurons and loss of available dopamine lead to an excess of excitatory acetylcholine at the synapse and consequent rigidity, tremors, and bradykinesia. Other nondopaminergic neurons may be affected, possibly contributing to depression and other nonmotor symptoms. Also, the basal ganglia are interconnected to the hypothalamus, potentially affecting autonomic and endocrine function as well.

Current research on the pathogenesis of Parkinson's disease focuses on damage to the substantia nigra from oxidative stress. Oxidative stress is believed to diminish brain iron content, impair mitochondrial function, inhibit antioxidant and protective systems, reduce glutathione secretion, and damage lipids, proteins, and deoxyribonucleic acid. Brain cells are less capable of repairing oxidative damage than are other tissues. (See *Neurotransmitter action in Parkinson's disease.*)

ASSESSMENT FINDINGS

The six cardinal signs of Parkinson's disease are:

- tremor
- slowed motion (bradykinesia)
- rigid muscles
- impaired posture and balance
- loss of automatic movements
- speech changes.

Dementia can occur in the later stages of the disease, and some people develop problems with memory and mental clarity.

Other findings include:

- oculogyric crisis (eyes fixed upward with involuntary tonic movements, or closed as in blepharospasm; usually accompanied by a delay in initiating movement to perform a purposeful action)
- dysphagia
- muscle cramps of the legs, neck, and trunk
- increased perspiration
- insomnia

- dysarthria and speaking in a high-pitched monotone
- drooling
- masklike facial expression
- difficulty walking (gait lacks normal parallel motion; may be retropulsive or propulsive)
- cognitive changes (dementia)
- depression and emotional changes
- urinary problems and constipation.

Parkinson's disease itself doesn't impair the intellect, but a coexisting disorder, such as arteriosclerosis, may do so.

COMPLICATIONS

- Injury from falls
- Aspiration
- Urinary tract infections
- Complications of immobility
- Depression
- Skin breakdown

TREATMENT

Because Parkinson's disease has no cure, the primary aim of treatment is to relieve signs and symptoms and keep the patient functional as long as possible. Treatment generally consists of medications to control signs and symptoms, physical therapy and, when drug treatments fail, surgery.

Several drug and drug combinations may be prescribed:

- Levodopa-carbidopa (Sinemet) halts peripheral dopamine synthesis.
- Entacapone (Comtan) or tolcapone (Tasmar) potentiate the effects of levodopa-carbidopa so that the patient needs less-frequent doses.
- The combination therapy of levodopa-carbidopa-entacapone (Stalevo) may be given to patients with no dyskinesia who experience end-of-dose "wearing off" when taking a total daily levodopa dose of

NEUROTRANSMITTER ACTION IN PARKINSON'S DISEASE

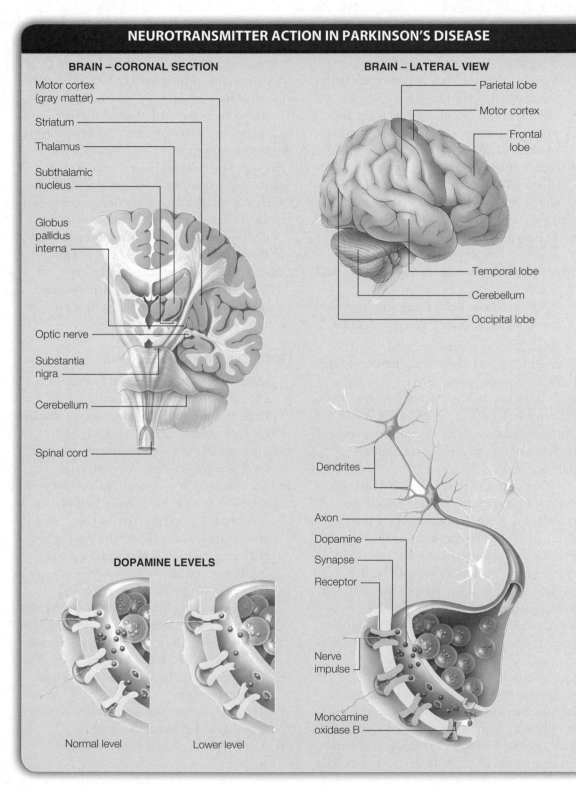

BRAIN – CORONAL SECTION

Motor cortex (gray matter)

Striatum

Thalamus

Subthalamic nucleus

Globus pallidus interna

Optic nerve

Substantia nigra

Cerebellum

Spinal cord

BRAIN – LATERAL VIEW

Parietal lobe

Motor cortex

Frontal lobe

Temporal lobe

Cerebellum

Occipital lobe

DOPAMINE LEVELS

Normal level   Lower level

Dendrites

Axon

Dopamine

Synapse

Receptor

Nerve impulse

Monoamine oxidase B

600 mg or less, replacing individual doses or immediate-release levodopa.

- Selegiline (Atapryl) or rasagiline (Azilect) conserve dopamine and enhance the therapeutic effect of levodopa.
- Selegiline and tocopherols delay the time when the patient with Parkinson's disease becomes disabled.
- Apomorphine (Apokyn), ropinirole (Requip), and bromocriptine (Parlodel) reduce the development of motor fluctuations and dyskinesias.
- Trihexyphenidyl (Artane), diphenhydramine (Benadryl), and amantadine (Symmetrel) decrease tremors, rigidity, and akinesia.
- Antidepressants help relieve the depression that commonly occurs with this disorder.

When drug treatment fails, stereotactic neurosurgery, including subthalamotomy and pallidotomy, may provide relief from signs and symptoms. In these procedures, electrical coagulation, freezing, radioactivity, or ultrasound destroys the ventrolateral nucleus of the thalamus to prevent involuntary movement.

Other surgical interventions include brain stimulator implantation, which alters the activity of the area in the brain where Parkinson's disease symptoms originate, and pacemaker implantation. In this procedure, the surgeon implants a pacemaker into the patient's chest wall and threads the electrode (using magnetic resonance imaging for guidance) to the thalamus, pallidum, or subthalamic nucleus. A successful procedure reduces the need for medication, which reduces medication-related adverse effects.

Neurotransplantation techniques, including the use of nerve cells from other parts of the patient's body, have also been attempted, with varying results. In a controversial surgical treatment called fetal cell transplantation, the physician injects fetal brain tissue into the patient's brain. If the injected cells grow within the brain, they allow the brain to process dopamine, which halts or reverses disease progression.

Individually planned physical therapy complements drug treatment and neurosurgery to maintain normal muscle tone and function. Appropriate physical therapy includes both active and passive range-of-motion (ROM) exercises, routine daily activities, walking, and baths and massage to help relax muscles.

Older adult patients may need smaller doses of antiparkinsonian drugs because of reduced tolerance. In these patients, watch carefully for and report orthostatic hypotension, irregular pulse, blepharospasm, and anxiety or confusion.

NURSING CONSIDERATIONS

- Monitor drug treatment and evaluate for effectiveness or adverse effects.
- If the patient has undergone surgery, watch for signs of hemorrhage and increased intracranial pressure by frequently checking level of consciousness and vital signs.
- Encourage independence. The patient with excessive tremor may achieve partial control of his body by sitting on a chair and using its arms to steady himself. Advise the patient to change position slowly and dangle his legs before getting out of bed.
- Encourage active ROM exercises and participation in physical therapy. Assist with exercises to maintain muscle tone and joint mobility, decrease spasticity, improve coordination, and boost morale.
- Help establish a daily routine to maintain optimal function.
- Help the patient overcome problems related to eating and elimination.
- Assist with meals and assess for signs of aspiration.

- Help establish a regular bowel routine by encouraging the patient to drink at least 2 qt (about 2 L) of liquids daily and to eat high-fiber foods. Provide an elevated toilet seat to help the patient maneuver from a standing to sitting position. Evaluate the need for bowel and bladder training.
- Show the family how to prevent pressure ulcers and contractures with proper positioning and passive ROM exercises.
- Inform the family of the dietary restrictions levodopa imposes, and explain household safety measures to prevent accidents.
- Provide emotional support. Teach the patient and family members about the disease, its progressive stages, and drug adverse effects. Help them to express their feelings and frustrations about the progressively debilitating effects of the disease.
- Establish long- and short-term treatment goals, and be aware of the patient's need for intellectual stimulation and diversion.
- Refer the patient and his family to the National Parkinson Foundation or the United Parkinson Foundation for more information.

Seizures

Seizure disorder, or epilepsy, has always been considered a disorder of early childhood that can last into adulthood. However, seizure disorder can affect anyone at any age, and statistics show that it's as likely to begin after age 60 as it is during the first decade of life. Because seizures in older adults can also be a signs of other disorders, such as head trauma and brain tumor, the diagnosis of seizure disorder is often missed.

Nonepileptic seizures (NES) are involuntary episodes of movement, sensation, or behaviors that don't result from abnormal cortical discharges.

CAUSES AND INCIDENCE

In older adults, the cause of seizures is usually unknown, although they may be associated with stroke, neurodegenerative diseases such as Alzheimer's disease, trauma, tumors, alcohol withdrawal, infection, or metabolic disorders such as uremia, hyperglycemia, hypoglycemia, and hyponatremia. Risk factors include dementia, depression, trauma, and alcohol abuse.

NES seizures may be related to syncopal episodes, complicated migraines, panic attacks, or transient ischemic attacks. They can also a physical manifestation of psychological distress.

PATHOPHYSIOLOGY

Some neurons in the brain may depolarize easily or be hyperexcitable; this epileptogenic focus fires more readily than normal when stimulated. In these neurons, the membrane potential at rest is less negative, or inhibitory connections are missing, possibly because of decreased gamma-aminobutyric acid activity or localized shifts in electrolytes.

On stimulation, the epileptogenic focus fires and spreads electrical current toward the synapse and surrounding cells. These cells fire in turn, and the impulse cascades to one side of the brain (a partial seizure), both sides of the brain (a generalized seizure), or the cortical, subcortical, or brain stem area.

The brain's metabolic demand for oxygen increases dramatically during a seizure. If this demand isn't met, hypoxia and brain damage ensue. Firing of inhibitory neurons causes the excitatory neurons to slow their firing and eventually stop.

If this inhibitory action doesn't occur, the result is status epilepticus: one prolonged seizure, or one seizure occurring right after another and another. Without treatment, this may be fatal.

ASSESSMENT FINDINGS

Depending on the type and cause of the seizure, signs and symptoms vary. (See *Differentiating seizures.*) The assessment may yield normal physical findings if the patient isn't having a seizure at the time and the cause is idiopathic. If the seizure is associated with an underlying problem, the patient's history and the physical examination should reveal signs and symptoms of that problem— unless the seizure resulted from a brain tumor, which sometimes produces no other symptoms.

In many cases, the patient's history reveals that seizure occurrence is unpredictable and unrelated to activities. Occasionally, a patient may report precipitating factors or events—for example, that the seizures always take place at a particular time, such as during sleep, or after a particular circumstance, such as lack of sleep or emotional stress. The patient may also report nonspecific changes, such as headache, mood changes, lethargy, and myoclonic jerking, occurring up to several hours before the onset of a seizure.

Patients who experience a generalized seizure may describe an aura, which represents the beginning of abnormal electrical discharges within a focal area of the brain. Typical auras may include a pungent smell, GI distress (nausea or indigestion), a rising or sinking feeling in the stomach, a dreamy feeling, an unusual taste, or a visual disturbance such as a flashing light that precedes seizure onset by a few seconds or minutes.

The patient may describe the effect the seizures have on his lifestyle, activities of daily living, and coping mechanisms. He may also have a history of status epilepticus. (See *Understanding status epilepticus*, page 212.)

If you observe the patient during a seizure, be sure to note the type of seizure he's experiencing. Otherwise, details of what occurs during a seizure—obtained from a family member or friend, if necessary—may help to identify the seizure type.

In an older adult with NES, signs include an altered mental state, staring, blackouts, and confusion. An older adult may also have a simple partial seizure, with only numbness in a hand or a leg. After a 1-minute seizure, it's not unusual for an older patient to be in a prolonged state of confusion, be prone to falls, or experience temporary paralysis that can last for days or even weeks.

COMPLICATIONS

- Anoxia
- Traumatic brain injury
- Fractures from falls
- Death from status epilepticus

TREATMENT

Typically, treatment for epilepsy consists of drug therapy specific to the type of seizure. The most commonly prescribed drugs include phenytoin, carbamazepine, phenobarbital, valproic acid, and primidone administered individually for generalized tonic-clonic seizures and complex partial seizures. Valproic acid, clonazepam, and ethosuximide are commonly prescribed for absence (petit mal) seizures. Lamotrigine is also prescribed as adjunct therapy for partial seizures. Fosphenytoin is a new I.V. preparation that effectively treats status epilepticus.

If drug therapy fails, treatment may include surgical removal of a demonstrated focal lesion to attempt to bring an end to seizures. Surgery is also performed when seizures result from an underlying problem, such as an intracranial tumor, a brain abscess or cyst, or vascular abnormalities.

DIFFERENTIATING SEIZURES

Seizures are classified into two major categories—partial and generalized—depending on the area of the brain affected by the abnormal electrical activity. Each type can be further classified based on the clinical manifestations described here.

Partial Seizures

Partial seizures arise from a localized area in the brain and cause specific symptoms. In some patients, partial seizure activity spreads to the entire brain, causing a generalized seizure. Partial seizures include simple partial (Jacksonian motor-type and sensory-type), complex partial (psychomotor or temporal lobe), and secondarily generalized partial seizures.

Simple partial (Jacksonian motor-type) seizure
This type of seizure begins as a localized motor seizure, which is characterized by a spread of abnormal activity to adjacent areas of the brain. Typically, the patient experiences a stiffening or jerking in one extremity, accompanied by a tingling sensation in the same area. For example, the seizure may start in the thumb and spread to the entire hand and arm. The patient seldom loses consciousness, although the seizure may secondarily progress to a generalized tonic-clonic seizure.

Simple partial (sensory-type) seizure
Perception is distorted in a simple partial (sensory-type) seizure. Symptoms can include hallucinations, flashing lights, tingling sensations, sensing a foul odor, vertigo, or déjà vu.

Complex partial seizure
Symptoms of complex partial seizure vary but usually include purposeless behavior. The patient may experience an aura and exhibit overt signs, including a glassy stare, picking at his clothes, aimless wandering, lip-smacking or chewing motions, and unintelligible speech. A seizure may last for a few seconds or as long as 20 minutes. Afterward, mental confusion may last for several minutes; as a result, an observer may mistakenly suspect psychosis or intoxication with alcohol or drugs. The patient has no memory of his actions during the seizure.

Secondarily generalized partial seizure
This type of seizure can be either simple or complex and can progress to generalized seizures. An aura may precede the progression. Loss of consciousness occurs immediately or within 1 or 2 minutes of the start of the progression.

Generalized Seizures

As the term suggests, these seizures cause a generalized electrical abnormality in the brain. They include several distinct types.

Absence (Petit mal) seizure
An absence seizure occurs most often in children but may also affect adults. It usually begins with a brief change in level of consciousness, indicated by blinking or rolling of the eyes, a blank stare, and slight mouth movements. The patient retains his posture and continues preseizure activity without difficulty. Typically, a seizure lasts from 1 to 10 seconds. The impairment is so brief that the patient is sometimes unaware of it. If not properly treated, these seizures can recur as often as 100 times a day. An absence seizure can progress to a generalized tonic-clonic seizure.

Myoclonic seizure
Also called *bilateral massive epileptic myoclonus,* a myoclonic seizure is marked by brief, involuntary muscular jerks of the body or extremities, which may occur in a rhythmic manner, and a brief loss of consciousness.

Generalized tonic-clonic (Grand mal) seizure
Typically, this seizure begins with a loud cry, precipitated by air rushing from the lungs through the vocal cords. The patient falls to the ground, losing consciousness. The body stiffens (tonic phase) and then alternates between episodes of muscle spasm and relaxation (clonic phase). Tongue biting, incontinence, labored breathing, apnea, and subsequent cyanosis may also occur. The seizure stops in 2 to 5 minutes, when abnormal electrical conduction of the neurons is completed. The patient then regains consciousness but is somewhat confused and may have difficulty talking. If he can talk, he may complain of drowsiness, fatigue, headache, muscle soreness, and arm or leg weakness. He may fall into a deep sleep after the seizure.

Akinetic seizure
An akinetic seizure is characterized by a general loss of postural tone and a temporary loss of consciousness. This type of seizure occurs in young children. Sometimes it's called a *drop attack* because it causes the child to fall.

UNDERSTANDING STATUS EPILEPTICUS

Status epilepticus—which can occur in all seizure types—is a potentially life-threatening condition in which the patient has an abnormally prolonged seizure (lasting longer than 5 minutes) or doesn't fully regain consciousness between seizures. The most life-threatening form is generalized tonic-clonic status epilepticus, a continuous generalized tonic-clonic seizure without an intervening return of consciousness.

Status epilepticus, always an emergency, is accompanied by respiratory distress. It can result from abrupt withdrawal of anticonvulsant medications, hypoxic or metabolic encephalopathy, acute head trauma, or septicemia secondary to encephalitis or meningitis.

Emergency treatment for status epilepticus usually consists of diazepam, phenytoin, or Phenobarbital; dextrose 50% I.V. (when seizures are secondary to hypoglycemia), and thiamine I.V. (in the presence of chronic alcoholism or withdrawal).

NURSING CONSIDERATIONS

Take the following steps for patients experiencing seizures:

- Provide emotional support. Encourage the patient and family to express their fears and concerns. Suggest counseling to help them cope.
- If the patient is taking anticonvulsants, constantly monitor him for signs and symptoms of toxicity, such as slurred speech, ataxia, lethargy, dizziness, drowsiness, nystagmus, irritability, nausea, and vomiting.

 Many older patients take several drugs, increasing the risk of toxicity and drug interactions. Check the patient's medication history, and note any drugs that can cause the signs and symptoms of anticonvulsant toxicity.

- When administering phenytoin I.V., use a large vein, administer at a slow rate (not to exceed 50 mg/minute), and monitor the patient frequently.

- Provide adequate patient support by developing an understanding of epilepsy and the myths and misconceptions that surround it. Answer any questions the patient and family members have about the condition. Help them to cope by dispelling myths. For example, assure them that epilepsy isn't contagious and is controllable for most patients who follow a prescribed regimen of medication. Provide assurance that most patients maintain a normal lifestyle.
- Explain to the patient and family the need to follow the prescribed drug schedule. Assure the patient that anticonvulsant drugs are safe when taken as ordered. Reinforce dosage instructions, and find methods to help the patient remember to take medications. Stress the importance of taking the medication regularly at the scheduled time. Caution the patient to monitor the amount of medication he has left so that he doesn't run out.

R_x Medication Alert Caution the patient not to add any new medications—including supplements—without consulting his health care provider first for possible drug interactions.

- Teach the patient about possible adverse effects, including drowsiness, lethargy, hyperactivity, confusion, and visual and sleep disturbances. All of these may indicate the need for dosage adjustment.
- Explain that phenytoin may lead to hyperplasia of the gums, which may be relieved by conscientious oral hygiene. Instruct the patient to report adverse reactions immediately.
- Explain the importance of having anticonvulsant blood levels and liver enzymes checked at regular intervals even if the seizures are under control.
- Instruct the patient to eat regular meals and to check with his physician before dieting.

Explain that maintaining adequate glucose levels provides the necessary energy for central nervous system neurons to work normally.

- If your patient drives, refer him to his state's motor vehicle department for information about driver's licenses. In most states, he'll need to be free from seizures for a specified period of time before he can have his driver's license back.
- Know which social agencies in your community can help epileptic patients. Refer the patient to the Epilepsy Foundation for general information.

If the patient will undergo surgery, take the following steps.

- Prepare the patient for surgery.
- Provide preoperative and postoperative care appropriate for the type of surgery the patient will undergo.
- Provide appropriate preoperative teaching. Explain the care that the patient can expect postoperatively.

Teach the patient's family how to care for the patient during a seizure. This is especially important if the patient experiences generalized tonic-clonic seizures, which may necessitate first aid. Instruct family members to do the following:

- Avoid restraining the patient during a seizure.
- Help the patient to a side-lying position, loosen any tight clothing, and place something flat and soft, such as a pillow, jacket, or hand, under his head.
- Clear the area of hard objects.
- Avoid forcing anything into the patient's mouth if his teeth are clenched—a tongue blade or spoon could lacerate his mouth and lips or displace teeth, precipitating respiratory distress.
- If necessary, turn his head to the side to maintain an open airway.

- Reassure the patient after the seizure subsides by telling him that he's all right. Orient him to time and place, and explain that he's had a seizure.

Stroke

A stroke, also called a brain attack, is a sudden impairment of cerebral circulation in one or more of the blood vessels supplying the brain. A stroke interrupts or diminishes oxygen supply and commonly causes serious damage or necrosis in brain tissues. The sooner circulation returns to normal after a stroke, the better chances are for complete recovery. However, about half of those who survive a stroke remain permanently disabled and experience a recurrence within weeks, months, or years.

Strokes are broadly classified as ischemic or hemorrhagic, depending on the cause of impaired circulation. (See *Types of stroke*, page 214.)

CAUSES AND INCIDENCE

A stroke results from obstruction of a blood vessel, typically in extracerebral vessels but occasionally in intracerebral vessels. Factors that increase the risk of stroke include a history of transient ischemic attacks (TIAs), atherosclerosis, hypertension, kidney disease, arrhythmias (specifically atrial fibrillation), electrocardiogram changes, rheumatic heart disease, diabetes mellitus, postural hypotension, cardiac or myocardial enlargement, high serum triglyceride levels, lack of exercise, cigarette smoking, and family history of stroke.

The major causes of stroke are thrombosis, embolism, and hemorrhage. Thrombosis is the most common cause in middle-aged and older adults, who have a higher incidence of atherosclerosis, diabetes, and hypertension. Thrombosis causes ischemia in brain tissue supplied

TYPES OF STROKE

Strokes are typically classified as ischemic or hemorrhagic, depending on the underlying cause. This chart describes the major types of stroke.

TYPE OF STROKE	DESCRIPTION
ISCHEMIC	
Thrombotic	• Most common type of stroke
	• Commonly the result of atherosclerosis; also associated with hypertension, smoking, or diabetes (disease process similar to myocardial infarction [MI])
	• Thrombus in extracranial or intracranial vessel blocks blood flow to the cerebral cortex
	• Carotid artery most commonly affected extracranial vessel
	• Common intracranial sites include bifurcation of carotid arteries, distal intracranial portion of vertebral arteries, and proximal basilar arteries
	• May occur during sleep or shortly after awakening, during surgery, or after an MI
Embolic	• Second most common type of stroke
	• Embolus from heart or extracranial arteries floats into cerebral bloodstream and lodges in middle cerebral artery or branches
	• Embolus commonly originates during atrial fibrillation
	• Typically occurs during activity
	• Develops rapidly
Lacunar	• Subtype of thrombotic stroke
	• Hypertension creates cavities deep in white matter of the brain, affecting the internal capsule, basal ganglia, thalamus, and pons
	• Lipid coating lining of the small penetrating arteries thickens and weakens wall, causing microaneurysms and dissections
HEMORRHAGIC	
	• Third most common type of stroke
	• Typically caused by hypertension or aneurysm rupture
	• Blood supply to area from the ruptured artery diminished and surrounding tissue compressed by accumulated blood

by the affected vessel as well as congestion and edema; the latter may produce more clinical effects than thrombosis itself, but these symptoms subside with the edema. Thrombosis may develop while the patient sleeps or shortly after he awakens; it can also occur during surgery or after a myocardial infarction. The risk increases with obesity and with smoking. (See *Ischemic stroke.*)

Overall, more men suffer from stroke than women; however, more women die from stroke. African-American men have a higher incidence and death rate than African-American women. Although stroke may occur at any age, 75% of strokes occur in patients over age 64.

PATHOPHYSIOLOGY

Regardless of the cause, the underlying event is deprivation of oxygen and nutrients. Normally, if the arteries become blocked, autoregulatory mechanisms help maintain cerebral circulation until collateral circulation develops to deliver blood to the affected area. If the compensatory mechanisms become overworked, or if cerebral blood flow remains impaired for more than a few minutes, oxygen deprivation leads to infarction of brain tissue.

A thrombotic or embolic stroke causes ischemia. Some of the neurons served by the occluded vessel die from lack of oxygen and nutrients, resulting in cerebral infarction.

ISCHEMIC STROKE

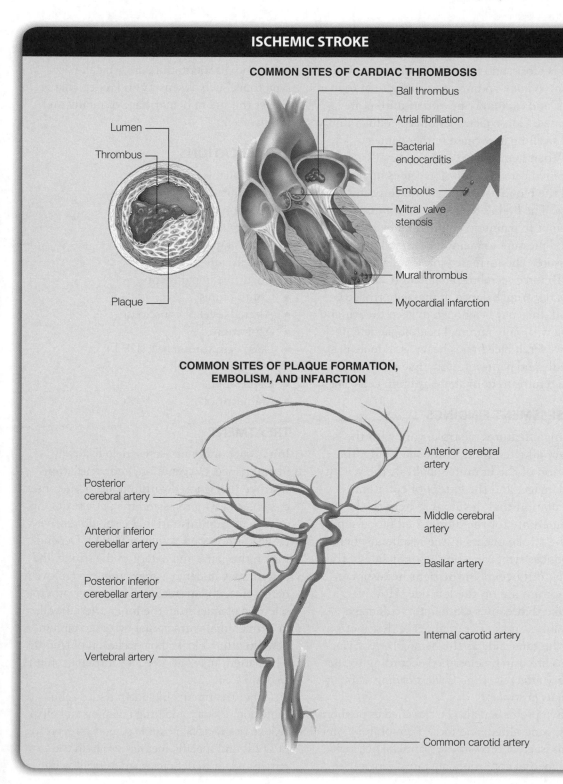

COMMON SITES OF CARDIAC THROMBOSIS

Lumen

Thrombus

Plaque

Ball thrombus

Atrial fibrillation

Bacterial endocarditis

Embolus

Mitral valve stenosis

Mural thrombus

Myocardial infarction

COMMON SITES OF PLAQUE FORMATION, EMBOLISM, AND INFARCTION

Posterior cerebral artery

Anterior inferior cerebellar artery

Posterior inferior cerebellar artery

Vertebral artery

Anterior cerebral artery

Middle cerebral artery

Basilar artery

Internal carotid artery

Common carotid artery

Injury to surrounding cells disrupts metabolism and leads to changes in ionic transport, localized acidosis, and free radical formation. Calcium, sodium, and water accumulate in injured cells, and excitatory neurotransmitters are released. Consequent continued cellular injury and swelling may cause further damage.

When hemorrhage is the cause of stroke, impaired cerebral perfusion causes infarction, and the blood itself acts as a space-occupying mass. The brain's regulatory mechanisms attempt to maintain equilibrium by increasing blood pressure to maintain cerebral perfusion pressure. The increased intracranial pressure (ICP) forces cerebrospinal fluid (CSF) out, thus restoring balance. If the hemorrhage is small, this may be enough to keep the patient alive with only minimal neurologic deficits. However, if bleeding is heavy, ICP increases rapidly and perfusion stops. Even if the pressure returns to normal, many brain cells die.

ASSESSMENT FINDINGS

Clinical features of stroke vary with the artery affected (and, consequentially, the portion of the brain it supplies), the severity of damage, and the extent of collateral circulation that develops to help the brain compensate for the diminished blood supply. If the stroke occurs in the left hemisphere, it produces symptoms on the right side of the body; if it occurs in the right hemisphere, symptoms are on the left side. However, a stroke that causes cranial nerve damage produces signs of cranial nerve dysfunction on the same side as the hemorrhage. Symptoms are usually classified according to the artery affected. (See *Understanding neurologic deficits in stroke.*)

Symptoms can also be classified as premonitory, generalized, and focal. Premonitory symptoms, such as drowsiness, dizziness, headache, and mental confusion, are rare. Generalized

symptoms, such as headache, vomiting, mental impairment, seizures, coma, nuchal rigidity, fever, and disorientation, are typical. Focal symptoms, such as sensory and reflex changes, reflect the site of hemorrhage or infarct and may worsen.

COMPLICATIONS

- Unstable blood pressure
- Fluid imbalances
- Infection
- Sensory impairment
- Motor impairment
- Speech impairment
- Cognitive impairment
- Contractures
- Altered level of consciousness
- Aspiration
- Deep vein thrombosis (DVT)
- Pulmonary emboli
- Depression
- Malnutrition

TREATMENT

Initial supportive measures include airway maintenance, oxygenation, and ventilation. If stroke is diagnosed within hours of the onset of signs and symptoms and the patient fits the criteria for administration, he should receive tissue plasminogen activator (TPA). Depending on the cause and extent of the stroke, the patient may undergo a craniotomy to remove a hematoma, endarterectomy to remove atherosclerotic plaques from the inner arterial wall, or extracranial-intracranial bypass to circumvent an artery blocked by occlusion or stenosis. The patient may also need a ventricular shunt to drain CSF.

Other treatments include physical rehabilitation, dietary and drug regimens to help reduce risk factors, possible surgery, prevention of DVT, and specific measures to help the patient adapt to deficits, such as swallowing

UNDERSTANDING NEUROLOGIC DEFICITS IN STROKE

This chart shows the common neurologic signs and symptoms that occur with a stroke.

ARTERY AFFECTED	SIGNS AND SYMPTOMS
Middle cerebral artery	• Aphasia, • Dysphasia • Visual field cuts • Hemiparesis on affected side (more severe in the face and arm than in the leg)
Carotid artery	• Weakness • Paralysis • Numbness • Sensory changes • Amaurosis fugax on affected side • Altered level of consciousness • Bruits • Headaches • Aphasia • Ptosis
Vertebrobasilar artery	• Weakness on affected side • Numbness around lips and mouth • Visual field cuts • Diplopia • Poor coordination • Dysphasia • Slurred speech • Dizziness • Amnesia • Ataxia
Anterior cerebral artery	• Confusion • Weakness and numbness (especially in the leg) on affected side • Incontinence • Loss of coordination • Impaired motor and sensory functions • Personality changes
Posterior cerebral arteries	• Visual field deficits • Sensory impairment • Dyslexia • Coma • Cortical blindness • Absence of paralysis

difficulties, speech impairment, and paralysis. The patient may also need counseling and drug therapy for depression.

Commonly prescribed medications include alteplase (Activase), a TPA that dissolves clots when administered within 3 hours of the onset of symptoms; heparin and warfarin (Coumadin) to provide anticoagulation, especially for patients with atrial fibrillation or other high-risk cardiac conditions; aspirin or clopidogrel (Plavix) for the antiplatelet effect to help prevent atherosclerotic strokes and TIAs; phenytoin (Dilantin) or fosphenytoin (Cerebyx) to treat or prevent seizures; docusate (Colace) to soften stool and prevent straining, which increases ICP; dexamethasone (Decadron) to minimize associated cerebral edema; and acetaminophen (Tylenol) to relieve headache, which typically follows hemorrhagic stroke.

NURSING CONSIDERATIONS

During a stroke, take the following steps:

- Maintain a patent airway and oxygenation. Watch for increasing respiratory distress or decreasing respiratory effort. Look for ballooning of the cheek with respirations; the side that balloons is the side affected by the stroke.
- If the patient is unconscious, place him in a lateral position to allow secretions to drain naturally or suction the secretions, as needed. Insert an artificial airway and start mechanical ventilation or supplemental oxygen, if necessary.
- Check vital signs and neurologic status, record observations, and report any significant changes to the physician. Monitor blood pressure, LOC, pupillary changes, motor function (voluntary and involuntary movements), sensory function, speech, skin color, temperature, signs of increased ICP, and nuchal rigidity or flaccidity. Remember, if stroke is impending, the patient's blood pressure will rise suddenly; he'll have a rapid, bounding pulse; and he may complain of a headache.

After a stroke, take the following steps:

- Apply compression sleeves to the lower extremities to help prevent DVT formation. Watch for signs of pulmonary emboli, such as chest pain, shortness of breath, dusky color, tachycardia, fever, and changed sensorium. If the patient is unresponsive, monitor his blood gas levels often; report increased partial pressure of carbon dioxide and decreased partial pressure of oxygen.

- Maintain fluid and electrolyte balance. If the patient can take liquids orally, offer them as often as fluid limitations permit. Administer I.V. fluids as ordered; never give too much, too fast because this can increase ICP. Offer the urinal or bedpan every 2 hours. If the patient is incontinent, he may need an indwelling urinary catheter, but avoid this if possible because of the risk of infection.

- Ensure adequate nutrition. Check for the gag reflex before offering small oral feedings of semisolid foods. Place the food tray within the patient's visual field because loss of peripheral vision is common. If oral feedings aren't possible, insert a nasogastric tube.

- Manage GI problems. Watch for signs that the patient is straining during elimination because this increases ICP. Modify his diet, administer stool softeners as indicated, and give laxatives if necessary. If the patient vomits (usually during the first few days), keep him positioned on his side to prevent aspiration.

- Provide careful mouth care. Clean and irrigate the patient's mouth to remove food particles. Care for his dentures as needed.

- Provide meticulous eye care. Remove secretions with a cotton ball and sterile normal saline solution. Instill eyedrops as ordered. Patch the patient's affected eye if he can't close the lid.

- Position the patient and align his extremities correctly. Use high-topped sneakers to prevent footdrop and contracture; a convoluted foam, flotation, or pulsating mattress or sheepskin can help prevent pressure ulcers. To prevent pneumonia, turn the patient at least every 2 hours. Elevate the affected hand to control dependent edema, and place it in a functional position.

- Assist the patient with exercise. Perform range-of-motion exercises for both the affected and unaffected sides. Teach and encourage the patient to use his unaffected side to exercise his affected side.
- Give medications as ordered, and watch for and report adverse effects.
- Establish and maintain communication with the patient. If he is aphasic, set up a simple method of communicating basic needs. Then, remember to phrase your questions so he'll be able to answer using this system. Repeat yourself quietly and calmly, and use gestures if necessary to help him understand. Even an unresponsive patient may be able to hear, so don't say anything in his presence that you wouldn't want him to hear and remember.
- Provide psychological support. Set realistic short-term goals. Involve the patient's family in his care when possible, and explain his deficits and strengths.
- If the patient has a visual field deficit, make sure caregivers and family members approach the patient from his visually intact side.
- Begin the patient's rehabilitation at the time of admission. The amount of teaching you'll have to do depends on the extent of neurologic deficit. To reinforce teaching, involve the patient's family in all aspects of rehabilitation. With their cooperation and support, devise a realistic discharge plan, and let them help decide when the patient can return home.
- If necessary, teach the patient to comb his hair, dress, and wash. With the aid of a physical therapist and an occupational therapist, obtain appliances (such as walking frames, hand bars by the toilet, and ramps) as needed. The patient may fail to recognize that he has a paralyzed side (called unilateral neglect) and must be taught to inspect that side of his body for injury and to protect it from harm.
- If speech therapy is indicated, encourage the patient to begin as soon as possible and to follow through with the speech pathologist's suggestions.
- Before discharge, warn the patient and his family to report any premonitory signs of a stroke, such as severe headache, drowsiness, confusion, and dizziness. Emphasize the importance of regular follow-up visits.
- If aspirin has been prescribed to minimize the risk of embolic stroke, tell the patient to watch for possible GI bleeding. Make sure the patient and his family realize that acetaminophen isn't a substitute for aspirin

Transient ischemic attacks

Transient ischemic attacks (TIAs) are sudden, brief episodes of neurologic deficit caused by focal cerebral ischemia. They usually last 5 to 20 minutes and are followed by rapid clearing of neurologic deficits (typically within 24 hours). Often called a mini-stroke, a TIA can signal an impending stroke.

CAUSES AND INCIDENCE

Causes of a TIA can include narrowing of a blood vessel, a blood clot that develops within an artery of the brain, a blood clot that travels to the brain from somewhere else in the body (for example, the heart), injury to blood vessels, and hypertension. If the patient has atherosclerosis—a condition in which fatty deposits occur on the inner lining of the arteries—he has a dramatically increased risk for both TIAs and stroke.

Less common causes of TIAs include blood disorders (including polycythemia, sickle cell anemia, and hyperviscosity syndromes), spasm of the small arteries in the brain, and problems with blood vessels caused by disorders such as fibromuscular dysplasia, inflammation of the arteries (arteritis, polyarteritis, and granulomatous angiitis), systemic lupus erythematosus, and syphilis.

About one in three people who have a TIA eventually have a stroke, and about 50% occur within a year after the transient ischemic attack.

PATHOPHYSIOLOGY

When TIA occurs, it's believed that microemboli released from a thrombus temporarily interrupt blood flow, especially in the small distal branches of the arterial tree in the brain. Small spasms in those arterioles may impair blood flow; these spasms may also precede a TIA. Predisposing factors for TIAs are the same as for thrombotic stroke.

The most distinctive characteristic of a TIA is the transient duration of neurologic deficits. The patient may appear to return to full function but may actually have developed small, difficult-to-detect deficits, which can lead to vascular dementia.

Signs and symptoms of a TIA correlate with the location of the affected artery. These include double vision, speech deficits (slurring or thickness), unilateral blindness, staggering or uncoordinated gait, unilateral weakness or numbness, falling because of weakness in the legs, and dizziness.

ASSESSMENT FINDINGS

The signs and symptoms of a TIA or stroke are the same and depend on the area of the brain that is affected. While stoke symptoms are permanent, symptoms of a TIA are transient and my resolve in their own. Signs and symptoms may include:

- dizziness
- loss of speech
- difficulty following commands
- confusion

- difficulty saying words
- loss of balance and coordination
- difficulty walking
- loss of vision in one eye (amaurosis fugax)

COMPLICATIONS

- Injuries due to falls
- Seizures
- Stroke

TREATMENT

During an active TIA, treatment aims to prevent a completed stroke and consists of aspirin or anticoagulants to minimize the risk of thrombosis. After or between attacks, preventive treatment includes carotid endarterectomy or cerebral microvascular bypass.

Underlying disorders should be treated appropriately, including such disorders as hypertension, heart disease, diabetes, arteritis, and blood disorders.

Treatment of symptoms of blood disorders may include phlebotomy and hydration; the underlying blood disorder should also be treated. Antihypertensive medications may be used to control high blood pressure. Medications to lower cholesterol may help reduce high blood cholesterol levels. Platelet inhibitors and anticoagulant medications (blood thinners) may be used to reduce clotting. Aspirin is the most commonly used medication for this purpose; others include dipyridamole, clopidogrel, aspirin/extended-release dipyridamole (Aggrenox), heparin, warfarin (Coumadin), and similar medications. Treatment may be continued for an indefinite time period.

NURSING CONSIDERATIONS

- Give medications as ordered, and watch for and report adverse effects.
- Help the patient understand that he must take his medications to treat hypertension as ordered.

- Administer cholesterol-lowering medications as ordered, and teach the patient how to eat a cholesterol-lowering diet.
- As appropriate, encourage the patient to quit smoking and provide information on smoking-cessation classes.

Musculoskeletal System

The aging process creates profound changes in the musculoskeletal system. The number of muscle fibers decreases, and the muscles become smaller and weaker. Muscle tone, strength, and endurance decline. Ligaments and tendons stiffen, reducing joint mobility, especially in the knees, hips, and spine. Wear and tear on the articular surfaces of the joints increases, resulting in the loss of synovial elasticity. Bone density decreases, weakening the bones. The intervertebral disks thin, causing older adults to lose close to ½" (1.3 cm) of height every 20 years. Pronounced curvature of the thoracic and cervical curves of the spine results in a stooped posture, with the head and neck thrust forward. The hips and stance widen. Movement typically becomes more cautious and deliberate, and walking and maintaining balance become more difficult.

In the bones and joints, osteoarthritis begins to develop from prolonged molecular changes in the articular cartilage (typically a genetic change, although it can also result from traumatic joint injury), and osteoporosis occurs as bone loss begins to exceed bone deposits. Hip fractures become more common, the result of falls, metastatic cancer, and other skeletal diseases. Gout can result from urate deposits, a disorder that occurs more frequently in men and postmenopausal women.

By understanding the kinds of changes the musculoskeletal system goes through with aging, you'll more easily recognize the signs of musculoskeletal disorders in your older patients. You can also help your patients understand these changes and take the necessary steps to maintain optimal functioning and health.

Fractures

Fractures related to osteoporosis are the main cause or morbidity and mortality in older adults. Reduction in bone density is the major cause of stress fractures involving the spine and pelvis. Falls can also contribute to fractures in weakened bones.

The most common fractures in older adults are hip fractures, pelvic fractures, and spinal compression fractures. Osteoporosis can lead to fractures of the proximal femur, proximal humerus, vertebrae, distal radius, and pelvis.

A fracture can result in substantial muscle, nerve, and other soft-tissue damage. The prognosis varies with the extent of disability or deformity, the amount of tissue and vascular damage, the adequacy of reduction and immobilization, and the patient's age, health, and nutritional status. The bones of adults in poor health or those with osteoporosis or impaired circulation may never heal properly.

CAUSES AND INCIDENCE

Most arm and leg fractures in older adults result from major trauma, such as a fall on an outstretched arm or elder abuse; abuse may result in multiple fractures or repeated episodes of fracture. However, in a person with a pathologic bone-weakening condition—such as osteoporosis, bone tumor, or metabolic disease—a simple cough or sneeze can cause a fracture. Prolonged standing, walking, or running can cause stress fractures of the foot and ankle in older adults.

PATHOPHYSIOLOGY

A fracture disrupts the periosteum and blood vessels in the cortex, marrow, and surrounding soft tissue. A hematoma forms between the broken ends of the bone and beneath the periosteum, and granulation tissue eventually replaces the hematoma.

Damage to bone tissue triggers an intense inflammatory response in which cells from surrounding soft tissue and the marrow cavity invade the fracture area, and blood flow to the entire bone increases. Osteoblasts in the periosteum, endosteum, and marrow produce osteoid (collagenous young bone that hasn't yet calcified, also called callus). The osteoid hardens along the outer surface of the shaft and over the broken ends of the bone. Osteoclasts resorb material from previously formed bones, and osteoblasts rebuild bone. Osteoblasts then transform into osteocytes (mature bone cells).

ASSESSMENT FINDINGS

The patient's history usually reveals what caused the fracture. The patient typically reports pain that increases with movement and an inability to intentionally move the part of the arm or leg distal to the injury. The severity of the pain depends on the fracture type and the amount of soft-tissue damage. The patient may also complain of a tingling sensation distal to the injury, possibly indicating nerve and vessel damage.

Inspection may disclose soft-tissue edema, an obvious deformity or shortening of the injured limb, and discoloration over the fracture site. Open fractures produce an obvious skin wound and bleeding. Gentle palpation usually reveals warmth, crepitus and, possibly, dislocation. Numbness distal to the injury and cool skin at the end of the extremity may indicate nerve and vessel damage.

Palpation may reveal loss of pulses distal to the injury, an indication of possible arterial compromise or nerve damage.

COMPLICATIONS

- Arterial damage
- Nonunion
- Fat embolism
- Infection
- Shock
- Avascular necrosis
- Peripheral nerve damage.

TREATMENT

The primary goals of treatment are to return the injured limb to maximal function, prevent complications, and obtain the best possible cosmetic results.

Emergency treatment consists of splinting the limb above and below the suspected fracture where it lies, applying a cold pack, and elevating the limb, all of which reduce edema and pain. A severe fracture that causes blood loss calls for direct pressure to control bleeding. The patient with a severe fracture may also need fluid replacement (including blood products) to prevent or treat hypovolemic shock.

After a fracture is confirmed, treatment begins with reduction (restoring displaced bone segments to their normal position). This is followed by immobilization with a splint, a cast, traction, or surgical repair.

In closed reduction (manual manipulation), a local anesthetic such as lidocaine and an analgesic such as morphine I.M. minimize pain; a muscle relaxant such as I.V. lorazepam or a sedative such as midazolam facilitates the muscle stretching necessary to realign the bone. An X-ray confirms reduction and proper bone alignment. General anesthesia may be needed for closed reduction.

When closed reduction isn't possible, open reduction during surgery reduces and immobilizes the fracture with rods, plates, or screws. Afterward, the patient usually must wear a cast.

When a splint or cast fails to maintain the reduction, immobilization requires skin or skeletal traction, using a series of weights and pulleys. In skin traction, elastic bandages and moleskin coverings are used to attach the traction devices to the patient's skin. In skeletal traction, a pin or wire inserted through the bone distal to the fracture and attached to a weight allows more prolonged traction. Skin traction may not be possible in an older patient because his skin may be too fragile.

Treatment for an open fracture also requires careful wound cleaning, tetanus prophylaxis, prophylactic antibiotics and, possibly, additional surgery to repair soft-tissue damage.

NURSING CONSIDERATIONS

- Reassure the patient with a fracture, who will probably be frightened and in pain. Ease pain with analgesics as needed.
- If the patient has a severe open fracture of a large bone such as the femur, watch for signs of shock. Monitor his vital signs; a rapid pulse, decreased blood pressure, pallor, and cool, clammy skin may indicate shock. Administer I.V. fluids and blood products as ordered.
- If the fracture requires long-term immobilization with traction, reposition the patient often to increase comfort and prevent pressure ulcers. Assist with active range-of-motion exercises to prevent muscle atrophy. Encourage deep breathing and coughing to avoid hypostatic pneumonia.
- In long-term immobilization, urge adequate fluid intake to prevent urinary stasis and constipation. Watch for signs of renal calculi (flank pain, nausea, and vomiting).

- Arrange for diversional activities. Allow the patient to express his concerns over lengthy immobilization and the problems it creates.
- Provide good cast care. While the cast is wet, support it with pillows. Observe for skin irritation near cast edges, and check for foul odors or discharge, particularly after open reduction, compound fracture, or skin lacerations and wounds on the affected limb.
- Encourage the patient to start moving around as soon as possible, and assist with walking. (Remember, the patient who has been bedridden for some time may be dizzy at first.)
- After cast removal, refer the patient to physical therapy to restore limb mobility.
- Show the patient how to use crutches properly.
- Tell the patient with a cast to report signs of impaired circulation (skin coldness, numbness, tingling, or discoloration) immediately. Tell the patient to make sure the plaster cast doesn't get wet, and instruct him not to insert foreign objects under the cast.
- Tell the patient not to walk on a leg cast or foot cast without the physician's permission. The patient with a fiberglass cast may be able to walk immediately, but plaster casts require 48 hours to dry and harden.
- Emphasize the importance of returning for follow-up care.

Gout

Gout—also known as gouty arthritis—is a metabolic disease marked by monosodium urate deposits that cause red, swollen, and acutely painful joints. Gout can affect any joint but mostly affects joints in the feet, especially the great toe, ankle, and midfoot.

Primary gout typically occurs in men over age 30 and in postmenopausal women who take diuretics. It follows an intermittent course that may leave patients symptom-free for years between attacks. Secondary gout occurs in older people.

In asymptomatic patients, serum urate levels rise but produce no symptoms. In symptom-producing gout, the first acute attack strikes suddenly and peaks quickly. Although it may involve only one or a few joints, this attack causes extreme pain. Mild acute attacks usually subside quickly and tend to recur at irregular intervals. Severe attacks may persist for days or weeks.

Intercritical periods are the symptom-free intervals between attacks. Most patients have a second attack between 6 months and 2 years after the first; in some patients, the second attack doesn't occur for 5 to 10 years. Delayed attacks, which may be polyarticular, are more common in untreated patients. These attacks tend to last longer and produce more symptoms than initial episodes. A migratory attack strikes various joints and the Achilles tendon sequentially and may be associated with olecranon bursitis.

Eventually, chronic polyarticular gout develops in patients who don't receive treatment to lower their uric acid. This final, unremitting stage of the disease (also known as tophaceous gout) is marked by persistent painful polyarthritis. An increased concentration of uric acid leads to urate deposits—called tophi—in cartilage, synovial membranes, tendons, and soft tissue.

Tophi form in the fingers, hands, knees, feet, ulnar sides of the forearms, pinna of the ear, Achilles tendon and, rarely, in such internal organs as the kidneys and myocardium. Renal involvement may adversely affect renal function.

Patients who receive treatment for gout have a good prognosis.

CAUSES AND INCIDENCE

Although the underlying cause of primary gout is unknown, it appears to be linked to a genetic defect in purine metabolism that causes overproduction of uric acid (hyperuricemia), retention of uric acid, or both.

Secondary gout develops during the course of another disease, such as obesity, diabetes mellitus, hypertension, polycythemia, leukemia, myeloma, sickle cell anemia, and renal disease. Secondary gout can also follow treatment with such drugs as hydrochlorothiazide or pyrazinamide.

PATHOPHYSIOLOGY

When uric acid becomes supersaturated in blood and other body fluids, it crystalizes and forms tophi—accumulations of urate salts in connective tissue throughout the body. The presence of the crystals triggers an acute inflammatory response in which neutrophils begin to attempt to ingest the crystals. Tissue damage begins when the neutrophils release their lysosomes, which not only damage the tissues but also perpetuate the inflammation.

ASSESSMENT FINDINGS

The patient's history may reveal that he has a sedentary lifestyle and a history of hypertension and renal calculi. He may report waking during the night with pain in his great toe or another location in the foot. He may complain that initially moderate pain has grown so intense that eventually he can't bear the weight of bed sheets or the vibrations of a person walking across the room. He may report accompanying chills and a mild fever.

Inspection typically reveals a swollen, dusky red or purple joint with limited movement. You may also notice tophi, especially in the outer ears, hands, and feet. (See *Recognizing gouty tophi*.)

Late in the chronic stage of gout, the skin over the tophi may ulcerate and release a chalky white exudate or pus. Chronic inflammation and tophaceous deposits prompt secondary joint degeneration. Erosions, deformity, and disability may develop.

Palpation may reveal warmth over the joint and extreme tenderness. The vital signs assessment may disclose fever and hypertension. If the patient has a fever, he may have a possible occult infection.

COMPLICATIONS

- Renal calculi
- Atherosclerotic disease
- Cardiovascular lesions
- Stroke
- Coronary thrombosis
- Hypertension
- Infection with tophi rupture and nerve entrapment

TREATMENT

Correct management has three goals:

- First, terminate the acute attack.
- Next, treat hyperuricemia to reduce urine uric acid levels.
- Finally, prevent recurrent gout and renal calculi.

Treatment for an acute attack consists of bed rest; immobilization and protection of the inflamed, painful joints; and local application of cold. Analgesics such as acetaminophen relieve the pain associated with mild attacks. Acute inflammation requires nonsteroidal anti-inflammatory drugs or I.M. corticotropin. Oral corticosteroids or intra-articular corticosteroid injections are occasionally necessary to treat acute attacks.

Treatment for chronic gout involves decreasing the serum uric acid level to less than 6.5 mg/dl. To determine the right medica-

RECOGNIZING GOUTY TOPHI

In advanced gout, urate crystal deposits develop into hard, irregular yellow-white nodules called *tophi*. These bumps commonly protrude from the pinna and great toe.

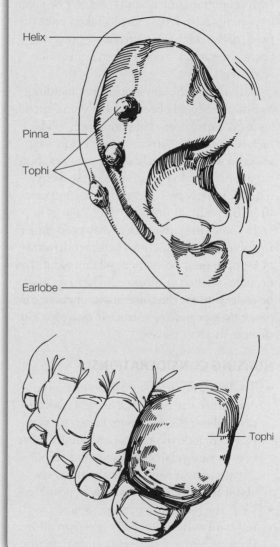

tion regimen, the patient should first undergo a 24-hour urinalysis to determine how much uric acid he excretes. If he excretes too little uric acid, he may receive allopurinol to reduce uric acid production (in reduced doses if he has decreased renal function).

Uricosuric agents promote uric acid excretion and inhibit the accumulation of uric acid. However, they have less value for patients with renal impairment and shouldn't be given to patients with renal calculi. Taken once or twice daily, colchicine effectively prevents acute gout attacks, but it doesn't affect uric acid levels.

Adjunctive therapy emphasizes avoiding alcohol (especially beer and wine) and cutting back on consumption of purine-rich foods, such as anchovies, liver, sardines, kidneys, sweetbreads, and lentils. Obese patients should begin a weight-loss program because weight reduction decreases uric acid levels and eases stress on painful joints.

In some cases, the patient may need surgery to improve joint function or correct deformities. Tophi must be excised and drained if they become infected or ulcerated. They can also be excised to prevent ulceration, improve the patient's appearance, or make it easier for him to wear shoes or gloves.

NURSING CONSIDERATIONS

- To diffuse anxiety and promote coping, encourage the patient to express his concerns about his condition. Listen supportively. Include the patient and family members in care-related decisions and all phases of care. Answer the patient's questions about his disorder as honestly as possible.
- Urge the patient to perform as much self-care as his immobility and pain allow. Provide him with adequate time to perform these activities at his own pace.
- Encourage bed rest, but use a bed cradle to keep bed linens off of sensitive, inflamed joints.
- Carefully evaluate the patient's condition after joint aspiration. Provide emotional

support during diagnostic tests and procedures.

- Give pain medication as needed, especially during acute attacks. Monitor the patient's response to this medication. Apply cold packs to inflamed joints to ease discomfort and reduce swelling.
- To promote sleep, administer pain medication at times that allow for maximum rest. Provide the patient with sleep aids, such as a bath, a back rub, or an extra pillow.
- Help the patient identify techniques and activities that promote rest and relaxation. Encourage him to perform them.
- Administer anti-inflammatory medication and other drugs as ordered. Watch for adverse reactions. Be alert for GI disturbances if the patient takes colchicine.
- When encouraging fluids, record intake and output accurately. Be sure to monitor serum uric acid levels regularly. As ordered, administer sodium bicarbonate or other agents to alkalinize the patient's urine.
- Provide a nutritious, but purine-poor diet.
- Watch for acute gout attacks 24 to 96 hours after surgery. Even minor surgery can trigger an attack. Before and after surgery, administer colchicine to help prevent gout attacks, as ordered.
- Urge the patient to drink plenty of fluids (as much as 2 qt [2 L] a day) to prevent renal calculi.
- Explain all treatments, tests, and procedures. Warn the patient before his first needle aspiration that it will be painful.
- Make sure the patient understands the rationale for evaluating serum uric acid levels periodically.
- Teach the patient relaxation techniques. Encourage him to perform them regularly.
- Instruct the patient to avoid purine-rich foods, such as anchovies, liver, sardines,

kidneys, luncheon meats, and lentils, because these substances raise the urate level.

- Discuss the principles of gradual weight reduction with an obese patient. Explain the advantages of a diet containing moderate amounts of protein and little fat.
- If the patient receives allopurinol or other drugs, instruct him to report any adverse reactions immediately. (Reactions may include nausea, vomiting, drowsiness, dizziness, urinary frequency, and dermatitis.) Warn the patient taking probenecid or sulfinpyrazone to avoid aspirin and other salicylates. Their combined effect causes urate retention.
- Inform the patient that long-term colchicine therapy is essential during the first 3 to 6 months of treatment with uricosuric drugs or allopurinol. Stress the importance of compliance.
- Urge the patient to control hypertension, especially if he has tophaceous renal deposits. Keep in mind that diuretics aren't advised for the gout patient; alternative antihypertensives are preferred.

Osteoarthritis

Osteoarthritis is the most common form of arthritis. It causes deterioration of the joint cartilage and formation of reactive new bone at the margins and subchondral areas of the joints. This chronic degeneration results from a change in the articular cartilage, most often in the hips and knees.

Depending on the site and severity of joint involvement, disability can range from minor limitation of the fingers to near immobility in people with hip or knee disease. Progression rates vary; joints may remain stable for years in the early stage of deterioration.

CAUSES AND INCIDENCE

Primary osteoarthritis may result from metabolic, genetic, chemical, and mechanical factors. Secondary osteoarthritis usually follows an identifiable event—most commonly a traumatic injury or a congenital abnormality such as hip dysplasia. Endocrine disorders such as diabetes mellitus, metabolic disorders such as chondrocalcinosis, and other types of arthritis also can lead to secondary osteoarthritis. (See *Understanding osteoarthritis*, page 228.)

Osteoarthritis occurs equally in both sexes and typically develops after age 40, with the earliest symptoms beginning in middle age and progressing as the patient ages.

PATHOPHYSIOLOGY

Osteoarthritis occurs in synovial joints. The joint cartilage deteriorates, and reactive new bone forms at the margins and subchondral areas of the joints. With age, cartilage hardens and there's less fluid in the joints, narrowing the joint space. Mechanical injury erodes articular cartilage, leaving the underlying bone unprotected. This causes sclerosis, or thickening and hardening of the bone underneath the cartilage.

Cartilage particles irritate the synovial lining, which becomes fibrotic and limits joint movement. Synovial fluid may be forced into defects in the bone. New bone (osteophyte or bone spur) forms at joint margins as the articular cartilage erodes, causing gross alteration of the bony contours and enlargement of the joint. These bone spurs also cause pain by traumatizing nearby soft tissue.

ASSESSMENT FINDINGS

The patient usually complains of gradually increasing signs and symptoms. He may report a predisposing event such as a traumatic injury. Most commonly, the patient has deep, aching joint pain, particularly after exercise or weight bearing on the affected joint. Rest may relieve the pain.

Additional complaints include stiffness in the morning (usually for less than 30 minutes

UNDERSTANDING OSTEOARTHRITIS

The characteristic breakdown of articular cartilage is a gradual response to aging or predisposing factors, such as joint abnormalities or traumatic injury. These illustrations will help you understand how osteoarthritis progresses.

Normal Anatomy

Normally, bones fit together. Cartilage—a smooth, fibrous tissue—cushions the end of each bone, and synovial fluid fills the joint space. This fluid lubricates the joint and eases movement, much like brake fluid in a car.

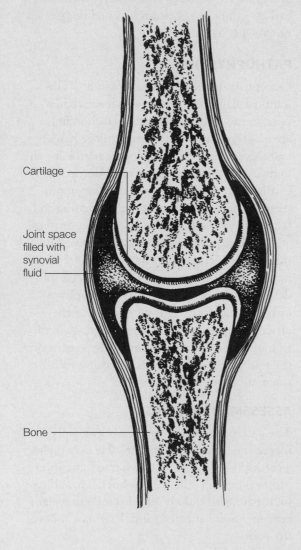

Cartilage

Joint space filled with synovial fluid

Bone

Early Stage

Cartilage may begin to break down long before symptoms surface. In early osteoarthritis, the patient typically has no symptoms or a mild, dull ache when he uses the joint. Rest relieves the discomfort. Or he may feel stiffness in the affected joint, especially in the morning. The stiffness usually lasts 15 minutes or less.

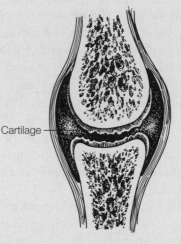

Cartilage

Later Stages

As the disease progresses, whole sections of cartilage may disintegrate, osteophytes (bony spurs) form, and fragments of cartilage and bone float freely in the joint. More common now, pain may be present even during rest. It typically worsens throughout the day. Movement becomes increasingly limited, and stiffness may persist even after limbering exercises.

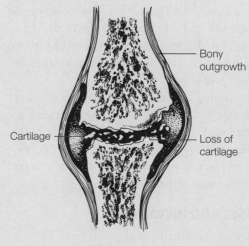

Bony outgrowth

Cartilage

Loss of cartilage

and after exercise), aching during changes in weather, a grating feeling when the joint moves, contractures, and limited movement. These symptoms tend to be worse in patients with poor posture, obesity, or occupational stress.

Inspection may reveal joint swelling, muscle atrophy, deformity of the involved areas, and gait abnormalities (when arthritis affects the hips or knees). Osteoarthritis of the interphalangeal joints (more common in women but also seen in men) produces hard nodes on the distal and proximal joints. Painless at first, these nodes eventually become red, swollen, and tender. The fingers may become numb and lose their dexterity. (*See Signs of osteoarthritis.*)

Palpation may reveal joint tenderness and warmth without redness, grating with movement, joint instability, muscle spasms, and limited movement.

COMPLICATIONS

- Flexion contractures
- Subluxation and deformity
- Ankylosis
- Bony cysts
- Gross bony overgrowth
- Central cord syndrome (with cervical spine osteoarthritis)
- Nerve root compression
- Cauda equina syndrome

TREATMENT

To relieve pain, improve mobility, and minimize disability, treatment includes medications, rest, physical therapy, assistive mobility devices and, possibly, surgery.

Medications include nonsteroidal anti-inflammatory drugs. In some patients, intra-articular injections of corticosteroids may be necessary. Such injections, given every 4 to 6 months, may delay nodal development in

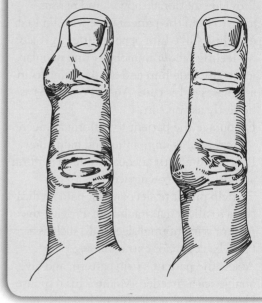

SIGNS OF OSTEOARTHRITIS

Heberden's nodes may appear on the dorsolateral aspect of the distal interphalangeal joints. These bony and cartilaginous enlargements are usually hard and painless. They typically occur in middle-aged and elderly osteoarthritis patients. Bouchard's nodes are similar to Heberden's nodes but are less common and appear on the proximal interphalangeal joints.

HEBERDEN'S NODES   **BOUCHARD'S NODES**

the hands. Injecting artificial joint fluid into the knee can provide relief of pain for up to 6 months.

Adequate rest is essential and should be balanced with activity. Physical therapy includes massage, moist heat, paraffin dips for the hands, supervised exercise to decrease muscle spasms and atrophy, and protective techniques for preventing undue joint stress. Some patients may reduce stress and increase stability by using crutches, braces, a cane, a walker, a cervical collar, or traction. Weight reduction may help an obese patient.

In some cases, a patient with severe disability or uncontrollable pain may undergo surgery. Arthroplasty (partial or total) involves replacing the deteriorated part of a joint with a prosthetic appliance. Arthrodesis is surgical fusion of bones; it's used primarily in the spine (laminectomy).

NURSING CONSIDERATIONS

- Provide emotional support and reassurance to help the patient cope with limited mobility. Give him opportunities to voice his feelings about immobility and nodular joints. Include him and family members in all phases of his care. Answer questions as honestly as you can.
- Encourage the patient to perform as much self-care as his immobility and pain allow. Provide him with adequate time to perform activities at his own pace.
- To help promote sleep, adjust pain medications to allow maximum rest. Provide the patient with normal sleep aids, such as a bath, back rub, or extra pillow.
- Assess the patient's pain pattern, and give analgesics as needed. Monitor his response.
- Help the patient identify techniques and activities that promote rest and relaxation. Encourage him to perform them.
- Administer anti-inflammatory medication and other drugs as ordered. Watch for adverse reactions.
- For joints in the hand, provide hot soaks and paraffin dips to relieve pain as ordered.
- For lumbosacral spinal joints, provide a firm mattress (or bed board) to decrease morning pain.
- For cervical spinal joints, adjust the patient's cervical collar to avoid constriction; watch for irritated skin with prolonged use.
- For the hip, use moist heat pads to relieve pain. Administer antispasmodic drugs as ordered.

- For the knee, assist with prescribed range-of-motion (ROM) exercises twice daily to maintain muscle tone. Help perform progressive resistance exercises to increase the patient's muscle strength.
- Check the patient's crutches, cane, braces, or walker for proper fit
- Instruct the patient to plan for adequate rest during the day, after exertion, and at night. Encourage him to learn and use energy-conservation methods, such as pacing, simplifying work procedures, and protecting joints.
- Instruct him to take medications exactly as prescribed. Tell him which adverse reactions to report immediately.
- Advise against overexertion. Tell the patient that he should take care to stand and walk correctly, to minimize weight-bearing activities, and to be especially careful when stooping or picking up objects.
- Tell the patient to wear well-fitting support shoes and to repair worn heels.
- Recommend having safety devices installed in the home, such as grab bars in the bathroom.
- Teach the patient to do ROM exercises, performing them as gently as possible.
- Advise maintaining proper body weight to minimize strain on joints.
- Teach the patient how to use crutches or other orthopedic devices properly. Stress the importance of proper fitting and regular professional readjustment of such devices. Warn that impaired sensation might allow tissue damage from these aids without discomfort.
- Recommend using cushions when sitting. Also suggest using an elevated toilet seat. Both reduce stress when rising from a seated position.
- Positively reinforce the patient's efforts to adapt. Point out improving or stabilizing physical functioning.

- As necessary, refer the patient to an occupational therapist or a home health nurse to help him cope with activities of daily living.

Osteoporosis

In osteoporosis, a metabolic bone disorder, the rate of bone resorption accelerates, and the rate of bone formation decelerates. The result is decreased bone mass. Bones affected by this disease lose calcium and phosphate and become porous, brittle, and abnormally vulnerable to fracture.

Osteoporosis may be primary, or it may or secondary to an underlying disease or other cause, such as prolonged steroid use. Primary osteoporosis can be classified as idiopathic, type I, or type II. Idiopathic osteoporosis affects both children and adults. Related to the loss of estrogen's protective effect on bone, type I osteoporosis results in trabecular bone loss and some cortical bone loss; patients with this type of osteoporosis may experience vertebral and wrist fractures. Type II osteoporosis is characterized by trabecular and cortical bone loss and consequent fractures of the proximal humerus, proximal tibia, femoral neck, and pelvis.

CAUSES AND INCIDENCE

The cause of primary osteoporosis is unknown, but contributing factors may include:

- mild but prolonged negative calcium balance resulting from inadequate dietary intake
- declining gonadal adrenal function
- faulty protein metabolism caused by estrogen deficiency
- a sedentary lifestyle
- inadequate vitamin D intake.

Secondary osteoporosis may result from prolonged therapy with steroids or heparin, bone immobilization or disuse (as occurs with hemiplegia), alcoholism, malnutrition, rheumatoid arthritis, liver disease, malabsorption, scurvy, lactose intolerance, hyperthyroidism, osteogenesis imperfecta, and Sudeck's atrophy (localized in hands and feet, with recurring attacks).

Approximately 75% to 80% of patients with osteoporosis are women. White and Asian women are at greater risk than African-American women. Type I (or postmenopausal) osteoporosis usually affects women ages 51 to 75. Type II (or senile) osteoporosis occurs most commonly between ages 70 and 85 in both men and women.

PATHOPHYSIOLOGY

In normal bone, the rates of bone formation and resorption are about constant; replacement follows absorption immediately, and the amount of bone replaced equals the amount of bone resorbed. The endocrine system maintains plasma and bone calcium metabolism by stimulating osteoblastic activity and limiting the osteoclastic-stimulating effects of parathyroid hormones.

Osteoporosis develops when new bone formation falls behind resorption. For example, heparin promotes bone resorption by inhibiting collagen synthesis or enhancing collagen breakdown. Elevated levels of cortisone, either endogenous or exogenous, inhibit GI absorption of calcium and suppress osteoblastic action.

ASSESSMENT FINDINGS

The history may typically disclose a postmenopausal patient or one with a condition known to cause secondary osteoporosis. The patient (usually an elderly woman) may report that she bent down to lift something, heard a snapping sound, and felt a sudden pain in her lower back. Or she may say that the pain developed slowly over several years. If the patient has

DETECTING HEIGHT LOSS

A patient with osteoporosis typically loses height gradually. A condition known as dowager's hump (shown below) develops when repeated vertebral fractures increase the spinal curvature. (Although a hallmark of osteoporosis, this malformation may occur apart from the disease.)

Reduced thoracic and abdominal volumes, decreased exercise tolerance, pulmonary insufficiency, and abdominal protrusion may accompany height loss.

To assess height loss, have the patient stand with her arms raised laterally and parallel to the floor. A measured difference exceeding 1½" (about 4 cm) between the patient's height and the distance across the outstretched arms (from longest fingertip to longest fingertip) suggests height loss.

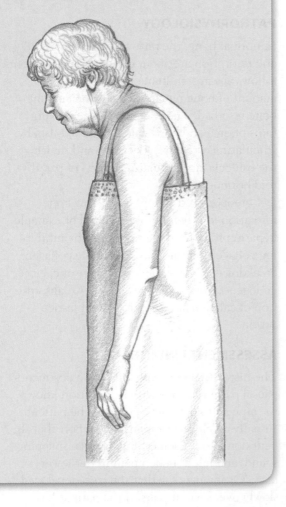

vertebral collapse, she may describe a backache and pain radiating around the trunk. Any movement or jarring aggravates the pain.

Inspection may reveal that the patient has a humped back and a markedly aged appearance. She may report a loss of height. (See *Detecting height loss.*)

Palpation may reveal muscle spasm. The patient may also have decreased spinal movement, with flexion more limited than extension.

COMPLICATIONS

- Compression fracture of the spine
- Hip and wrist fractures
- Loss of mobility

TREATMENT

To control bone loss, prevent additional fractures, and control pain, treatment is focused on a physical therapy program of gentle exercise and activity and drug therapy to slow disease progress. Other treatment measures include supportive devices and, possibly, surgery.

Medications may include bisphosphonates, such as alendronate and risedronate, to prevent bone loss and reduce the risk of fractures. Calcium and vitamin D supplements may help to support normal bone metabolism. Raloxifene and calcitonin may be used to reduce bone resorption and slow the decline in bone mass.

Surgery (open reduction and internal fixation) can correct pathologic fractures of the femur. Colles' fracture requires reduction and immobilization (with a cast) for 4 to 10 weeks.

To help prevent primary osteoporosis, older adults should consume adequate dietary calcium—including calcium supplements as appropriate—and exercise regularly. Fluoride treatments may also offer some preventive benefit. Hormone replacement therapy (HRT) with estrogen and progesterone may retard bone loss and prevent the occurrence of fractures; however, this therapy remains controversial. HRT decreases bone reabsorption and increases bone mass but is association with an increased risk of breast cancer.

Secondary osteoporosis can be prevented through effective treatment of the underlying disease, early mobilization after surgery or trauma, careful observation for signs of malabsorption, and prompt treatment of hyperthyroidism. Decreased alcohol consumption and caffeine use, as well as smoking cessation, can also help prevent secondary osteoporosis.

NURSING CONSIDERATIONS

- Design your plan of care to consider the patient's fragility. Concentrate on careful positioning, ambulation, and prescribed exercises.
- Provide emotional support and reassurance to help the patient cope with limited mobility. Give her opportunities to voice her feelings. If possible, arrange for her to interact with others who have similar problems.
- Include the patient and family members in all phases of care. Answer questions as honestly as you can.
- Encourage the patient to perform as much self-care as her immobility and pain allow. Allow her adequate time to perform these activities at her own pace.
- Check the patient's skin daily for redness, warmth, and new sites of pain, which may indicate new fractures.
- Provide the patient with activities that involve mild exercise; help her to walk several times daily. As appropriate, perform passive range-of-motion exercises, or encourage her to perform active exercises. Make sure she attends scheduled physical therapy sessions.

- Impose safety precautions. Keep bed rails up. Move the patient gently and carefully at all times. Discuss with ancillary facility personnel how easily an osteoporotic patient's bones can fracture.
- Provide a balanced diet rich in nutrients that support skeletal metabolism: vitamin D, calcium, and protein.
- Administer analgesics and heat to relieve pain as ordered. Assess the patient's response.
- Explain all treatments, tests, and procedures. For example, if the patient is undergoing surgery, explain all preoperative and postoperative procedures and treatments to the patient and family members.
- Make sure the patient and family members clearly understand the prescribed drug regimen. Tell them how to recognize significant adverse reactions. Instruct them to report them immediately.
- Teach the patient taking estrogen to perform breast self-examination. Tell her to perform this examination at least once a month and to report any lumps right away. Emphasize the need for regular gynecologic examinations. Also instruct her to report abnormal vaginal bleeding promptly.
- If the patient takes a calcium supplement, encourage liberal fluid intake to help maintain adequate urine output and thereby avoid renal calculi, hypercalcemia, and hypercalciuria.
- Tell the patient to report any new pain sites immediately, especially after trauma.
- Advise the patient to sleep on a firm mattress and to avoid excessive bed rest.
- Teach the patient how to use a back brace properly, if appropriate.
- Thoroughly explain osteoporosis to the patient and family members. If they don't understand the disease process, they may

feel needless guilt, thinking that they could have acted to prevent bone fractures.

- Demonstrate proper body mechanics. Show the patient how to stoop before lifting anything and how to avoid twisting movements and prolonged bending.
- Encourage the patient to install safety devices, such as grab bars and railings, at home.
- Advise the patient to eat a diet rich in calcium. Give her a list of calcium-rich foods. Explain that type II osteoporosis may be prevented by adequate dietary calcium intake and regular exercise. Hormonal and fluoride treatments also may help prevent osteoporosis.
- Explain that secondary osteoporosis may be prevented by effectively treating underlying disease, early mobilization after surgery or trauma, decreased alcohol consumption, careful observation for signs of malabsorption, and prompt treatment of hyperthyroidism.
- Reinforce the patient's efforts to adapt, and show her how her condition is improving or stabilizing. As necessary, refer her to an occupational therapist or a home health nurse to help her cope with activities of daily living.

Paget's disease

Paget's disease—also known as osteitis deformans—is a slowly progressive metabolic bone disease characterized by an initial phase of excessive bone resorption (osteoclastic phase) followed by a reactive phase of excessive abnormal bone formation (osteoblastic phase). The new bone structure, which is chaotic, fragile, and weak, causes painful deformities of the external contour and the internal structures.

Paget's disease usually affects one or several skeletal areas (most commonly the spine, pelvis, femur, and skull). Occasionally, a patient has widely distributed skeletal deformity. In

about 5% of patients, the involved bone undergoes malignant changes.

The disease can be fatal, particularly when associated with heart failure (widespread disease creates a continuous need for high cardiac output), bone sarcoma, or giant cell tumors.

CAUSES AND INCIDENCE

Although the exact cause of Paget's disease isn't known, one theory suggests that a slow or dormant viral infection (possibly mumps) causes a dormant skeletal infection, which surfaces many years later as the disease. It occurs most often in men over age 40, with a higher incidence in adults over age 80.

PATHOPHYSIOLOGY

In this disorder, repeated episodes of accelerated osteoclastic resorption of spongy bone occur. The trabeculae diminish, and vascular fibrous tissue replaces marrow. This is followed by short periods of rapid, abnormal bone formation. The collagen fibers in this new bone are disorganized, and glycoprotein levels in the matrix decrease. The partially resorbed trabeculae thicken and enlarge because of excessive bone formation, and the bone becomes soft and weak. Eventually, Paget's disease progresses to an inactive phase in which abnormal remodeling is minimal or absent.

ASSESSMENT FINDINGS

Clinical effects vary. The patient with early disease may be asymptomatic. As the disease progresses, he may report severe, persistent pain. If abnormal bone impinges on the spinal cord or sensory nerve root, he may complain of impaired mobility and pain that increases with weight bearing.

If the patient's head is involved, inspection may reveal characteristic cranial enlargement over the frontal and occipital areas. The patient may comment that his hat size has increased, and he may have headaches. Other deformities include kyphosis (spinal curvature caused by compression fractures of affected vertebrae) accompanied by a barrel-shaped chest and asymmetrical bowing of the tibia and femur, which typically reduces height. Palpation may disclose warmth and tenderness over affected sites.

COMPLICATIONS

- Blindness and hearing loss
- Pathologic fractures
- Hypertension
- Renal calculi
- Hypercalcemia
- Gout
- Heart failure
- Respiratory failure

TREATMENT

If the patient is asymptomatic, treatment isn't needed. The patient with symptoms requires drug therapy.

The hormone calcitonin may be given subcutaneously, intranasally, or I.M. The patient requires long-term maintenance therapy with calcitonin; noticeable improvement occurs after the first few weeks of treatment. The patient also may receive oral bisphosphonates (such as etidronate, alendronate, pamidronate, tiludronate, and risedronate) to retard bone resorption (and relieve bone lesions) and to reduce serum alkaline phosphatase and urinary hydroxyproline excretion. Bisphosphonates produce improvement after 1 to 3 months.

Plicamycin (a cytotoxic antibiotic used to decrease serum calcium, urinary hydroxyproline, and serum alkaline phosphatase levels) produces remission of symptoms within 2 weeks and biochemically detectable improvement in 1 to 2 months. Plicamycin can destroy platelets or compromise renal function, so it's usually given only to patients who have severe disease, require rapid relief, or don't respond to other treatment.

Self-administration of calcitonin and bisphosphonates helps patients with Paget's disease lead nearly normal lives. Even so, these patients may need surgery to reduce or prevent pathologic fractures, correct secondary deformities, and relieve neurologic impairment. To decrease the risk of excessive bleeding caused by hypervascular bone, drug therapy with calcitonin and bisphosphonates or plicamycin must precede surgery. Joint replacement is difficult because polymethylmethacrylate (a gluelike bonding material) doesn't set properly on bone affected by Paget's disease. Other treatments vary according to symptoms.

NURSING CONSIDERATIONS

- Assess the patient's pain level daily to evaluate the effectiveness of analgesic therapy. Watch for new areas of pain or newly restricted movements—which may indicate new fracture sites—and sensory or motor disturbances, such as difficulty in hearing, seeing, or walking.
- Monitor serum calcium and alkaline phosphatase levels.
- If bed rest confines the patient for prolonged periods, prevent pressure ulcers with meticulous skin care. Reposition the patient frequently, and use a flotation mattress. Provide high-topped sneakers or a footboard to manage footdrop.
- Monitor intake and output. Encourage adequate fluid intake to minimize renal calculi formation.
- Help the patient adjust to lifestyle changes imposed by Paget's disease. Teach him to pace activities and, if necessary, to use assistive devices.
- Encourage the patient to follow a recommended exercise program. Urge him to avoid both immobilization and excessive activity.

- Suggest a firm mattress or a bed board to minimize spinal deformities.
- Explain all medications to the patient. Instruct him to use analgesic medications cautiously.
- To prevent falls at home, urge the patient to remove throw rugs and small obstacles from the floor.
- Emphasize the importance of regular check-ups, including eye and ear checkups, to assess for complications.
- Demonstrate how to inject calcitonin properly and how to rotate injection sites. Caution the patient that adverse reactions may occur (including nausea, vomiting, local inflammatory reaction at the injection site, facial flushing, itchy hands, and fever). Reassure him that these reactions are usually mild and occur infrequently.
- Tell the patient receiving etidronate to take this medication with fruit juice 2 hours before or after meals (milk or other calcium-rich fluids impair absorption), divide the daily dosage to minimize adverse reactions, and watch for and report stomach cramps, diarrhea, fractures, and new or increasing bone pain.
- Instruct the patient receiving plicamycin to watch for signs of infection (including elevated temperature), easy bruising, and bleeding. Urge him to schedule and report for regular follow-up laboratory tests.
- Refer the patient and family members to community support resources, such as a home health care agency and the Paget's Disease Foundation.

GI System

As the body ages, the GI system goes through several changes. With age, peristalsis and smooth muscle tone decrease, mucosal lining atrophies, and liver size decreases. These changes result in delayed esophageal and gastric emptying, causing a feeling of fullness after ingesting smaller amounts of food. Altered gastric acid secretion may cause discomfort, indigestion, and appetite loss, and gastric acid reflux can result from medication use or disease. Other complications include constipation and fecal incontinence.

A common complaint in older adults, constipation can result when slower peristalsis reduces transit time in the large intestine, possibly causing water reabsorption and hardening of the stool. Other factors that contribute to constipation include reduced fluid intake, weakened anal sphincter control, a diminished defecation reflex, inactivity, immobility, laxative dependence, and adverse drug effects.

Fecal incontinence may result from age or disease-related changes in GI function or, less commonly, from musculoskeletal or neurologic changes (such as weakened pelvic floor muscles and prostate enlargement in men). If severe, fecal incontinence can have serious psychosocial effects and threaten the older adult's ability to function and survive.

Other GI problems commonly seen in older adults include colorectal cancer, diverticular disease, esophageal cancer, and peptic ulcer.

Colorectal cancer

Malignant tumors of the colon or rectum are almost always adenocarcinomas. About half of these are sessile lesions of the rectosigmoid area; the rest are polypoid lesions.

Colorectal cancer progresses slowly, remaining localized for a long time. With early diagnosis, the 5-year survival rate is 50%. It's potentially curable in 75% of patients if an early diagnosis allows resection before nodal involvement.

TYPES OF COLORECTAL CANCER

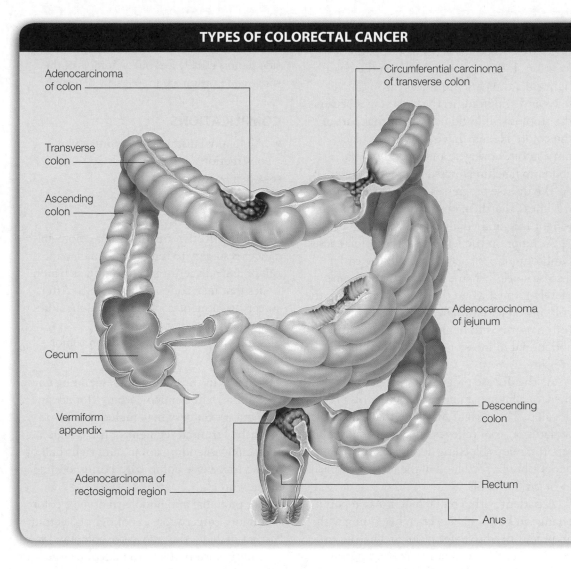

Adenocarcinoma of colon

Transverse colon

Ascending colon

Cecum

Vermiform appendix

Adenocarcinoma of rectosigmoid region

Circumferential carcinoma of transverse colon

Adenocarocinoma of jejunum

Descending colon

Rectum

Anus

CAUSES AND INCIDENCE

Although the exact cause of colorectal cancer is unknown, studies show a greater incidence in areas of higher economic development, suggesting a relationship to a diet that includes excess animal fat, especially from beef, and low fiber.

Colorectal cancer is the second most common visceral neoplasm in the United States and Europe. It's equally distributed between men and women and is more common after age 40.

PATHOPHYSIOLOGY

Most lesions of the large bowel are moderately differentiated adenocarcinomas. These tumors tend to grow slowly and remain asymptomatic for long periods. Tumors in the sigmoid and descending colon grow circumferentially and constrict the intestinal lumen. At diagnosis, tumors in the ascending colon are usually large and are palpable on physical examination. (See *Types of colorectal cancer*.)

ASSESSMENT FINDINGS

Signs and symptoms depend on the tumor's location. If the tumor develops on the colon's right side, the patient probably won't have signs and symptoms in the early stages because the stool is still in liquid form in that part of the colon. He may have a history of black, tarry stools, however, and report anemia, abdominal aching, pressure, and dull cramps. As the disease progresses, he may complain of weakness, diarrhea, obstipation, anorexia, weight loss, and vomiting.

A tumor on the left side of the colon causes symptoms of obstruction even in the early disease stages because stools are more completely formed when they reach this part of the colon. The patient may report rectal bleeding (often ascribed to hemorrhoids), intermittent abdominal fullness or cramping, and rectal pressure.

As the disease progresses, obstipation, diarrhea, or ribbon- or pencil-shaped stools may develop. The patient may note that the passage of flatus or stool relieves his pain. He may also report obvious bleeding during defecation and dark or bright red blood in the feces and mucus in or on the stools.

A patient with a rectal tumor may report a change in bowel habits, often beginning with an urgent need to defecate on arising (morning diarrhea) or obstipation alternating with diarrhea. He may also notice blood or mucus in the stools and complain of a sense of incomplete evacuation. Late in the disease, he may complain of pain that begins as a feeling of rectal fullness and progresses to a dull, sometimes constant ache confined to the rectum or sacral region.

Inspection of the abdomen may reveal distention or visible masses. Abdominal veins may appear enlarged and visible from portal obstruction. The inguinal and supraclavicular nodes may also appear enlarged. You may note abnor-mal bowel sounds on abdominal auscultation. Palpation may reveal abdominal masses. Right-side tumors usually feel bulky; tumors of the transverse portion are more easily detected.

COMPLICATIONS

- Abdominal distention and intestinal obstruction
- Anemia

TREATMENT

The most effective treatment for colorectal cancer is surgery to remove the malignant tumor and adjacent tissues, as well as lymph nodes that may contain cancer cells. After surgery, treatment continues with chemotherapy, radiation therapy, or both.

The type of surgery depends on tumor location:

- Tumors in the cecum and ascending colon call for right hemicolectomy (for advanced disease). Surgery may include resection of the terminal segment of the ileum, cecum, ascending colon, and right half of the transverse colon with corresponding mesentery.
- For proximal and middle transverse colon tumors, surgery consists of right colectomy that includes the transverse colon and mesentery corresponding to midcolic vessels, or segmental resection of the transverse colon and associated midcolic vessels.
- For tumors in the sigmoid colon, surgery usually is limited to the sigmoid colon and mesentery.
- Tumors in the upper rectum usually require anterior or low anterior resection. A newer method, using a stapler, allows for much lower resections than previously possible.
- Tumors in the lower rectum require abdominoperineal resection and permanent sigmoid colostomy.

If metastasis has occurred or if the patient has residual disease or a recurrent inoperable tumor, he needs chemotherapy. Drugs used in such treatment commonly include fluorouracil combined with levamisole or leucovorin.

Radiation therapy, used before or after surgery, induces tumor regression.

NURSING CONSIDERATIONS

- Before colorectal surgery, monitor the patient's diet modifications and administer laxatives, enemas, and antibiotics, as ordered. These measures help clean the bowel and decrease abdominal and peritoneal cavity contamination during surgery.
- After surgery, monitor the patient's visual signs, intake and output, and fluid and electrolyte balance. Also monitor for complications, including anastomotic leaks, hemorrhage, irregular bowel function, phantom rectum, ruptured pelvic peritoneum, stricture, urinary dysfunction, and wound infection.
- Care for the patient's incision and, if appropriate, the stoma. To decrease discomfort, administer ordered analgesics as necessary and perform comfort measures such as repositioning.
- Encourage the patient to look at the stoma and to participate in caring for it as soon as possible. Teach good hygiene and skin care. Allow him to shower or bathe as soon as the incision heals.
- Consult with an enterostomal therapist, if available, for questions on setting up a postoperative regimen for the patient.
- Watch for adverse effects of radiation therapy (including nausea, vomiting, hair loss, and malaise), and provide comfort measures and reassurance.
- During chemotherapy, watch for complications (such as infection) and expected adverse effects. Prepare the patient for these problems. Take steps to reduce these effects; for example, have the patient rinse his mouth with normal saline mouthwash to deter ulcers.
- To help prevent infection, use strict aseptic technique when caring for I.V. catheters and providing wound care. Change I.V. tubing and sites as directed by facility policy. Have the patient wash his hands before and after meals and after going to the bathroom.
- Listen to the patient's fears and concerns, and stay with him during periods of severe stress and anxiety.
- Encourage the patient to identify actions and care measures that will promote his comfort and relaxation. Try to perform these measures, and encourage the patient and family members to do so as well.
- Whenever possible, include the patient and family members in care decisions.
- If appropriate, explain that the stoma will be red, moist, and swollen; reassure the patient that postoperative swelling eventually subsides.
- Show the patient a diagram of the intestine before and after surgery, stressing how much of the bowel remains intact. Supplement your teaching with instruction booklets (available for a fee from the United Ostomy Association and free from various companies that manufacture ostomy supplies). If possible, arrange a postoperative visit from a recovered ostomy patient.
- Explain to the patient's family members that their positive reactions foster the patient's adjustment.
- If appropriate, instruct the patient with a sigmoid colostomy to perform his own irrigation as soon as he's able after surgery. Advise him to schedule irrigation for the time of the day when he normally evacuates. Many patients find that irrigating

GUIDELINES FOR DETECTING COLORECTAL CANCER

The following recommendations from the American Cancer Society detail screening tests that will allow for the early detection of colorectal cancer. These guidelines apply to men and women age 50 and older.

SCREENING TEST	FREQUENCY RECOMMENDATIONS
Fecal occult blood test (FOBT)	• Every year
Flexible sigmoidoscopy	• Every 5 years
FOBT plus flexible sigmoidoscopy	• FOBT every year • Flexible sigmoidoscopy every 5 years *
Colonoscopy	• Every 10 years
Double-contrast barium enema	• Every 5 years

* Most clinicians prefer the combination of FOBT and flexible sigmoidoscopy over either test alone.

every 1 to 3 days is necessary for regular evacuation.

- Direct the patient to follow a high-fiber diet.
- If flatus, diarrhea, or constipation occurs, tell the patient to eliminate suspected causative foods from his diet. Explain that he may reintroduce them later. Teach him which foods may alleviate constipation, and encourage him to increase his fluid and fiber intake.
- If diarrhea is a problem, advise the patient to try eating applesauce, bananas, or rice. Caution him to take laxatives or antidiarrheal medications only as prescribed by his physician.
- When appropriate, explain that after several months, many patients with an ostomy establish control with irrigation and no longer need to wear a pouch. A stoma cap or gauze sponge placed over the stoma protects it and absorbs mucoid secretions. Explain that before achieving such control, the patient can resume physical activities—including sports—provided he isn't at risk for injuring the stoma or surrounding abdominal muscles.
- If the patient wants to swim, he can place a pouch or stoma cap over the stoma.

He should avoid heavy lifting, which can cause herniation or prolapse through weakened muscles in the abdominal wall. Suggest that he consider a structured, gradually progressive exercise program to strengthen abdominal muscles. Such a program can be instituted under a physician's supervision.

- Emphasize the need for keeping follow-up appointments. Anyone who has had colorectal cancer runs an increased risk of developing another primary cancer. The patient should have yearly screenings (sigmoidoscopy, digital rectal examination, and stool test for blood) and follow-up testing.
- If the patient is to undergo radiation therapy or chemotherapy, explain the treatment to him. Make sure he understands the adverse effects that usually occur and the measures he can take to decrease their severity or prevent their occurrence.
- Instruct the patient and family members about the American Cancer Society's guidelines for colorectal cancer screening, including an annual digital rectal examination as part of a routine physical. (See *Guidelines for detecting colorectal cancer.*)
- Refer the patient to a home health care agency that can check on his physical care at home.

Diverticular disease

Diverticular disease is a disorder in which bulging pouches (diverticula) in the GI wall push the mucosal lining through the surrounding muscle. The most common site for diverticula is in the sigmoid colon, but they may develop anywhere, from the proximal end of the pharynx to the anus. Other typical sites include the duodenum, near the pancreatic border or the ampulla of Vater, and the jejunum. Although diverticular disease of the stomach is rare, it may be a precursor of peptic or neoplastic disease.

Diverticular disease has two clinical forms. In diverticulosis, diverticula are present but don't cause symptoms. In diverticulitis—a far more serious disorder—diverticula become inflamed and can such cause complications as obstruction, infection, and hemorrhage.

CAUSES AND INCIDENCE

Diet, especially highly refined foods, may be a contributing factor. Lack of fiber reduces fecal residue, narrows the bowel lumen, and leads to higher intra-abdominal pressure during defecation.

Diverticular disease is most common in adults aged 45 and older and affects 30% of adults over age 60. It's less common in nations where the diet contains abundant natural bulk and fiber.

PATHOPHYSIOLOGY

A diverticulum develops when pressure in the intestinal lumen is exerted on a weak area, such as a point where blood vessels enter the intestine, causing a break in the muscular continuity of the GI wall. The pressure in the lumen forces the intestine out, creating a pouch (diverticulum).

Diverticulitis occurs when retained undigested food mixed with bacteria accumulates in the diverticulum, forming a hard mass (fecalith). This substance cuts off the blood supply to the diverticulum's thin walls, increasing its susceptibility to attack by colonic bacteria. Inflammation follows bacterial infection. (See *Diverticulosis of the colon*, page 242.)

ASSESSMENT FINDINGS

Usually, the patient with diverticulosis is symptom-free. Occasionally, the history reveals intermittent pain in the left lower abdominal quadrant, which may be relieved by defecation or the passage of flatus. The patient may report alternating bouts of constipation and diarrhea. The assessment usually reveals no clinical findings. Rarely, palpation discloses abdominal tenderness in the left lower quadrant.

The patient with diverticulitis may have a history of diverticulosis, diagnosed incidentally on radiography of the GI tract. Investigation of his dietary history commonly reveals low fiber consumption. He may report recently eating foods that contain seeds or kernels, such as tomatoes, nuts, popcorn, or strawberries, or indigestible roughage, such as celery or corn. Seeds and undigested roughage can block the neck of a diverticulum, causing diverticulitis.

The patient with diverticulitis typically complains of moderate pain in the left lower abdominal quadrant, which he may describe as dull or steady. Straining, lifting, or coughing may aggravate his pain. Other signs and symptoms include mild nausea, flatus, and intermittent bouts of constipation, sometimes accompanied by rectal bleeding. Some patients report diarrhea.

On inspection, the patient with diverticulitis may appear distressed. Palpation may confirm his reports of left lower quadrant abdominal pain. He may have a low-grade fever.

In acute diverticulitis, the patient may report muscle spasms and show signs of

DIVERTICULOSIS OF THE COLON

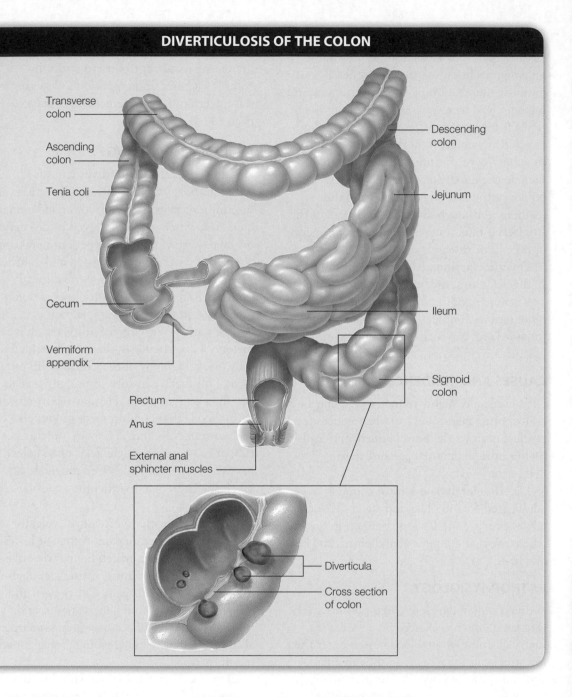

Transverse colon

Ascending colon

Tenia coli

Cecum

Vermiform appendix

Rectum

Anus

External anal sphincter muscles

Descending colon

Jejunum

Ileum

Sigmoid colon

Diverticula

Cross section of colon

peritoneal irritation. Palpation may reveal guarding and rebound tenderness. Rectal examination may disclose a tender mass if the inflamed area is close to the rectum.

COMPLICATIONS

- Rectal hemorrhage
- Portal pyemia from artery or vein erosion
- Fistula

- Obstruction
- Perforation
- Abscess
- Peritonitis

TREATMENT

Patient management depends on the type of diverticular disease and the severity of symptoms. Asymptomatic diverticulosis generally requires no treatment except a high-fiber diet and the avoidance of nuts, seeds, and popcorn. Intestinal diverticulosis that causes pain, mild GI distress, constipation, or difficult defecation may respond to a liquid or low-residue diet, stool softeners, and occasional doses of mineral oil. These measures relieve symptoms, minimize irritation, and lessen the risk of progression to diverticulitis. After pain subsides, patients also benefit from increased water consumption (eight glasses per day), a high-residue diet, and bulk medication such as psyllium.

Treatment for patients with mild diverticulitis without signs of perforation is intended to prevent constipation and combat infection. Therapy may include bed rest, a liquid diet, stool softeners, a broad-spectrum antibiotic, meperidine to control pain and relax smooth muscle, and an antispasmodic such as propantheline to control muscle spasms.

For patients with more severe diverticulitis, treatment consists of the above measures and I.V. therapy. The patient typically needs a nasogastric (NG) tube to relieve intra-abdominal pressure and is allowed nothing by mouth.

Patients who hemorrhage need blood replacement and careful monitoring of fluid and electrolyte balance. Such bleeding usually stops spontaneously. If it continues, angiography for catheter placement and infusion of vasopressin into the bleeding vessel is effective.

Occasionally, surgery may be required. A patient with diverticulitis that doesn't respond to medical treatment or that causes severe recurrent attacks in the same area may need a colon resection to remove a diseased segment of intestine.

NURSING CONSIDERATIONS

When caring for patients with diverticular disease, take the following steps:

- Keep in mind that diverticulitis, which produces more serious symptoms and complications, usually requires more interventions than diverticulosis.
- If the patient is anxious, provide psychological support. Listen to his concerns, and offer reassurance when appropriate.
- Administer medications (antibiotics, stool softeners, and antispasmodics) as ordered. Monitor the patient for the desired effects, and observe for possible adverse reactions. If pain is severe, administer analgesics as ordered.
- Inspect all stools carefully for color and consistency. Note the frequency of bowel movements.
- Maintain bed rest for the patient with acute diverticulitis. Don't permit him to perform any actions that increase intra-abdominal pressure, such as lifting, straining, bending, and coughing.
- Maintain diet as ordered. The patient experiencing an acute attack usually requires a liquid diet. If the patient has severe symptoms or if he experiences nausea and vomiting or abdominal distention, insert an NG tube and attach it to intermittent suction as ordered. Make sure he receives nothing by mouth, and administer ordered I.V. fluids. As symptoms subside, gradually advance the diet. Don't offer foods that could lodge in the diverticulum (such as seeds, nuts, and fruit with peels).

- Monitor the patient for signs and symptoms of complications. Watch for temperature elevation, increasing abdominal pain, blood in stools, and leukocytosis.
- If diverticular bleeding occurs, the patient may require angiography and catheter placement for vasopressin infusion. If so, inspect the insertion site frequently for bleeding, check pedal pulses often, and keep the patient from flexing his legs at the groin. Also watch for vasopressin-induced fluid retention (signaled by apprehension, abdominal cramps, seizures, and oliguria or anuria) and severe hyponatremia (signaled by hypotension; rapid, thready pulse; cold, clammy skin; and cyanosis).
- If surgery is scheduled, provide routine preoperative care. Also perform any special required procedures, such as administering antibiotics and providing a specific diet for several days preoperatively.

After colon resection, take the following steps:

- Watch for signs of infection. Provide meticulous wound care because perforation may have already infected the area. Check drainage sites frequently for signs of infection (pus on dressings and foul odor) or fecal drainage. Change dressings as necessary.
- Watch for signs of postoperative bleeding, such as hypotension and decreased hemoglobin and hematocrit level.
- Record intake and output accurately. Administer I.V. fluids and medications as ordered.
- Keep the NG tube patent. If it dislodges, notify the surgeon at once; don't attempt to reposition it. After the NG tube is removed, advance the patient's diet as ordered, and note how he tolerates diet changes.
- If the patient has a colostomy, provide care and give the patient an opportunity to express his feelings.

- Be sure the patient understands the desired actions and possible adverse effects of his prescribed medications.
- Review recommended dietary changes. Encourage the patient to drink 2 to 3 L of fluid per day. Emphasize the importance of dietary roughage and the harmful effects of constipation and straining during a bowel movement. Advise increasing the intake of foods high in undigestible fiber, such as fresh vegetables, whole grain breads, and wheat or bran cereals. Warn that a high-fiber diet may temporarily cause flatulence. Advise the patient to relieve constipation with stool softeners or bulk-forming cathartics.
- Tell the patient to notify the physician if he has a temperature over 101° F (38.3° C); abdominal pain that is severe or that lasts for more than 3 days; or blood in his stools. Emphasize that these symptoms indicate complications.
- Postoperatively, teach the patient to care for his colostomy as needed. Arrange for a visit by an enterostomal therapist.

Esophageal cancer

Esophageal cancer is a malignant tumor of the esophagus that has various subtypes, primarily squamous cell cancer and adenocarcinoma. The disease is nearly always fatal.

CAUSES AND INCIDENCE

Although the cause of esophageal cancer is unknown, several predisposing factors have been identified. These include chronic irritation from heavy smoking or excessive use of alcohol; stasis-induced inflammation, as in achalasia or stricture; previous head and neck tumors; and nutritional deficiency, as in untreated sprue and Plummer-Vinson syndrome.

Esophageal cancer occurs more frequently in men over age 60. It's found worldwide, but incidence varies geographically, with the disease occurring more frequently in Japan, Russia, China, the Middle East, and the Transkei region of South Africa.

PATHOPHYSIOLOGY

Most esophageal tumors are poorly differentiated squamous cell carcinomas. Adenocarcinomas occur less frequently and are contained to the lower third of the esophagus. Esophageal tumors are usually fungating and infiltrating and partially constrict the lumen of the esophagus.

Regional metastasis occurs early by way of submucosal lymphatics, often fatally invading adjacent vital intrathoracic organs. If the patient survives primary extension, the liver and lungs are the usual sites of distant metastases. Unusual metastasis sites include the bone, kidneys, and adrenal glands. (See *Common esophageal cancers*, page 246.)

ASSESSMENT FINDINGS

Early in the disease, the patient may report a feeling of fullness, pressure, indigestion, or substernal burning. He may also tell you he uses antacids to relieve GI upset. Later, he may complain of dysphagia and weight loss. The degree of dysphagia varies, depending on the extent of disease. At first, the dysphagia is mild, occurring only after the patient eats solid foods, especially meat. Later, the patient has difficulty swallowing coarse foods and, in some cases, liquids.

The patient may complain of hoarseness (from laryngeal nerve involvement), chronic cough (possibly from aspiration), anorexia, vomiting, and regurgitation of food, resulting from the tumor size exceeding the limits of the esophagus. He may also complain of pain on swallowing or pain that radiates to his back.

A patient in the late stages of the disease appears very thin, cachectic, and dehydrated.

COMPLICATIONS

- Inability to control secretions
- Obstruction of the esophagus
- Mediastinitis
- Loss of lower esophageal sphincter control
- Aspiration pneumonia
- Tracheoesophageal or bronchoesophageal fistula
- Aortic perforation

TREATMENT

Esophageal cancer usually is advanced when diagnosed, so surgery and other treatments can only relieve disease effects.

Palliative therapy consists of treatment to keep the esophagus open, including dilation of the esophagus, laser therapy, radiation therapy, and installation of prosthetic tubes (such as the Celestin tube) to bridge the tumor. Radical surgery can excise the tumor and resect either the esophagus alone or the stomach and esophagus. Chemotherapy and radiation therapy can slow the growth of the tumor. Gastrostomy or jejunostomy can help provide adequate nutrition. A prosthesis can be used to seal any fistulas that develop. Endoscopic laser treatment and bipolar electrocoagulation can help restore swallowing by vaporizing cancerous tissue. If the tumor is in the upper esophagus, however, the laser can't be positioned properly. Analgesics are used for pain control.

NURSING CONSIDERATIONS

- Monitor the patient's nutritional and fluid status, and provide him with high-calorie, high-protein foods. If he's having trouble swallowing solids, puree or liquefy his food, and offer a commercially available nutritional supplement. As ordered, provide tube feedings, and prepare him for supplementary parenteral nutrition.

COMMON ESOPHAGEAL CANCERS

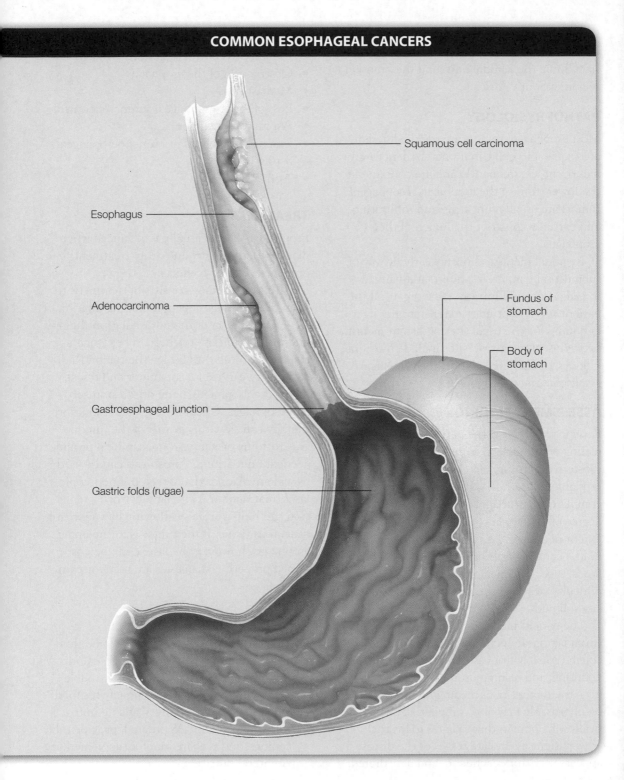

Squamous cell carcinoma

Esophagus

Adenocarcinoma

Gastroesphageal junction

Gastric folds (rugae)

Fundus of stomach

Body of stomach

- To prevent food aspiration, place the patient in Fowler's position for meals and allow plenty of time to eat. If he regurgitates food after eating, provide mouth care.
- If the patient has a gastrostomy tube, give food slowly (over 20 to 30 minutes) by gravity in prescribed amounts (usually 200 to 500 ml). Offer him something to chew before each feeding. This promotes gastric secretions and provides some semblance of normal eating.
- Administer ordered analgesics for pain relief as necessary. Provide comfort measures, such as repositioning and distractions.
- After surgery, monitor the patient's vital signs, fluid and electrolyte balance, and intake and output. Immediately report unexpected changes in the patient's condition. Monitor him for such complications as infection, fistula formation, pneumonia, empyema, and malnutrition.
- If an anastomosis to the esophagus was performed, position the patient flat on his back to prevent tension on the suture line. Watch for signs of an anastomotic leak.
- If the patient had a prosthetic tube inserted, make sure it doesn't become blocked or dislodged. This could cause a perforation of the mediastinum or precipitate tumor erosion.
- After radiation therapy, monitor the patient for such complications as esophageal perforation, pneumonitis and fibrosis of the lungs, and myelitis of the spinal cord.
- After chemotherapy, take steps to decrease adverse effects, such as providing normal saline mouthwash to help prevent mouth ulcers. Allow the patient plenty of rest, and administer medications as ordered to reduce adverse effects.
- Protect the patient from infection.
- Throughout therapy, answer the patient's questions and tell him what to expect from surgery and other therapies. Listen to his fears and concerns, and stay with him during periods of severe anxiety.
- Encourage the patient to identify actions and care measures that promote his comfort and relaxation. Try to perform these measures, and encourage the patient and family members to do so as well.
- Whenever possible, include the patient in care decisions.
- Explain the procedures the patient will undergo after surgery: closed chest drainage, nasogastric suctioning, and placement of gastrostomy tubes.
- If appropriate, instruct family members in gastrostomy tube care. This includes checking tube patency before each feeding, providing skin care around the tube, and keeping the patient upright during and after feedings.
- Stress the need to maintain adequate nutrition. Ask a dietitian to instruct the patient and family members. If the patient has difficulty swallowing solids, instruct him to puree or liquefy his food and to follow a high-calorie, high-protein diet to minimize weight loss. Also, recommend that he add a commercially available, high-calorie supplement to his diet.
- Encourage the patient to follow as normal a routine as possible after recovery from surgery and during radiation therapy and chemotherapy. Tell him that this will help him maintain a sense of control and reduce the complications associated with immobility.
- Advise the patient to rest between activities and to stop an activity that tires him or causes pain.
- Refer the patient and family members to appropriate organizations, such as the American Cancer Society.

Hiatal hernia

Hiatal hernia (also called hiatus hernia) is a defect in the diaphragm that permits a portion of the stomach to pass through the diaphragmatic opening into the chest. It commonly produces no symptoms.

CAUSES AND INCIDENCE

Hernias typically result when an organ protrudes through an abnormal opening in the muscle wall of the cavity that surrounds it. In a hiatal hernia, an increase in intra-abdominal pressure forces a portion of the stomach to protrude through the diaphragm. This increase in intra-abdominal pressure can result from ascites, pregnancy, obesity, wearing constrictive clothing, bending, straining, coughing; Valsalva's maneuver, or extreme physical exertion.

The incidence of this disorder increases with age. By age 60, about 60% of people have hiatal hernias. However, most have no symptoms; the hernia is an incidental finding during a barium swallow, or it may be detected by tests that follow the discovery of occult blood. The prevalence is higher in women than in men.

PATHOPHYSIOLOGY

Three types of hiatal hernia can occur: a sliding hernia, a paraesophageal (rolling) hernia, or a mixed hernia. A mixed hernia includes features of the sliding and rolling hernias. (See *Types of hiatal hernia.*)

The exact cause of a paraesophageal hiatal hernia isn't fully understood. One theory holds that the stomach isn't properly anchored below the diaphragm, permitting the upper portion of the stomach to slide through the esophageal hiatus when intra-abdominal pressure increases.

In a sliding hernia, the muscular collar around the esophageal and diaphragmatic junction loosens, permitting the lower portion of the esophagus and the upper portion of the stomach to rise into the chest when intra-abdominal pressure increases. This muscle weakening may be associated with normal aging, or it may be secondary to esophageal carcinoma, kyphoscoliosis, trauma, or surgery. A sliding hernia may also result from certain diaphragmatic malformations that can cause congenital weakness.

ASSESSMENT FINDINGS

When a sliding hernia causes symptoms, the patient typically complains of heartburn, indicating an incompetent lower esophageal sphincter (LES) and gastroesophageal reflux. The patient history usually reveals that heartburn occurs 1 to 4 hours after eating and is aggravated by reclining, belching, or conditions that increase intra-abdominal pressure. Heartburn may be accompanied by regurgitation or vomiting. The patient may complain of retrosternal or substernal chest pain (typically after meals or at bedtime), reflecting reflux of gastric contents, distention of the stomach, and spasm.

Keep in mind that the patient with a paraesophageal hernia is usually asymptomatic. Because this type of hernia doesn't disturb the closing mechanism of the LES, it doesn't usually cause gastric reflux and reflux esophagitis. Symptoms, when present, usually stem from incarceration of a stomach portion above the diaphragmatic opening. The symptomatic patient may report a feeling of excessive fullness after eating or, if the hernia interferes with breathing, a feeling of breathlessness or suffocation. The patient may also complain of chest pain resembling angina pectoris.

COMPLICATIONS

- Gastroesophageal reflux
- Esophagitis and esophageal ulcers

TYPES OF HIATAL HERNIA

These figures depict the normal stomach and the primary forms of hiatal hernia.

In a sliding hernia, both the stomach and the gastroesophageal junction slip up into the chest, so the gastoesophageal junction is above the diaphragmatic hiatus. This type of hernia causes symptoms if the lower esophageal sphincter (LES) is incompetent, which permits gastric reflux and heartburn.

In a paraesophageal, or rolling, hernia, a part of the greater curvature of the stomach rolls through the diaphragmatic defect. This type of hernia usually doesn't cause gastric reflux and heartburn because the closing mechanism of the LES is unaffected. However, it can cause displacement or stretching of the stomach or lead to strangulation of the herniated portion.

Sliding hernia

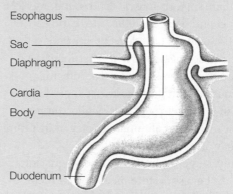

Esophagus
Sac
Diaphragm
Cardia
Body
Duodenum

Normal stomach

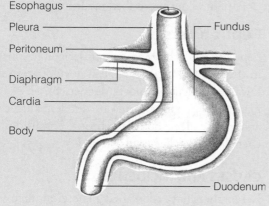

Esophagus
Pleura
Peritoneum
Diaphragm
Cardia
Body
Fundus
Duodenum

Paraesophageal or rolling hernia

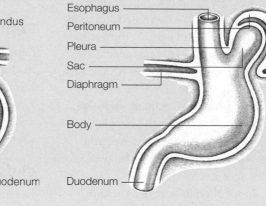

Esophagus
Peritoneum
Pleura
Sac
Diaphragm
Body
Duodenum

- Aspiration pneumonia
- Respiratory distress
- Esophageal stricture
- Esophageal incarceration
- Gastric ulcer
- Peritonitis

TREATMENT

The goal of therapy is to relieve symptoms by minimizing or correcting the incompetent LES (if present) and to manage and prevent complications. Drugs, activity modifications, and diet changes reduce gastroesophageal reflux.

Antacids neutralize refluxed fluids; using antacids is probably the best treatment for intermittent reflux. Intensive antacid therapy may call for hourly dosing; however, the choice of antacids should take into account the patient's bowel function. Histamine-2 receptor antagonists also modify the acidity of fluid refluxed into the esophagus.

Drug therapy to strengthen LES tone may consist of a cholinergic agent such as bethanechol. Metoclopramide has also been used to stimulate smooth-muscle contraction, increase LES tone, and decrease reflux after eating.

Other measures to reduce intermittent reflux include restricting any activity that increases intra-abdominal pressure and discouraging smoking because it stimulates gastric acid production. Modifying the diet to include smaller, more frequent meals and eliminating spicy or irritating foods may also reduce reflux.

Rarely, surgery is required when signs and symptoms persist despite medical treatment or if complications develop. Indications for surgery include esophageal stricture, significant bleeding, pulmonary aspiration, or incarceration or strangulation of the herniated stomach portion. Techniques vary, but most forms of surgery create an artificial closing mechanism at the gastroesophageal junction to strengthen the barrier function of the LES. The surgeon may use an abdominal or a thoracic approach. Laparoscopic surgery to repair the hernia is now commonplace. A newer treatment involves thorascopic surgery, with the hernia repaired microscopically.

Rare postsurgical complications include mucosal erosion, ulcers, and bleeding of the gastric pouch; pressure on the left lung due to the size and placement of the pouch; and formation of a volvulus.

A sliding hernia without an incompetent sphincter rarely produces reflux or symptoms and thus requires no treatment. A large rolling hernia and most paraesophageal hernias should be surgically repaired (even if no symptoms are produced) because of the high risk of complications, especially strangulation.

NURSING CONSIDERATIONS

- Prepare the patient for diagnostic tests. After endoscopy, watch for signs and symptoms of perforation (decreasing blood pressure, rapid pulse, shock, and sudden pain) caused by the endoscope.
- Administer prescribed antacids and other medications, and monitor the patient's response.
- To reduce intra-abdominal pressure and prevent aspiration, have the patient sleep in a reverse Trendelenburg position (with the head of the bed elevated 6″ to 12″ [15 to 30 cm]).
- If surgery is necessary, prepare the patient and provide appropriate preoperative and postoperative care.
- Explain significant symptoms, diagnostic tests, and prescribed treatments. Teach the patient about prescribed medications.

Peptic ulcers

Peptic ulcers, which are circumscribed lesions in the mucosal membrane, can develop in the lower esophagus, stomach, duodenum, or jejunum. The major forms are duodenal ulcer and gastric ulcer; both are chronic conditions. (See *Understanding peptic ulcers.*)

CAUSES AND INCIDENCE

Researchers have identified a bacterial infection with *Helicobacter pylori* as a leading cause of peptic ulcer disease. They also found that *H. pylori* release a toxin that promotes mucosal inflammation and ulceration.

In a peptic ulcer resulting from *H. pylori*, acid seems to be mainly a contributor to the consequences of the bacterial infection rather than its dominant cause. Other risk factors include the use of certain medications—nonsteroidal anti-inflammatory drugs (NSAIDs), for example—and pathologic hypersecretory states, such as Zollinger-Ellison syndrome.

Duodenal ulcers, which account for about 80 % of peptic ulcers, affect the proximal part of the small intestine. These ulcers, which

UNDERSTANDING PEPTIC ULCERS

A GI lesion isn't necessarily an ulcer. Lesions that don't extend below the mucosal lining (epithelium) are called erosions. Lesions of both acute and chronic ulcers can extend through the epithelium and perforate the stomach wall. Chronic ulcers also have scar tissue at the base.

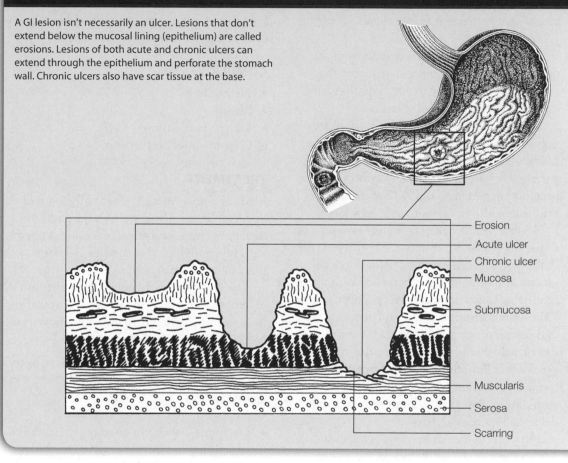

- Erosion
- Acute ulcer
- Chronic ulcer
- Mucosa
- Submucosa
- Muscularis
- Serosa
- Scarring

occur most commonly in men between ages 20 and 50, follow a chronic course characterized by remissions and exacerbations. About 5 % to 10 % of patients with duodenal ulcers develop complications that necessitate surgery.

Gastric ulcers, which affect the stomach mucosa, are most common in middle-aged and older men, especially among those who are poor and undernourished. They also tend to occur in chronic users of aspirin or alcohol. In older adults, peptic ulcer disease carries a mortality rate of 80%.

PATHOPHYSIOLOGY

Although the stomach contains acidic secretions that can digest substances, intrinsic defenses protect the gastric mucosal membrane from injury. A thick, tenacious layer of gastric mucus protects the stomach from autodigestion, mechanical trauma, and chemical trauma. Prostaglandins provide another line of defense. Gastric ulcers may be a result of destruction of the mucosal barrier.

The duodenum is protected from ulceration by the function of Brunner's glands. These glands produce a viscid, mucoid, alkaline secretion that neutralizes the acid chyme. Duodenal ulcers appear to result from excessive acid protection.

H. pylori release a toxin that destroys the gastric and duodenal mucosa, reducing the epithelium's resistance to acid digestion and causing gastritis and ulcer disease.

Salicylates and other NSAIDs inhibit the secretion of prostaglandins (substances that block ulceration). Certain illnesses, such as pancreatitis, hepatic disease, Crohn's disease, preexisting gastritis, and Zollinger-Ellison syndrome, also contribute to ulceration.

Several factors can also predispose a patient to peptic ulcers. For instance, blood type (type A for gastric ulcers and type O for duodenal ulcers) and other genetic factors make it more likely that a patient will develop a peptic ulcer. Exposure to irritants, such as tobacco, alcohol, and coffee, may contribute by accelerating gastric acid emptying and promoting mucosal breakdown. Emotional stress also contributes to ulcer formation because of the increased stimulation of acid and pepsin secretion and decreased mucosal defense.

Physical trauma and normal aging also add to the risk. As a person ages, his pyloric sphincter may wear down, permitting the reflux of bile into the stomach. This appears to be a common contributor to the development of gastric ulcers in older adults.

ASSESSMENT FINDINGS

Assessment findings may vary according to the type of ulcer. The patient with a gastric ulcer may report pain that worsens with eating, the result of food stretching the mucosa. He may also complain of nausea and vomiting secondary to mucosal stretching.

The patient with a duodenal ulcer may complain of gnawing, dull, aching, or hunger-like epigastric pain, the result of excessive acid production. Food or antacids may relieve the pain, but it usually recurs in 2 to 4 hours when food no longer acts as a buffer to acid.

COMPLICATIONS

- Hemorrhage
- Shock
- Gastric perforation
- Gastric outlet obstruction

TREATMENT

Medical management is essentially symptomatic, emphasizing drug therapy, physical rest, dietary changes, and stress reduction. Patients with severe signs and symptoms or complications may require surgery.

The goal of drug therapy is to eradicate *H. pylori*, reduce gastric secretions, protect the mucosa from further damage, and relieve pain. Medications may include:

- bismuth and two other antimicrobial agents, usually tetracycline or amoxicillin and metronidazole
- antacids to reduce gastric acidity
- histamine-2 receptor antagonists, such as cimetidine or ranitidine, to reduce gastric secretion for short-term therapy (up to 12 weeks), or a proton pump inhibitor such as lansoprazole for 12 weeks
- coating agents, such as sucralfate, for duodenal ulcers (sucralfate forms complexes with proteins at the base of an ulcer, forming a protective coat that prevents further digestive action of acid and pepsin)
- antisecretory agents such as misoprostol if the ulceration resulted from NSAID use and the NSAID must be continued for another condition such as arthritis
- sedatives and tranquilizers, such as chlordiazepoxide and phenobarbital, for patients with gastric ulcers

- anticholinergics such as propantheline to inhibit the vagus nerve effect on the parietal cells and to reduce gastrin production and excessive gastric activity in duodenal ulcers (these drugs are usually contraindicated in gastric ulcers).

Standard therapy also includes physical rest and decreased activity, which help decrease the amount of gastric secretion. Diet therapy may consist of eating six small meals daily (or small hourly meals) rather than three regular meals.

If GI bleeding occurs, emergency treatment begins with passage of a nasogastric (NG) tube to allow iced saline lavage, possibly containing norepinephrine. Gastroscopy allows visualization of the bleeding site and coagulation by laser or cautery to control bleeding. This therapy allows surgery to be postponed until the patient's condition stabilizes.

Surgery is indicated for perforation, unresponsiveness to conservative treatment, suspected cancer, and other complications. The type of surgery chosen for peptic ulcers depends on the location and extent of the disorder.

NURSING CONSIDERATIONS

When caring for a patient with a peptic ulcer, take the following steps:

- Administer prescribed medications. Monitor the patient for the desired effects and watch for adverse reactions. Most medications should alleviate the patient's discomfort, so ask whether his pain is relieved.
- Provide six small meals or small hourly meals as ordered. Advise the patient to eat slowly, chew thoroughly, and have small snacks between meals.
- Schedule the patient's care so that he can get plenty of rest.
- Continuously monitor the patient for complications: hemorrhage (sudden onset of weakness, fainting, chills, dizziness, thirst, the desire to defecate, and passage of loose, tarry, or even red stools); perforation (acute onset of epigastric pain followed by lessening of the pain and the onset of a rigid abdomen, tachycardia, fever, or rebound tenderness); obstruction (feeling of fullness or heaviness, copious vomiting containing undigested food after meals); and penetration (pain radiating to the back, night distress). If any of these occurs, notify the physician immediately.

After surgery, take the following steps:

- Keep the NG tube (that was inserted in the operating room) patent. If the tube isn't functioning, don't reposition it; you could damage the suture line or anastomosis. Notify the surgeon promptly.
- Monitor intake and output, including NG tube drainage. Also, check bowel sounds. Allow the patient nothing by mouth until peristalsis resumes and the NG tube is removed or clamped.
- Replace fluids and electrolytes. Assess for signs of dehydration, sodium deficiency, and metabolic alkalosis, which can occur secondary to gastric suction. Provide parenteral nutrition if ordered; it's usually given if the patient isn't allowed to eat for 1 week or more.
- Control postoperative pain with narcotics and analgesics as ordered.
- Watch for and report complications: hemorrhage; shock; iron, folate, or vitamin B_{12} deficiency anemia; and dumping syndrome.
- Teach the patient about peptic ulcer disease, and help him to recognize its signs and symptoms. Explain scheduled diagnostic tests and prescribed therapies. Review symptoms associated with complications, and urge him to notify the physician if any of these occur. Emphasize the importance

of complying with treatment, even after his symptoms are relieved.

- Review the proper use of prescribed medications, discussing the desired actions and possible adverse effects of each drug.
- Instruct the patient to take antacids 1 hour after meals. If he follows a sodium-restricted diet, advise him to take only low-sodium antacids. Caution him that antacids may cause changes in bowel habits (diarrhea with magnesium-containing antacids, constipation with aluminum-containing antacids).
- Check all medications the patient is using. Antacids inhibit the absorption of many other drugs, including digoxin. Work out a schedule for taking medications.
- Warn against excessive intake of coffee and alcoholic beverages during exacerbations.
- Encourage the patient to make appropriate lifestyle changes. Explain that emotional tension can precipitate an ulcer attack and prolong healing. Help the patient identify anxiety-producing situations, and teach him to perform relaxation techniques, such as distraction and meditation.
- If the patient smokes, urge him to stop because smoking stimulates gastric acid secretion. Refer him to a smoking-cessation program.
- Tell the patient to read labels of non-prescription medications and to avoid preparations that contain corticosteroids, aspirin, or other NSAIDs such as ibuprofen. Explain that these drugs inhibit mucus secretion and therefore leave the GI tract vulnerable to injury from gastric acid. Advise him to use alternative analgesics such as acetaminophen. Caution him to avoid systemic antacids such as sodium bicarbonate, because they're absorbed into the circulation and can cause an acid-base imbalance.
- Tell the patient that, although cimetidine, famotidine, and other histamine-receptor antagonists are available over-the-counter, he shouldn't take them without consulting his physician. These drugs may duplicate prescribed medications or suppress important symptoms.
- To avoid dumping syndrome after gastric surgery, advise the patient to lie down after meals, drink fluids between meals rather than with meals, avoid eating large amounts of carbohydrates, and eat four to six small high-protein, low-carbohydrate meals daily.

Endocrine System

The endocrine system consists of various tissues and glands that produce and secrete hormones into the bloodstream. With age, the rates of hormone secretion and metabolic degradation change, as does target tissue sensitivity to hormonal stimulation.

In older adults, endocrine disorders represent potentially hidden sources of illness and death. For example, diabetes mellitus or thyroid disease can progress silently until severe enough to cause significant complications. Often, these disorders are discovered incidentally during a routine examination or a workup for another condition.

Diabetes mellitus grows more prevalent with age. What's more, an older adult may lack the classic diabetes symptoms of polydipsia, polyphagia, and polyuria. Instead, diagnosis may not come until the patient has complications, such as cataracts, neuropathy, foot ulcers, peripheral vascular disease, or even hypoglycemic nonketotic coma.

In the thyroid, age-related changes diminish glandular substance and may cause fibrosis and lymphocyte infiltration. Nodules and small, firm goiters that could interfere with normal thyroid functioning also become more common with age. Hypothyroidism can be difficult to diagnose because its symptoms closely resemble the effects of normal aging.

Hyperthyroidism is seven times more common after age 60. As with diabetes, an older adult with hyperthyroidism may have few symptoms and lack the typical restlessness, hyperactivity, and nervous appearance. Symptoms of coexisting diseases may further confuse the clinical picture.

Make sure you understand what to look for to detect endocrine disorders in your older adult patients. By recognizing the differences in how endocrine disorders can present in older patients, you can help uncover potentially dangerous illnesses.

Diabetes mellitus

Diabetes mellitus is a chronic disease of absolute or relative insulin deficiency or resistance that produces a hyperglycemic state. It's characterized by disturbances in carbohydrate, protein, and fat metabolism.

Normally, insulin transports glucose into the cells for use as energy and storage as glycogen. It also stimulates protein synthesis and free fatty acid storage in the adipose tissues. Insulin deficiency compromises the body tissues' access to essential nutrients for fuel and storage.

Diabetes mellitus occurs in two primary forms: Type 1, characterized by absolute insufficiency, and the more prevalent type II, characterized by insulin resistance with varying degrees of insulin secretory defects.

Culture Certain tribes of Native North Americans have high rates of type 2 diabetes mellitus; in some tribes, the rate of disease is 154% higher than other groups in the United States. Some practices that may contribute to this high rate of disease include:

- diets high in calories, carbohydrates, and fats
- high rates of obesity
- a sedentary lifestyle
- viewing a heavier body as the ideal body type (thinness is viewed as not being healthy).

These populations—as well as other high-risk groups, such as Hispanics and African-Americans—require more frequent screenings for the disease.

CAUSES AND INCIDENCE

The etiology of both type 1 and type 2 diabetes remains unknown. Genetic factors may play a part in the development of all types. Autoimmune disease and viral infections may be risk factors in type I; a sedentary lifestyle and diet have been linked to the development of type II.

Other risk factors include:

- obesity, which contributes to the resistance to endogenous insulin
- physiologic or emotional stress, which can cause prolonged elevation of stress hormone levels (cortisol, epinephrine, glucagon, and growth hormone); this increases blood glucose levels, which in turn places increased demands on the pancreas
- metabolic syndrome, a precursor to the development of type II diabetes mellitus; the rate of metabolic syndrome in older adults is at least 42% higher than the general population for adults ages 60 to 69 and 43% higher for adults age 70 or older
- taking medications that can antagonize the effects of insulin, including thiazide diuretics, adrenal corticosteroids, and oral contraceptives.

The onset of type 1 usually occurs before age 30, although it may occur at any age; the patient usually is thin and requires exogenous insulin and dietary management to achieve control. Type 2 usually occurs in obese adults after age 40, although it's becoming more common in North American youths. It's typically treated with diet and exercise, in combination with antidiabetic drugs; treatment may include insulin therapy.

Diabetes mellitus is thought to affect about 6.3% of the population of the United States (18 million people); about one-third remains undiagnosed. Incidence is essentially the same between males and females and increases with age.

PATHOPHYSIOLOGY

Type 1 and type 2 diabetes mellitus are two separate, distinct pathophysiologic entities. In people genetically susceptible to type 1 diabetes, a triggering event, possibly a viral infection, causes the production of autoantibodies, which kill the beta cells of the pancreas. This leads to a decline in and an ultimate lack of insulin secretion. Insulin deficiency—when more than 90% of the beta cells have been destroyed—leads to hyperglycemia, enhanced lipolysis, and protein catabolism.

Type 2 diabetes mellitus is a chronic disease caused by impaired insulin production, inappropriate hepatic glucose production, peripheral insulin receptor insensitivity, or a combination of these factors. Antibodies may destroy insulin, impairing the body's ability to produce insulin and leading to uncontrolled glucose levels.

ASSESSMENT FINDINGS

The patient with type 1 diabetes usually reports rapidly developing signs and symptoms. The patient with type 2 diabetes typically has vague, long-standing signs and symptoms that develop gradually. Insulin deficiency causes hyperglycemia, which pulls fluid from body tissues, causing osmotic diuresis, polyuria, dehydration, polydipsia, dry mucous membranes, and poor skin turgor. These patients generally report a family history of diabetes mellitus, gestational diabetes or the delivery of a baby weighing more than 9 lb (4 kg), severe viral infection, other endocrine disease, recent stress or trauma, or use of drugs that increase blood glucose levels.

In ketoacidosis and hyperosmolar nonketotic state, dehydration can cause hypovolemia and shock. Wasting of glucose in the urine usually produces weight loss and hunger in uncontrolled type 1 diabetes, even if the patient eats voraciously. Patients may complain of weakness; vision changes; frequent skin and urinary tract infections; dry, itchy skin; sexual problems; and vaginal discomfort, all of which are symptoms of hyperglycemia. *Candida albicans*, a common fungal infection, occurs in folds of the skin under the breasts, around the nails, and between toes.

Inspection may show retinopathy or cataract formation. Skin changes, especially on the legs and feet, may indicate impaired peripheral circulation. Common findings include light brown, scaly patches (dermopathy) that result from small-vessel damage.

Muscle wasting and loss of subcutaneous fat may be evident in type 1 diabetes; type 2 is characterized by obesity, particularly in the abdominal area. Long-term effects produce signs of neuropathy, atherosclerosis, and peripheral and autonomic neuropathy. Peripheral neuropathy usually affects the hands and feet and may produce numbness or pain. The patient may also have an undetected injury or infected wound because of impaired sensation.

A patient with autonomic neuropathy may experience gastroparesis leading to delayed gastric emptying and a feeling of nausea or fullness after eating. He may also report nocturnal diarrhea and impotence.

Palpation may disclose poor skin turgor and dry mucous membranes related to dehydration. Decreased peripheral pulses, cool skin temperature, and decreased reflexes may also be palpable. Assessment of the feet using a monofilament and a tuning fork may disclose a loss of protective sensation. Auscultation may reveal orthostatic hypotension. Patients with ketoacidosis may have a characteristic fruity breath odor because of increased acetone production.

Older adults with type 2 diabetes often experience depression and memory problems; you may observe that he appears depressed and anxious and has poor short-term memory.

COMPLICATIONS

- Cardiovascular disease
- Nephropathy
- Retinopathy
- Ketoacidosis and hyperosmolar coma
- Infections
- Foot deformity

TREATMENT

For patients with type 1 diabetes, treatment includes insulin replacement, diet, and exercise. Current forms of insulin-replacement include single-dose, mixed-dose, split mixed-dose, and multiple-dose regimens. The multiple-dose regimens may include use of an insulin pump.

Patients may take rapid-acting (regular or lispro), intermediate-acting (NPH), long-acting (insulin glargine), or a combination of rapid-acting and intermediate-acting (70/30 or 50/50 of NPH and regular) human insulin mixed together.

Some patients may benefit from taking lispro in place of regular insulin because it has a rapid onset (15 minutes) and doesn't require waiting to eat after injection. The drug also has a short duration of action (4 hours), which decreases between-meal and nocturnal hypoglycemia. Islet cell or pancreas transplantation is available if the patient doesn't respond well to drug therapy and requires chronic immunosuppression.

Patients with type 2 diabetes may require oral antidiabetic drugs to stimulate endogenous insulin production, increase insulin sensitivity at the cellular level, suppress hepatic gluconeogenesis, and delay GI absorption of carbohydrates. Studies have shown that treatment with a lipase inhibitor (such as orlistat) combined with a low-calorie diet significantly decreases the weight of overweight patients with type 2 diabetes. Patients following this therapy also displayed improvements in glycemic control and cardiovascular risk profile; levels of glycosylated hemoglobin, fasting glucose, and postprandial glucose also improved significantly.

A patient with either type of diabetes requires a planned diet that meets nutritional needs, controls blood glucose levels, and allows him to reach and maintain an appropriate body weight. An obese patient with type 2 diabetes also needs to lose weight. A patient with type 1 diabetes may need a high-calorie diet, depending on his growth stage and activity level. For success, the patient must follow the diet consistently and eat meals at regular times.

Vitamin E is under investigation because its cellular effects may reduce the risk of macrovascular disease in patients with type 2 diabetes. Researchers have confirmed its antioxidant effects and discovered that, in high doses, it acts as an anti-inflammatory. It's also thought that, because vitamin E reduces plaque formation at the endothelial level, it may decrease the risk of heart disease and stroke. Vitamin E may also have an effect on the metabolic syndrome that causes type 2 diabetes and may prevent the disease from occurring, although the American Diabetic Association questions the efficacy and long-term safety of vitamin E.

NURSING CONSIDERATIONS

- Keep accurate records of vital signs, weight, fluid intake, urine output, and calorie intake. Monitor serum glucose and urine acetone levels.
- Monitor for acute complications of diabetic therapy, especially hypoglycemia (vagueness, slow cerebration, dizziness, weakness, pallor, tachycardia, diaphoresis, seizures, and coma); immediately give carbohydrates in the form of fruit juice, hard candy, honey or, if the patient is unconscious, glucagon or I.V. dextrose. Agencies identify specific protocols for management of hypoglycemia.
- Watch for signs of hyperosmolar coma (polyuria, thirst, neurologic abnormalities, and stupor). This hyperglycemic crisis requires I.V. fluids and insulin replacement.
- Monitor diabetic effects on the cardiovascular system, such as cerebrovascular, coronary artery, and peripheral vascular impairment, and on the peripheral and autonomic nervous systems.
- Provide meticulous skin care, especially to the feet and legs. Treat all injuries, cuts, and blisters. Avoid constricting hose, slippers, and bed linens. Refer the patient to a podiatrist.
- Observe for signs of urinary tract and vaginal infections. Encourage adequate fluid intake.
- Monitor the patient for signs of diabetic neuropathy (numbness or pain in the hands and feet, footdrop, and neurogenic bladder).
- Consult a dietitian to plan a diet with the recommended allowances of calories, protein, carbohydrates, and fats, based on the patient's particular requirements.
- Encourage the patient to verbalize feelings about diabetes and its effects on lifestyle and life expectancy. Offer emotional support and a realistic assessment of his condition. Stress that with proper treatment, he can have a near-normal lifestyle and life expectancy. Assist the patient to develop coping strategies. Refer him and his family to a counselor if necessary. Encourage them to join a support group.
- Stress the importance of carefully adhering to the prescribed program and blood glucose control. Tailor your teaching to the patient's needs and abilities. Discuss diet, medications, exercise, monitoring techniques, hygiene, and how to prevent and recognize hypoglycemia and hyperglycemia.
- To encourage compliance to lifestyle changes, emphasize how blood glucose control affects long-term health. Tell the patient he and his physician will need to determine appropriate A1C test goals based on the American Diabetes Association's current standards.
- For a willing older patient who is active, has good cognitive function, and is likely to live long enough to benefit from a regimen that helps to prevent complications, explain the benefits of intensive glycemic, blood pressure, and lipid control, using the goals for younger adults with diabetes. For an older patient with a history of severe hypoglycemia, limited life expectancy, comorbid conditions, or longstanding diabetes with minimal or stable complications, less stringent A1C goals may be appropriate.
- Monitory pharmacologic therapy closely for older patients, watching for signs of complications. Keep in mind that medications will start at the lowest dose and be titrated

up to achieve the target glycemic control without adverse effects. Use caution for patients with renal insufficiency receiving metformin. For patients taking thiazolidine-diones, watch for signs of fluid retention and heart failure. Be alert for signs of hypoglyce-mia for patients taking sulfonylureas, other insulin secretagogues, and insulin. Keep in mind that patients or caregivers using insu-lin must have the visual ability, motor skills, and cognitive functioning to administer the drug safely.

- Teach the patient how to care for his feet: He should wash them daily, carefully dry between his toes, and inspect for corns, calluses, redness, swelling, bruises, and breaks in the skin. Urge him to report any skin changes to the physician. Advise him to wear comfortable, nonconstricting shoes and never to walk barefoot.
- Urge annual regular ophthalmologic examinations for early detection of diabetic retinopathy. Describe the signs and symp-toms of diabetic neuropathy, and emphasize the need for safety precautions because decreased sensation can mask injuries.
- Teach the patient how to manage diabetes when he has a minor illness, such as a cold, flu, or upset stomach.
- To prevent diabetes, teach people at high risk to avoid risk factors; for example, they should maintain proper weight and exercise regularly.
- Teach the patient and his family how to monitor the patient's diet. Show them how to read labels in the supermarket to iden-tify fat, carbohydrate, protein, and sugar content.
- Encourage the patient and his family to contact the American Association of Diabetes Educators and the American Diabetes Association to obtain additional information.

Hypoglycemia

Hypoglycemia is a potentially dangerous abnormally low blood glucose level. It occurs when glucose burns up too rapidly, when the glucose release rate falls behind tissue demands, or when excessive insulin enters the bloodstream. As it does when deprived of oxygen, the brain stops functioning properly when deprived of glucose. Prolonged glucose deprivation can result in tissue damage, and even death.

Two types of hypoglycemia can occur: reactive and fasting. Reactive hypoglycemia results from the body's reaction to diges-tion or from the administration of excessive insulin. Fasting hypoglycemia causes discom-fort during periods of abstinence from food, with blood glucose levels decreasing gradu-ally. This rare type of hypoglycemia occurs most commonly in the early morning before breakfast.

Hypoglycemia tends to cause vague signs and symptoms that depend on how quickly the patient's glucose levels drop. Gradual onset of hypoglycemia produces predominantly central nervous system (CNS) signs and symptoms; a more rapid decline in plasma glucose levels results predominantly in adrenergic signs and symptoms.

CAUSES AND INCIDENCE

The two forms of hypoglycemia have differ-ent causes and occur in different types of patients. In a diabetic patient, reactive hypoglycemia may result from the administration of too much insulin or—less commonly—too much oral antidiabetic medi-cation. In a mildly diabetic patient (or one in the early stages of diabetes mellitus), reactive hypoglycemia may result from delayed and excessive insulin production after carbohy-drate ingestion.

A nondiabetic patient may also suffer reactive hypoglycemia from a sharp increase in insulin output after a meal. Sometimes called postprandial hypoglycemia, this type of reactive hypoglycemia usually disappears when the patient eats something sweet. In some patients, reactive hypoglycemia has no known cause (idiopathic reactive). It also may result from gastric dumping syndrome from total parenteral nutrition, or from impaired glucose tolerance.

Fasting hypoglycemia usually results from an excess of insulin or insulin-like substance or from a decrease in counterregulatory hormones. It can be exogenous, resulting from external factors, such as alcohol and drug ingestion, or endogenous, resulting from organic problems. Endogenous hypoglycemia may result from tumors or liver disease. Insulinomas—small islet cell tumors in the pancreas—secrete excessive amounts of insulin, which inhibits hepatic glucose production. The tumors are benign in 90% of patients.

Nonendocrine causes of fasting hypoglycemia include severe liver diseases, such as hepatitis, cancer, cirrhosis, and liver congestion associated with heart failure. All these conditions reduce the uptake and release of glycogen from the liver.

Endocrine causes include destruction of pancreatic islet cells; adrenocortical insufficiency, which contributes to hypoglycemia by reducing the production of cortisol and cortisone needed for gluconeogenesis; and pituitary insufficiency, which reduces corticotropin and growth hormone levels.

PATHOPHYSIOLOGY

Metabolism in the brain depends primarily on glucose from the blood supply. The brain can convert a limited amount of glucose from glycogen stored in brain cells, but it uses up this supply within minutes. As a result, the brain is one of the first organs affected by falling blood glucose levels. In most people, a subtle reduction of mental efficiency progresses to impairment of judgment, seizures, and coma. Prolonged hypoglycemia may result in permanent brain damage.

Nervous, hormonal, and metabolic responses also occur. Other changes include glycogenolysis in muscle and liver tissue, where glycogen is stored. This is a hormonal response to epinephrine and glucagon, a pancreatic peptide triggered by low blood glucose levels.

ASSESSMENT FINDINGS

The history of a patient with suspected hypoglycemia should include the pattern of food intake for the preceding 24 hours as well as drug and alcohol use. The medical or surgical history may disclose causative factors, such as gastrectomy and hepatic disease.

A patient with reactive hypoglycemia may report adrenergic symptoms, such as diaphoresis, anxiety, hunger, nervousness, and weakness, indicating a rapid decline in blood glucose levels. A patient with fasting hypoglycemia may report signs and symptoms of CNS disturbance, such as dizziness, headache, clouding of vision, restlessness, and mental status changes, indicating a slow decline in blood glucose levels. With prolonged glucose deprivation, the patient's history (obtained from family or friends, if necessary) may reveal seizures, decreasing level of consciousness (LOC), and coma. A patient with pharmacologic hypoglycemia may experience a rapid or slow decline in blood glucose levels.

Inspection may reveal adrenergic signs, such as diaphoresis, pallor, and tremor; or CNS signs, such as restlessness, loss of fine-motor skills, and altered LOC. Palpation may disclose tachycardia.

COMPLICATIONS

- Permanent brain damage
- Falls and injury
- Death

TREATMENT

Reactive hypoglycemia requires dietary modification to help delay glucose absorption and gastric emptying. Such modifications typically include small, frequent meals; avoiding simple carbohydrates (including alcohol and fruit drinks); and consuming complex carbohydrates, fiber, and fat. The patient may also receive anticholinergic drugs to slow gastric emptying and intestinal motility and to inhibit vagal stimulation of insulin release.

For fasting hypoglycemia, the patient may require surgery and drug therapy. A patient with insulinoma should have the tumor removed. Drug therapy may include nondiuretic thiazides such as diazoxide to inhibit insulin secretion, streptozocin and hormones such as glucocorticoids, and long-lasting glycogen.

For severe hypoglycemia (producing confusion or coma), initial treatment is usually I.V. administration of a bolus of dextrose 50% solution. This is followed by a constant infusion of glucose until the patient can eat a meal. A patient who experiences adrenergic reactions without CNS symptoms may receive oral carbohydrates (parenteral therapy isn't required).

NURSING CONSIDERATIONS

- Watch for and report signs of hypoglycemia in high-risk patients.
- Implement measures to protect the unconscious patient, such as maintaining a patent airway.
- Monitor infusion of hypertonic glucose to avoid hyperglycemia, circulatory overload, and cellular dehydration. Terminate glucose

solutions gradually to prevent hypoglycemia caused by hyperinsulinemia.

- Measure blood glucose levels as ordered.
- Monitor the effects of drug therapy, and watch for the development of any adverse reactions.
- Explain the purpose, preparation, and procedure for any diagnostic tests.
- Emphasize the importance of carefully following the prescribed diet to prevent a rapid drop in blood glucose levels. Advise the patient to eat small meals throughout the day, and mention that bedtime snacks may be necessary to keep blood glucose at an even level. Instruct the patient to avoid alcohol and caffeine because they may trigger severe hypoglycemic episodes.
- If the patient is obese and has impaired glucose tolerance, suggest ways he can restrict his caloric intake and lose weight. If necessary, help him find a weight-loss support group.
- Warn the patient with fasting hypoglycemia not to postpone or skip meals and snacks. Instruct the patient to call his physician for instructions if he doesn't feel well enough to eat.
- Discuss lifestyle and personal habits to help the patient identify precipitating factors, such as poor diet, stress, or noncompliance with diabetes mellitus treatment. Explain ways that he can change or avoid each precipitating factor. If necessary, teach him stress-reduction techniques, and encourage him to join a support group.
- Teach the patient about precautions to take when exercising; for example, tell him to consume extra calories and not to exercise alone or when his blood glucose level is likely to drop.
- Inform the patient that he should carry a source of fast-acting carbohydrates (such as hard candy) with him at all times. Advise him to wear a medical identification

MANAGING MYXEDEMA COMA

Myxedema coma is a medical emergency that is commonly fatal. Progression is usually gradual, but when stress aggravates severe or prolonged hypothyroidism, coma may develop abruptly. Examples of severe stress include infection, exposure to cold, and trauma. Other precipitating factors include thyroid medication withdrawal and the use of a sedative, an opioid, or an anesthetic.

Patients in myxedema coma have significantly depressed respirations, so their partial pressure of carbon dioxide in arterial blood may increase. Decreased cardiac output and worsening cerebral hypoxia may also occur. The patient is stuporous and hypothermic, and her vital signs reflect bradycardia and hypotension.

Lifesaving Interventions

If your patient becomes comatose, begin these interventions as soon as possible:

- Maintain airway patency with ventilatory support if necessary.
- Maintain circulation through I.V. fluid replacement.
- Provide continuous electrocardiogram monitoring.
- Monitor arterial blood gases to detect hypoxia and metabolic acidosis.
- Warm the patient by wrapping her in blankets. Don't use a warming blanket because it might increase peripheral vasodilation, causing shock.
- Monitor body temperature until stable with a low-reading thermometer.
- Replace thyroid hormone by administering large doses of I.V. levothyroxine as ordered. Monitor vital signs because rapid correction of hypothyroidism can cause adverse cardiac reactions.
- Monitor intake and output and daily weight. With treatment, urine output should increase and body weight should decrease; if not, report this to the physician.
- Replace fluids and other substances such as glucose. Monitor serum electrolyte levels.
- Administer a corticosteroid as ordered.
- Check for possible sources of infection, such as blood, sputum, or urine, which may have precipitated the coma. Treat infections or any other underlying illness.

bracelet or to carry a medical identification card that describes his condition and its emergency treatment measures.

- For the patient with pharmacologic hypoglycemia from insulin or oral antidiabetic agents, review the essentials of managing diabetes mellitus, if indicated.
- If warranted, teach the patient about prescribed drug therapy or surgery.
- Because hypoglycemia is a chronic disorder, encourage the patient to see his physician regularly.
- Encourage the patient and his family to discuss their concerns about the patient's condition and treatment.

Hypothyroidism

In hypothyroidism, metabolic processes slow down because of a deficiency of the thyroid hormones triiodothyronine (T_3) or thyroxine (T_4).

Hypothyroidism is classified as primary or secondary. Primary hypothyroidism stems from a disorder of the thyroid gland itself. Secondary hypothyroidism is caused by a failure to stimulate normal thyroid function or by a failure of target tissues to respond to normal blood levels of thyroid hormones. Either type may progress to myxedema, which is clinically much more severe and considered a medical emergency. (See *Managing myxedema coma.*)

CAUSES AND INCIDENCE

Hypothyroidism results from a variety of abnormalities that lead to insufficient synthesis of thyroid hormones. Common causes of hypothyroidism include thyroid gland surgery (thyroidectomy), irradiation therapy inflammation, chronic autoimmune thyroiditis (Hashimoto's disease), and inflammatory conditions, such as amyloidosis and sarcoidosis.

The disorder may also result from pituitary failure to produce thyroid-stimulating hormone (TSH), hypothalamic failure to produce thyrotropin-releasing hormone, inborn errors of thyroid hormone synthesis, inability to synthesize thyroid hormones because of iodine deficiency (usually dietary), or the use of antithyroid medications such as propylthiouracil.

The disorder is most prevalent in women; in the United States, incidence is increasing significantly in people ages 40 to 50. Older adults can also suffer from subclinical thyroid dysfunction. (See *Mild thyroid dysfunction in older adults*.)

Pathophysiology

Hypothyroidism may reflect a malfunction of the hypothalamus, pituitary, or thyroid gland, all of which are part of the same negative-feedback mechanism. However, disorders of the hypothalamus and pituitary gland rarely cause hypothyroidism.

Chronic autoimmune thyroiditis—also called chronic lymphocystic thyroiditis—occurs when autoantibodies destroy thyroid gland tissue. Chronic autoimmune thyroiditis associated with goiter is called Hashimoto's thyroiditis. The cause of this autoimmune process is unknown, although heredity plays a role, and specific human leukocytes antigen subtypes are associated with greater risk.

Outside the thyroid, antibodies can reduce the effect of thyroid hormone in two ways. First, antibodies can block the TSH receptor and prevent the production of TSH. Second, cytoxic antithyroid antibodies may trigger thyroid destruction.

MILD THYROID DYSFUNCTION IN OLDER ADULTS

Older adults may be at risk not just from hypothyroidism, but also from mild thyroid dysfunction, although further research is needed confirm the benefits of screening and treating such disorders. An older patient may have subclinical hypothyroidism when increased levels of thyrotropin-stimulating hormone (TSH) occur with normal T_4 levels. This disorder can progress to hypothyroidism and is associated with atherosclerotic cardiovascular disease. Indications include mild serum lipoprotein and cardiac function abnormalities.

A patient with subclinical hypothyroidism may receive levothyroxine to maintain serum TSH levels in a normal range, although the risks of such treatment must be balanced with benefits.

The older adult is also at risk for subclinical hyperthyroidism. Suppressed TSH levels are associated with an increased risk of atrial fibrillation and bone demineralization.

ASSESSMENT FINDINGS

The patient's history may reveal vague and varied symptoms that developed slowly over time. The patient may report energy loss, fatigue, forgetfulness, sensitivity to cold, unexplained weight gain, and constipation. As the disorder progresses, signs and symptoms may include anorexia, decreased libido, menorrhagia, paresthesia, joint stiffness, and muscle cramping.

Inspection reveals characteristic alterations in the patient's overall appearance and behavior. These changes include decreased mental stability (slight mental slowing to severe obtundation) and a thick, dry tongue, causing hoarseness and slow, slurred speech.

You'll probably note dry, flaky, inelastic skin; puffy face, hands, and feet; periorbital edema; and drooping upper eyelids. Hair may be dry and sparse, with patchy hair loss and loss of the outer third of the eyebrow. Nails may be thick and brittle with visible transverse and longitudinal grooves. You may also find ataxia, intention tremor, and nystagmus.

Palpation may reveal cool, doughy skin; a weak pulse and bradycardia; weak muscles; sacral or peripheral edema; and delayed reflex relaxation time (especially in the Achilles tendon). The thyroid tissue itself may not be easily palpable unless a goiter is present.

Auscultation may show absent or decreased bowel sounds, hypotension, a gallop or distant heart sounds, and adventitious breath sounds. Percussion and palpation may reveal abdominal distention or ascites.

COMPLICATIONS

- Myxedema coma
- Pernicious anemia
- Achlorhydria
- Anemia
- Goiter
- Psychiatric disturbances

TREATMENT

In hypothyroidism, recommended treatment consists of gradual thyroid hormone replacement with the synthetic hormone levothyroxine (T_4) and, occasionally, liothyronine (T_3). Treatment begins slowly, particularly in older patients, to avoid adverse cardiovascular effects; the dosage increases every 2 to 3 weeks until the desired response is obtained.

Rapid treatment may be necessary for patients with myxedema coma and those about to undergo emergency surgery (because of sensitivity to central nervous system depression). In these patients, both I.V. administration of levothyroxine and hydrocortisone therapy is warranted.

Culture In the United States, soil in the Great Lakes region has a low iodine content, resulting in low iodine levels in food grown there. People living in those areas should receive sufficient iodine if they use iodized salt. In underdeveloped countries, prophylactic iodine supplements have successfully decreased the incidence of iodine-deficient goiter.

NURSING CONSIDERATIONS

- Routinely monitor and keep accurate records of the patient's vital signs, fluid intake, urine output, and daily weight.
- Monitor the patient's cardiovascular status. Auscultate heart and breath sounds, and watch closely for chest pain or dyspnea. Provide rest periods, and gradually increase activity to avoid fatigue and to decrease myocardial oxygen demand. Observe for dependent and sacral edema, apply antiembolism stockings, and elevate extremities to assist venous return.
- Encourage the patient to cough and breathe deeply to prevent pulmonary complications. Maintain fluid restrictions and a low-salt diet.
- Auscultate for bowel sounds, check for abdominal distention, and monitor the frequency of bowel movements. Provide the patient with a high-bulk, low-calorie diet and encourage activity to combat constipation and promote weight loss. Administer cathartics and stool softeners as needed.
- Monitor mental and neurologic status. Observe the patient for disorientation, decreased LOC, and hearing loss. If needed, reorient the patient to person, place, and time and use alternative communication techniques for impaired hearing. Explain all procedures slowly and carefully and avoid sedation, if possible. Provide a consistent environment to decrease confusion and frustration. Offer support and encouragement to the patient and family.
- Provide meticulous skin care. Turn and reposition the patient every 2 hours for a patient on extended bed rest.

Use alcohol-free skin care products and an emollient lotion after bathing.

- Provide extra clothing and blankets for a patient with decreased cold tolerance. Dress the patient in layers and adjust room temperature if possible.
- During thyroid replacement therapy, watch for signs and symptoms of hyperthyroidism, such as restlessness, sweating, and excessive weight loss.
- Encourage the patient to verbalize her feelings and fears about changes in body image and possible rejection by others. Help her identify her strengths and use them to develop coping strategies, and encourage her to develop interests that foster a positive self-image and de-emphasize appearance. Reassure the patient that her appearance will improve with thyroid replacement.
- Help the patient and family members understand the patient's physical and mental changes. Teach them that hypothyroidism commonly causes mood changes and altered thought processes. Stress that these problems usually subside with proper treatment. Urge family members to encourage and accept the patient and to help her adhere to her treatment regimen. If necessary, refer the patient and family members to a mental health professional for additional counseling.
- Instruct the patient and family to identify and report the signs and symptoms of life-threatening myxedema. Stress the importance of obtaining prompt medical care for respiratory problems and chest pain.
- Teach the patient and family about long-term hormone replacement therapy. Emphasize that lifelong administration of this medication is necessary, that the patient should take it exactly as prescribed, and that she should never abruptly discontinue it. Advise the patient always to wear a medical identification bracelet and to carry her medication with her.
- Advise the patient and family members to keep accurate records of daily weight.
- Instruct the patient to eat a well-balanced diet high in fiber and fluids to prevent constipation, to restrict sodium to prevent fluid retention, and to limit calories to minimize weight gain.
- Tell the patient to schedule activities to avoid fatigue and to get adequate rest.
- Emphasize the importance of complying with periodic laboratory tests necessary to assess thyroid function.

Integumentary System

As the body ages, dramatic changes occur in all of the skin's layers. In younger adults, skin cells turn over roughly every 3 weeks. But in older adults, this turnover slows to once every 2 months. Skin elasticity declines from the progressive degeneration of collagen and elastin, increasing the risk of tears and epidermal stripping. Photosensitivity increases as the number of melanocytes declines. Melanocyte loss also results in graying hair and, when coupled with reduced capillary blood supply, fading of normal skin color.

Other changes take place, too. Diminished adhesion between the dermis and the epidermis causes increased wrinkling and slackness, especially in the extremities, neck, and face. Wrinkling is exacerbated by prolonged sun exposure. A diminishing blood supply reduces the skin's thermoregulatory function, causing older people to feel colder in the extremities. The blood vessels themselves also become more fragile, leading to easy bruising and formation of senile purpura.

Fat loss from subcutaneous tissue (as well as other body sites) predisposes older patients to pressure ulcer formation, especially of the scapulae, trochanters, knees, and other bony prominences. Older people are also more likely to suffer from herpes zoster, psoriasis, and dry skin and itching, which stem partly from diminished sweat gland secretions.

As a nurse, a good deal of your care for older patients includes maintaining skin integrity and managing skin injuries. Understanding what happens to the skin with aging and how advancing age affects the skin's ability to recover from injury and infection will help you whenever you change the dressings on an older patient's surgical wound, apply topical medications, provide treatment to relieve itching, or assess for the risk of pressure ulcers.

Pressure ulcers

Pressure ulcers are localized areas of cellular necrosis that occur most commonly in the skin and subcutaneous tissue over bony prominences, especially the sacrum, ischial tuberosities, greater trochanter, heels, malleoli, and elbows. These ulcers may be superficial, caused by local skin irritation with subsequent surface maceration, or deep, originating in underlying tissue. Deep lesions typically go undetected until they penetrate the skin but, by then, they've usually caused subcutaneous damage.

CAUSES AND INCIDENCE

Pressure, particularly over bony prominences, interrupts normal circulatory function and causes most pressure ulcers. The intensity and duration of such pressure govern the severity of the ulcer; pressure exerted over an area for a moderate period (1 to 2 hours) produces tissue ischemia and increased capillary pressure, leading to edema and multiple small-vessel thromboses. An inflammatory reaction gives way to ulceration and necrosis of ischemic

cells. In turn, necrotic tissue predisposes the body to bacterial invasion and infection. (See *Common sites of pressure ulcers*.)

Shearing force, the force applied when tissue layers move over one another, can also cause ulcerations. This force stretches the skin, compressing local circulation. For example, if the head of the patient's bed is raised, gravity tends to pull the patient downward and forward, creating a shearing force. The friction of the patient's skin against the bed, such as occurs when a patient slides himself up in bed rather than lifting his hips, compounds the problem.

Moisture, whether from perspiration or incontinence, can also cause pressure ulcers. Such moisture softens skin layers and provides an environment for bacterial growth, leading to skin breakdown.

Age also has a role in the incidence of pressure ulcers. Muscle and subcutaneous tissue is lost with ageing, and skin elasticity decreases. Both factors increase the risk of developing pressure ulcers.

Other factors that can predispose a patient to pressure ulcers and delay healing include poor nutrition, diabetes mellitus, paralysis, cardiovascular disorders, and aging. Added risks include obesity or insufficient weight, edema, anemia, poor hygiene, and exposure to chemicals.

PATHOPHYSIOLOGY

A pressure ulcer is caused by an injury to the skin and its underlying tissues. The pressure exerted on the area restricts blood flow to the site and causes ischemia and hypoxemia. As the capillaries collapse, thrombosis occurs and leads to tissue edema and necrosis. Ischemia also contributes to an accumulation of toxins. The toxins further break down the tissue and also contribute to tissue necrosis.

COMMON SITES OF PRESSURE ULCERS

Pressure ulcers may develop at any of these pressure points. To prevent sores, reposition the patient and check frequently and carefully for skin changes.

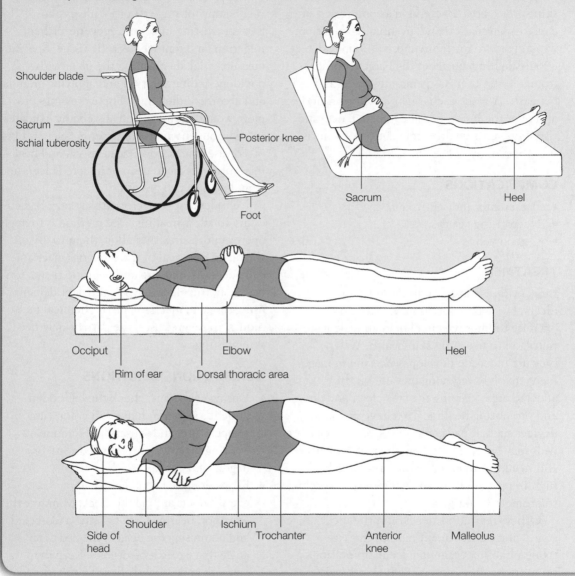

Shoulder blade

Sacrum

Ischial tuberosity

Posterior knee

Foot

Sacrum   Heel

Occiput   Elbow   Heel

Rim of ear   Dorsal thoracic area

Side of head   Shoulder   Ischium   Trochanter   Anterior knee   Malleolus

ASSESSMENT FINDINGS

The patient with a pressure ulcer has a history of one or more predisposing factors. Inspection of an early, superficial lesion reveals shiny, erythematous changes over the compressed area, caused by localized vasodilation when pressure is relieved. If the superficial erythema has progressed, you'll see small blisters or erosions and, ultimately, necrosis and ulceration.

In underlying damage from pressure between deep tissue and bone, you'll note an inflamed skin surface area. Bacteria in a compressed site cause inflammation and, eventually, infection, which leads to further necrosis. You may detect a foul-smelling, purulent discharge seeping from a lesion that has penetrated the skin from beneath. A black eschar may develop around and over the lesion because infected, necrotic tissue prevents healthy granulation of scar tissue. (See *Stages of pressure ulcers*.)

COMPLICATIONS

- Bacteremia and septicemia
- Necrotizing fasciitis
- Osteomyelitis

TREATMENT

Prevention is most important in pressure ulcers, by such means as movement and exercise to improve circulation and adequate nutrition to maintain skin health. When pressure ulcers do develop, successful management involves relieving pressure on the affected area, keeping the area clean and dry, and promoting healing. To relieve pressure, devices such as pads, mattresses, and special beds may be used, although the patient will still need turning and repositioning. A diet high in protein, iron, and vitamin C also helps to promote healing.

Other treatments depend on the ulcer stage. Stage I treatment aims to increase tissue pliability, stimulate local circulation, promote healing, and prevent skin breakdown. Specific measures include the use of lubricants (such as Lubriderm), clear plastic dressings (Op-Site), gelatin-type wafers (DuoDERM), vasodilator sprays (Proderm), and whirlpool baths.

For stage II ulcers, additional treatments include cleaning the ulcer with normal saline solution. This removes ulcer debris and helps prevent further skin damage and infection.

Therapy for stage III or IV ulcers aims to treat existing infection, prevent further infection, and remove necrotic tissue. Specific measures include cleaning the ulcer with povidone-iodine solution and applying granular and absorbent dressings. These dressings promote wound drainage and absorb any exudate. In addition, enzymatic ointments (such as Elase or Travase) break down dead tissue, and healing ointments clean deep or infected ulcers and stimulate new cell growth.

Debridement of necrotic tissue may be necessary to allow healing. One method is to apply open wet dressings and allow them to dry on the ulcer. Removal of the dressings mechanically debrides exudate and necrotic tissue. On occasion, the ulcer may require debridement using surgical, mechanical, or chemical techniques. In severe cases, the patient may need skin grafting.

NURSING CONSIDERATIONS

- During each shift, check the bedridden patient's skin for changes in color, turgor, temperature, and sensation. Examine an existing ulcer for any change in size or degree of damage.
- Reposition the bedridden patient at least every 2 hours around the clock. Minimize the effects of shearing force by using a footboard and not raising the head of the bed to an angle that exceeds 60 degrees. Keep the patient's knees slightly flexed for short periods.
- Perform passive range-of-motion (ROM) exercises or encourage the patient to do active exercises if possible.
- To prevent pressure ulcers in an immobilized patient, use pressure-relief aids on the bed.

STAGES OF PRESSURE ULCERS

These illustrations depict the various stages of pressure ulcer development.

Suspected deep tissue injury

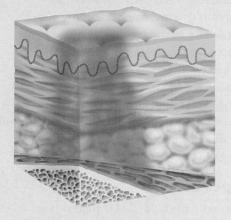

Stage I

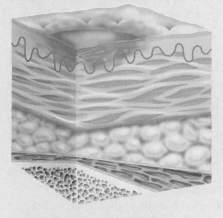

Stage II

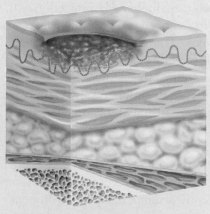

Stage III

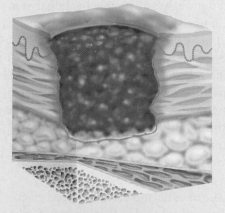

Stage IV

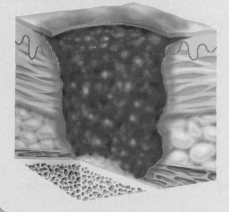

Unstageable

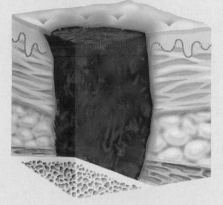

- Give the patient meticulous skin care. Keep the skin clean and dry without using harsh soaps. Gently massaging the skin around (not on) the affected area promotes healing. Rub moisturizing lotions into the skin thoroughly to prevent maceration of the skin surface. Change bed linens frequently for a diaphoretic or incontinent patient.
- If the patient is incontinent, offer a bedpan or commode frequently. Use only a single layer of padding for urine and fecal incontinence because excessive padding increases perspiration, which leads to maceration. Excessive padding may also wrinkle, irritating the skin.
- Clean open lesions with normal saline solution. If possible, expose the lesions to air and sunlight to promote healing. Dressings, if needed, should be porous and lightly taped to healthy skin.
- Encourage adequate food and fluid intake to maintain body weight and promote healing. Consult the dietitian to provide a diet that promotes granulation of new tissue. Encourage the debilitated patient to eat frequent, small meals that include protein- and calorie-rich supplements. Assist the weakened patient with meals.
- Because anemia and elevated blood glucose levels may lead to skin breakdown, monitor hemoglobin and blood glucose levels and hematocrit.
- Explain the function of pressure-relief aids and topical agents and demonstrate their proper use.
- Teach the patient and his family position-changing techniques and active and passive ROM exercises.
- Stress good hygiene. Teach the patient to avoid skin-damaging agents, such as harsh soaps, alcohol-based products, tincture of benzoin, and hexachlorophene.

- As indicated, explain debridement procedures and prepare the patient for skin-graft surgery.
- Teach the patient and his family to recognize and record signs of healing. Explain that treatment typically varies according to the stage of healing.
- Encourage the patient to eat a well-balanced diet and consume an adequate amount of fluids, explaining their importance for skin health. Point out dietary sources rich in vitamin C, which aids wound healing, promotes iron absorption, and helps in collagen formation.

Herpes zoster

Herpes zoster (also called shingles) is an acute unilateral and segmental inflammation of the dorsal root ganglia caused by infection with the herpesvirus varicella-zoster, which also causes chickenpox. This infection usually occurs in adults. It produces localized vesicular skin lesions, confined to a dermatome, and severe neuralgic pain in peripheral areas innervated by the nerves arising in the inflamed root ganglia.

The prognosis is good unless the infection spreads to the brain. Eventually, most patients recover completely, except for possible scarring and, in corneal damage, visual impairment. Occasionally, neuralgia may persist for months or years.

CAUSES AND INCIDENCE

Herpes zoster results from reactivation of varicella virus that has lain dormant in the cerebral ganglia (extramedullary ganglia of the cranial nerves) or the ganglia of posterior nerve roots since a previous episode of chickenpox. Exactly how or why this reactivation occurs isn't clear.

Herpes zoster occurs primarily in adults, especially those older than age 50. It seldom recurs. It's also seen in patients with human immunodeficiency virus and other immunodeficiency disorders.

PATHOPHYSIOLOGY

Some believe that the virus multiplies as it's reactivated and that antibodies remaining from the initial infection neutralize it. However, if effective antibodies aren't present, the virus continues to multiply in the ganglia, destroy the host neuron, and spread down the sensory nerves to the skin.

ASSESSMENT FINDINGS

Herpes zoster begins with fever and malaise. Within 2 to 4 days, severe deep pain, pruritus, and paresthesia or hyperesthesia develop, usually on the trunk and occasionally on the arms and legs in a dermatomal distribution. Pain may be continuous or intermittent and usually lasts from 1 to 4 weeks. Up to 2 weeks after the first symptoms, small red nodular skin lesions erupt on the painful areas. (These lesions typically spread unilaterally around the thorax or vertically over the arms or legs.) Sometimes nodules don't appear at all, but when they do, they quickly become vesicles filled with clear fluid or pus. About 10 days after they appear, the vesicles dry and form scabs. When ruptured, such lesions usually become infected and, in severe cases, may lead to the enlargement of regional lymph nodes; they may even become gangrenous. Intense pain may occur before the rash appears and after the scabs form.

Occasionally, herpes zoster involves the cranial nerves, especially the trigeminal and geniculate ganglia or the oculomotor nerve. Geniculate zoster may cause vesicle formation in the external auditory canal, ipsilateral facial palsy, hearing loss, dizziness, and loss of taste. Trigeminal ganglion involvement causes eye pain and, possibly, corneal and scleral damage

and impaired vision. Rarely, oculomotor involvement causes conjunctivitis, extraocular weakness, ptosis, and paralytic mydriasis.

In rare cases, herpes zoster leads to generalized central nervous system infection, muscle atrophy, motor paralysis (usually transient), acute transverse myelitis, and ascending myelitis. More commonly, generalized infection causes acute urine retention and unilateral diaphragm paralysis. In postherpetic neuralgia, most common in older patients, intractable neurologic pain may persist for years. Scars may be permanent.

Patients with immunodeficiency disorders may develop disseminated zoster. Lesions are bilateral and not limited to dermatomal distribution.

COMPLICATIONS

- Postherpetic neuralgia
- Permanent scarring

TREATMENT

Antiviral therapy is the mainstay of treatment. Acyclovir seems to stop the rash's progression and prevent visceral complications. Capsaicin, transcutaneous electrical nerve stimulation, and low-dose amitriptyline are the current treatments of choice for postherpetic neuralgia. Topical antiviral ointment is helpful if started early in the disease process.

Herpes zoster can resolve spontaneously and may require only symptomatic treatment. Such treatment aims to relieve itching and neuralgic pain with calamine lotion or another antipruritic; aspirin, possibly with codeine or another analgesic; and, occasionally, collodion or compound benzoin tincture applied to unbroken lesions. If bacteria have infected ruptured vesicles, the treatment plan usually includes an appropriate systemic antibiotic.

Trigeminal zoster with corneal involvement calls for instillation of idoxuridine ointment or another antiviral agent. To help a patient cope with the intractable pain of postherpetic neuralgia, the physician may order systemic corticosteroids—such as cortisone or possibly corticotropin—to reduce inflammation (although their use is controversial). The physician may also prescribe tranquilizers, sedatives, or tricyclic antidepressants with phenothiazines. In some immunocompromised patients, acyclovir I.V. appears to prevent disseminated, life-threatening disease. High doses of interferon (an antiviral glycoprotein) have been used in patients with cancer when the herpetic lesions are limited to the dermatome.

NURSING CONSIDERATIONS

Your care plan should emphasize keeping the patient comfortable, maintaining meticulous hygiene, and preventing further infection. During the acute phase, adequate rest and supportive care can promote proper healing of lesions.

Take the following steps:

- If calamine lotion has been ordered, apply it liberally to the lesions. If lesions are severe and widespread, apply a wet dressing. Drying therapies, such as oxygen or air-loss bed, and silver sulfadiazine (Silvadene) ointment may also be used.
- Instruct the patient to avoid scratching the lesions.
- If vesicles rupture, apply a cold compress as ordered.
- To decrease the pain of oral lesions, tell the patient to use a soft toothbrush, eat soft foods, and use a saline or bicarbonate mouthwash.
- To minimize neuralgic pain, never withhold or delay administration of analgesics. Give them exactly on schedule because the pain of herpes zoster can be severe. In postherpetic neuralgia, consult a pain specialist to

maximize pain relief without risking tolerance to the analgesic.
- Repeatedly reassure the patient that herpetic pain will eventually subside. Encourage diversionary or relaxation activity.
- Institute droplet and contact precautions. Disseminated zoster requires the same isolation precautions as primary varicella.

Genitourinary and Reproductive Systems

Aging brings many changes in the genitourinary (GU) and reproductive systems. As bladder muscles weaken and bladder capacity decreases, an older adult may have difficulty emptying his bladder, resulting in more residual bladder urine. With age, the micturition reflex is delayed and the pelvic diaphragm weakens, especially in women who have delivered twins or triplets.

In aging men, benign prostatic hyperplasia is common and typically leads to urinary tract problems. Nursing interventions focus on treating symptoms and caring for the patient after prostate surgery.

Among older adults, chronic renal failure can arise as a complication of age-related diseases, such as chronic glomerulonephritis, diabetes mellitus, and hypertension. Drugs used to treat other conditions also can contribute to chronic renal failure. Instead of experiencing azotemia (failure of the kidneys to remove urea from the blood) and other classic signs and symptoms, an older adult may present with worsening preexisting medical conditions.

Urinary incontinence, also common among older adults, can cause embarrassment, social isolation, depression, and institutionalization. Because the patient may be too embarrassed to report the problem or may think it's a normal part of aging, you'll need to provide careful, compassionate assessment to detect incontinence.

Urinary tract infection (UTI) may cause only vague signs and symptoms in older adults. As with many other GU problems, UTIs will challenge your assessment skills and may require you to adapt interventions and your teaching style to help treat the problem and prevent recurrences.

In women, menopause signals the end of the reproductive years and ushers in changes in sexual function and body image. Estrogen level decreases, which raises the risk of heart disease, osteoporosis, and certain cancers. Older women have a significantly higher risk for breast cancer; 70% of new cases occur after age 50. The best test for detecting breast cancer is regular breast self-examination, followed by annual mammography. A mammogram can detect tumors too small to palpate during self-examination.

For many GU and reproductive disorders, older adults may lack classic signs and symptoms. You'll need expert assessment skills to detect such problems.

Benign prostatic hyperplasia

Although most men over age 50 have some prostatic enlargement, in benign prostatic hyperplasia (BPH) the prostate gland enlarges sufficiently to compress the urethra and cause some overt urinary obstruction. Depending on the size of the enlarged prostate, the age and health of the patient, and the extent of the obstruction, BPH may be treated surgically or symptomatically.

CAUSES AND INCIDENCE

Age-associated changes in hormone activity, arteriosclerosis, inflammation, and metabolic or nutritional disturbances can all contribute to BPH.

The incidence of BPH increases with age. After age 40, the incidence increases sharply, with men in their 50s having a 50% incidence of the disease and those age 70 and older having an 80% incidence of BPH.

PATHOPHYSIOLOGY

Androgenic hormone production decreases with age, causing an imbalance in androgen and estrogen levels and resulting in high levels of dihydrotestosterone, the main prostatic intracellular androgen. The shift in hormone balance induces the early, nonmalignant changes of BPH in periurethral glandular tissue. Fibroadenomatosis nodules (masses of fibrous glandular tissue) continue to grow, compressing the remaining normal gland (nodular hyperplasia). The hyperplastic tissue is mostly glandular, with some fibrous stroma and smooth muscle.

As the prostate enlarges, it may push into the bladder and obstruct urine outflow by compressing or distorting the prostatic urethra. Progressive bladder distention may lead to the formation of a pouch that retains urine when the rest of the bladder empties. This retained urine may lead to calculus formation or cystitis. (See *Prostatic enlargement in BPH*, page 274.)

ASSESSMENT FINDINGS

Clinical features of BPH depend on the extent of prostatic enlargement and on the lobes affected. Characteristically, the patient complains of a group of signs and symptoms known as prostatism: decreased urine stream caliber and force, an interrupted stream, urinary hesitancy, and difficulty starting urination, which results in straining and a feeling of incomplete voiding. As the obstruction increases, the patient may report frequent urination with nocturia, dribbling, urine retention, incontinence and, possibly, hematuria.

PROSTATIC ENLARGEMENT IN BPH

This illustration shows an enlarged prostrate in a patient with benign hyperplasia (BPH)

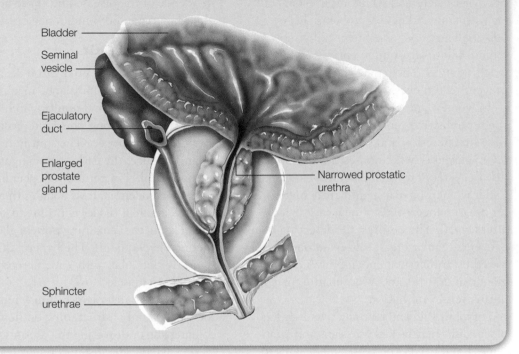

Physical examination reveals a visible midline mass above the symphysis pubis, which represents an incompletely emptied bladder. Palpation discloses a distended bladder; rectal palpation reveals an enlarged prostate.

COMPLICATIONS

- Urinary stasis, urinary tract infection (UTI), or calculi
- Bladder wall trabeculation
- Detrusor muscle hypertrophy
- Bladder diverticula and saccules
- Urethral stenosis
- Hydronephrosis
- Paradoxic (overflow) incontinence
- Acute or chronic renal failure
- Acute postobstructive diuresis

TREATMENT

Conservative therapy includes prostatic massages, sitz baths, short-term fluid restriction (to prevent bladder distention) and, if infection develops, antimicrobials. Regular sexual intercourse may help relieve prostatic congestion. Treatment with terazosin and finasteride has also proven effective. Terazosin (tamsulosin and prazosin) and alpha-adrenergic blockers release the prostate and bladder muscles, reducing straining with urination. Finasteride inhibits the action of 5-alpha-reductase, thereby preventing conversion of testosterone to dihydrotestosterone. This may lead to reduced prostate size over time.

Surgery is the only effective therapy for relief of acute urine retention, hydronephrosis, severe hematuria, and recurrent UTI or for palliative relief of intolerable symptoms. A transurethral resection may be performed if the prostate weighs less than 2 oz (57 g). In this procedure, a resectoscope removes tissue with a wire loop and an electric current. For high-risk patients, continuous drainage with an indwelling urinary catheter alleviates urine retention. Other transurethral procedures include vaporizing the prostate or a prostate incision with a scalpel or laser.

Other operations involve open surgical removal of the prostate. One of the following procedures may be appropriate:

- Suprapubic (transvesical) prostatectomy is the most common procedure and is especially useful when prostatic enlargement remains within the bladder area.
- Perineal prostatectomy usually is performed for a large gland in an older patient. The operation commonly results in impotence and incontinence.
- Retropubic (extravesical) prostatectomy allows direct visualization; potency and continence usually are maintained.
- Transurethral microwaves (heat therapy) are now being used in some patients. The procedure is more effective than alpha-adrenergic blockers but less effective than surgery.

NURSING CONSIDERATIONS

Take the following actions for patients with BPH:

- Prepare the patient for diagnostic tests and surgery as appropriate.
- Monitor and record the patient's vital signs, intake and output, and daily weight. Watch closely for signs of postobstructive diuresis (such as increased urine output and hypotension), which may lead to dehydration, lowered blood volume, shock, electrolyte losses, and anuria.

- Administer antibiotics as ordered for UTI, urethral procedures that involve instruments, and cystoscopy.
- If urine retention occurs, try to insert an indwelling urinary catheter. If the catheter can't be passed transurethrally, assist with suprapubic cystostomy. Watch for rapid bladder decompression.
- Avoid giving a patient with BPH decongestants, tranquilizers, antidepressants, or anticholinergics because these drugs can worsen the obstruction.

After prostatic surgery, take the following steps:

- Maintain the patient's comfort, and watch for and prevent postoperative complications. Observe for signs of shock and hemorrhage. Check the catheter frequently (every 15 minutes for the first 2 to 3 hours) for patency and urine color; check the dressings for bleeding.
- Postoperatively, many urologists insert a three-way catheter and establish continuous bladder irrigation. If the patient is undergoing bladder irrigation, keep the solution flowing at a rate sufficient to maintain patency and ensure that returns are clear and light pink. Watch for fluid overload from absorption of the irrigating fluid into the systemic circulation. If a regular catheter is used, observe it closely. If drainage stops because of clots, irrigate the catheter as ordered, usually with 80 to 100 ml of normal saline solution, while maintaining aseptic technique.
- Watch for septic shock, the most serious complication of prostatic surgery. Immediately report severe chills, sudden fever, tachycardia, hypotension, or other signs of shock. Start rapid infusion of I.V. antibiotics as ordered. Watch for pulmonary embolism, heart failure, and acute renal

failure. Monitor vital signs, central venous pressure, and arterial pressure.

- Administer belladonna and opium suppositories or other anticholinergics, as ordered, to relieve bladder spasms that can occur after transurethral resection.
- Make the patient comfortable after an open procedure. Administer suppositories (except after perineal prostatectomy), and give analgesics to control incisional pain. Change dressings frequently.
- Continue infusing I.V. fluids until the patient can drink enough on his own (2 to 3 qt [2 to 3 L]/day) to maintain adequate hydration.
- Administer stool softeners and laxatives as ordered to prevent straining. Don't check for fecal impaction because a rectal examination can cause bleeding.
- After the catheter is removed, the patient may experience urinary frequency, dribbling and, occasionally, hematuria. Reassure him and family members that he'll gradually regain urinary control.
- Reinforce prescribed limits on activity. Warn the patient against lifting, performing strenuous exercises, and taking long automobile rides for at least 1 month after surgery because these activities increase the tendency to bleed. Also caution him not to have sexual intercourse for several weeks after discharge.
- Teach the patient to recognize the signs and symptoms of UTI. Urge him to immediately report these to the physician because infection can worsen the obstruction.
- Instruct the patient to follow the prescribed oral antibiotic regimen, and tell him the indications for using gentle laxatives.
- Urge the patient to seek medical care immediately if he can't void at all, if he passes bloody urine, or if he develops a fever.

Breast cancer

Breast cancer is the most common cancer that affects women. It's estimated that 1 in 8 women in the United States will develop breast cancer during her lifetime. Male breast cancer accounts for 1% of all male cancers and less than 1% of all breast cancers.

The 5-year survival rate for localized breast cancer is 98% because of early diagnosis and a variety of treatments. Lymph node involvement is the most valuable prognostic predictor. With adjuvant therapy, 70% to 75% of women with negative nodes will survive 10 years or more, compared with 20% to 25% of women with positive nodes.

CAUSES AND INCIDENCE

The cause of breast cancer isn't known, but its high incidence in women implicates estrogen. It may develop anytime after puberty but is most common after age 50. Certain predisposing factors are clear; women at high risk include those who have a family history of breast cancer, particularly first-degree relatives (mother, sister, and maternal aunt).

Other women at high risk include those who:

- have long menstrual cycles or began menses early (before age 12) or menopause late (after age 55)
- have taken hormonal contraceptives
- used hormone replacement therapy for more than 5 years
- who took diethylstilbestrol to prevent miscarriage
- have never been pregnant
- were first pregnant after age 30
- have had unilateral breast cancer
- have had ovarian cancer, particularly at a young age
- were exposed to low-level ionizing radiation.

Recently, scientists have discovered the BRCA1 and BRCA2 genes. Mutations in these genes are thought to be responsible for less than 10% of breast cancers. However, these discoveries have made genetic predisposition testing an option for women at high risk for breast cancer.

Women at lower risk include those who:

- were pregnant before age 20
- have had multiple pregnancies
- are Native American or Asian.

PATHOPHYSIOLOGY

Breast cancer occurs more commonly in the left breast than the right and more commonly in the outer upper quadrant. Growth rates vary. Theoretically, slow-growing breast cancer may take up to 8 years to become palpable at 1 cm. It spreads by way of the lymphatic system and the bloodstream, through the right side of the heart to the lungs, and eventually to the other breast, the chest wall, liver, bone, and brain.

Most breast cancers arise from the ductal epithelium. Tumors of the infiltrating ductal type don't grow to a large size but metastasize early (70% of breast cancers).

Breast cancer is classified by histologic appearance and location of the lesion:

- Adenocarcinoma arises from the epithelium.
- Intraductal cancer develops within the ducts (includes Paget's disease).
- Infiltrating cancer occurs in parenchyma of the breast.
- Inflammatory cancer (rare) reflects rapid tumor growth, in which the overlying skin becomes edematous, inflamed, and indurated.
- Lobular carcinoma in situ reflects tumor growth involving lobes of glandular tissue.
- Medullary or circumscribed cancer consists of a large tumor with a rapid growth rate.

The descriptive terms should be coupled with a staging or nodal status classification system for a clearer understanding of the extent of the

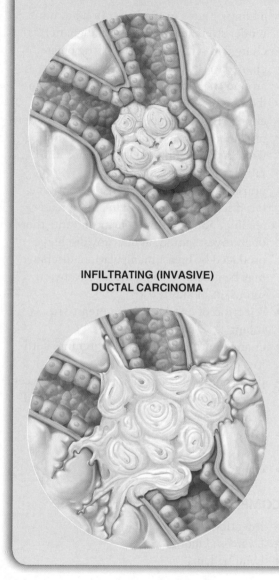

UNDERSTANDING BREAST CANCER

DUCTAL CARCINOMA IN SITU

INFILTRATING (INVASIVE) DUCTAL CARCINOMA

cancer. The most commonly used system for staging cancer, both before and after surgery, is the TNM staging (tumor size, nodal involvement, metastatic progress) system. (See *Understanding breast cancer*.)

ASSESSMENT FINDINGS

Warning signals of possible breast cancer include:

- a lump or mass in the breast (a hard, non-tender stony mass is usually malignant)
- change in symmetry or size of the breast
- change in skin, thickening, scaly skin around the nipple, dimpling, edema (peau d'orange), or ulceration
- change in skin temperature (a warm, hot, or pink area; suspect cancer in a nonlactating woman older than childbearing age until proven otherwise)
- unusual drainage or discharge (a spontaneous discharge of any kind in a nonbreast-feeding, nonlactating woman warrants thorough investigation, as does any discharge produced by breast manipulation; discharge may be greenish black, white, creamy, serous, or bloody)
- rejection of one breast by a breast-fed infant
- change in the nipple, such as itching, burning, erosion, or retraction
- pain (not usually a symptom of breast cancer unless the tumor is advanced, but it should be investigated)
- bone metastasis, pathologic bone fractures, and hypercalcemia
- edema of the arm.

COMPLICATIONS

- Infection
- Decreased mobility
- Lymphedema

TREATMENT

Much controversy exists over breast cancer treatments. In choosing therapy, the patient and practitioner should take into consideration the stage of the disease, the woman's age and menopausal status, and the disfiguring effects of the surgery. Treatment of breast cancer may include surgery, chemotherapy, radiation therapy, drug therapy, or a combination of treatments.

Surgery involves either mastectomy or lumpectomy. A lumpectomy may be performed on an outpatient basis and may be the only surgery needed, especially if the tumor is small and there's no evidence of axillary node involvement. In many cases, radiation therapy is combined with this surgery.

A two-stage procedure, in which the surgeon removes the lump and confirms that it's malignant and then discusses treatment options with the patient, is desirable because it allows the patient to participate in her treatment plan. Sometimes, if the tumor is diagnosed as clinically malignant, such planning can be done before surgery. In lumpectomy and dissection of the axillary lymph nodes, the tumor and the axillary lymph nodes are removed, leaving the breast intact. A simple mastectomy removes the breast but not the lymph nodes or pectoral muscles. Modified radical mastectomy removes the breast and the axillary lymph nodes. Radical mastectomy, the performance of which has declined, removes the breast, pectoralis major and minor, and the axillary lymph nodes.

The spread of breast cancer to regional lymph nodes is considered a vital prognostic indicator. Sentinel lymph-node biopsy, a reliable and minimally invasive procedure, is used to identify and sample the sentinel lymph node closest to the breast tumor. During the patient's surgery, the axillary node is injected with dye to help with identification and then sent to the pathologist to assess for cancer spread. If the node is negative, the patient can be spared an axillary node dissection, which carries its own risks and the potential for long-term complications.

Reconstructive breast surgery can be performed at the same time as mastectomy or it can be planned for a later date. Several options are available for breast reconstruction, including the insertion of breast implants or a transverse rectus abdominis musculocutaneous flap.

Chemotherapy, involving various cytotoxic drug combinations, is used as either adjuvant or primary therapy, depending on several factors, including the TNM staging and estrogen receptor status. The most commonly used antineoplastic drugs are cyclophosphamide, fluorouracil, methotrexate, doxorubicin, vincristine, and paclitaxel. A common drug combination used in both premenopausal and postmenopausal women is cyclophosphamide, doxorubicin, and paclitaxel.

Tamoxifen, an estrogen antagonist, is the adjuvant treatment of choice for postmenopausal patients with positive estrogen receptor status. It's also been found to reduce the risk of breast cancer in women at high risk.

Peripheral stem cell therapy is an option, but it's rarely used for advanced breast cancer.

Primary radiation therapy before or after tumor removal is effective for small tumors in early stages with no evidence of distant metastasis; it's also used to prevent or treat local recurrence. Presurgical radiation to the breast in inflammatory breast cancer helps make tumors more surgically manageable.

Estrogen, progesterone, androgen, or antiandrogen aminoglutethimide therapy may also be given to breast cancer patients. The success of these drug therapies—along with growing evidence that breast cancer is a systemic, not local, disease—has led to a decline in ablative surgery.

NURSING CONSIDERATIONS

To provide good care for a patient with breast cancer, begin with a history, assess the patient's feelings about her illness, and determine what she knows about it and what she expects. Preoperatively, make sure you know what kind of surgery is scheduled so you can prepare her properly. If a mastectomy is scheduled, in addition to the usual preoperative preparation (for example, skin preparations and not allowing the patient anything by mouth), provide the following information:

- Teach the patient how to deep-breathe and cough to prevent pulmonary complications and how to rotate her ankles to help prevent thromboembolism.
- Tell her she can ease her pain by lying on the affected side or by placing a hand or pillow on the incision. Preoperatively, show her where the incision will be. Inform her that she'll receive pain medication and that she need not fear addiction. Remember, adequate pain relief encourages coughing and turning and promotes general well-being. Positioning a small pillow anteriorly under the patient's arm provides comfort.
- Encourage her to get out of bed as soon as possible (even as soon as the anesthesia wears off or the first evening after surgery).
- Explain that, after mastectomy, an incisional drain or suction device will be used to remove accumulated serous or sanguineous fluid, thereby promoting healing.

After surgery, provide the following care:

- Inspect the dressing anteriorly and posteriorly, reporting bleeding promptly.
- Measure and record the amount of drainage; also note the color. Expect drainage to be bloody during the first 4 hours and afterward to become serous.
- Check circulatory status (blood pressure, pulse, respirations, and bleeding).
- Monitor intake and output for at least 48 hours after general anesthesia.
- Inform the patient to not let anyone draw blood, start an I.V., give an injection, or

take a blood pressure on the affected side because these activities will also increase the chances of developing lymphedema.

- Inspect the incision. Encourage the patient and her partner to look at her incision as soon as possible, perhaps when the first dressing is removed.
- Advise the patient to ask her practitioner about reconstructive surgery or to call the local or state medical society for the names of plastic reconstructive surgeons who regularly perform surgery to create breast mounds. In many cases, reconstructive surgery may be planned before the mastectomy.
- Instruct the patient about breast prostheses. The American Cancer Society's Reach to Recovery group can provide instruction, emotional support and counseling, and a list of area stores that sell prostheses.
- Give psychological and emotional support. Most patients fear cancer and possible disfigurement and worry about loss of sexual function. Explain that breast surgery doesn't interfere with sexual function and that the patient may resume sexual activity as soon as she desires after surgery.
- Also explain to the patient that she may experience phantom breast syndrome (a phenomenon in which the patient experiences a tingling or a pins-and-needles sensation in the area of the amputated breast tissue) or depression following mastectomy. Listen to the patient's concerns, offer support, and refer her to an appropriate organization such as Reach to Recovery, which offers caring and sharing groups to help breast cancer patients in the hospital and at home.

Chronic renal failure

Chronic renal failure is usually the end result of a gradually progressive loss of renal function. It also occasionally results from a rapidly progressive disease of sudden onset that gradually destroys the nephrons and eventually causes irreversible renal damage. Few symptoms develop until after more than 75% of glomerular filtration is lost. Then, the remaining normal parenchyma deteriorate progressively and symptoms worsen as renal function decreases.

Progressive stages of chronic renal failure include:

- reduced renal reserve (glomerular filtration rate [GFR] 35% to 50% of normal)
- renal insufficiency (GFR 20% to 35% of normal)
- renal failure (GFR 20% to 25% of normal)
- end-stage renal disease (GFR less than 20% of normal).

This syndrome is fatal without treatment, but maintenance dialysis or a kidney transplant can sustain life.

CAUSES AND INCIDENCE

Chronic renal failure may result from:

- chronic glomerular disease, such as glomerulonephritis
- chronic infections, such as chronic pyelonephritis or tuberculosis
- congenital anomalies, such as polycystic kidney disease
- vascular diseases, such as renal nephrosclerosis or hypertension
- obstructive processes, such as calculi or benign prostatic hypertrophy
- collagen diseases, such as systemic lupus erythematosus
- nephrotoxic agents, such as long-term aminoglycoside therapy
- endocrine diseases, such as diabetic nephropathy
- disorders that impair circulation, such as sickle cell disease.

PATHOPHYSIOLOGY

Chronic renal failure results from nephron destruction which eventually causes irreversible renal damage. The nephron damage is progressive; damaged nephrons can't function and don't recover. The kidneys can maintain relatively normal function until about 75% of the nephrons are nonfunctional. Surviving nephrons hypertrophy and increase their rate of filtration, reabsorption, and secretion. Compensatory excretion continues as the GFR diminishes.

ASSESSMENT FINDINGS

The patient's history may include a disease or condition that can cause renal failure, but he may not have any symptoms for a long time. Signs and symptoms usually occur by the time the GFR is 20% to 35% of normal, and almost all body systems are affected. Assessment findings reflect the involved system; many findings reflect involvement of more than one system.

Renal

In certain fluid and electrolyte imbalances, the kidneys can't retain salt, and hyponatremias occur. The patient may complain of dry mouth, fatigue, and nausea. You may note hypotension, loss of skin turgor, and listlessness that may progress to somnolence and confusion. Later, as the number of functioning nephrons decreases, so does the kidneys' capacity to excrete sodium and potassium. Urine output decreases, and the urine is very dilute, with casts and crystals present. Accumulation of potassium causes muscle irritability and then muscle weakness, irregular pulses, and life-threatening cardiac arrhythmias as serum potassium levels increase. Sodium retention causes fluid overload, and edema is palpable. Metabolic acidosis also occurs.

Cardiovascular

When the cardiovascular system is involved, assessment reveals hypertension and an irregular pulse. Life-threatening cardiac arrhythmias can occur. With pericardial involvement, you may auscultate a pericardial friction rub. Uremic toxins cause the pericardial sac to become inflamed and irritated. You may note distant heart sounds if pericardial effusion is present. You may auscultate bibasilar crackles and palpate peripheral edema if heart failure occurs.

Respiratory

Pulmonary changes include reduced pulmonary macrophage activity with increased susceptibility to infection. If pneumonia is present, you may note decreased lung sounds over areas of consolidation. Bibasilar crackles indicate pulmonary edema. With pleural involvement, the patient may complain of pleuritic pain, and you may auscultate a pleural friction rub. Crackles may indicate pleural effusion. Kussmaul's respirations occur with metabolic acidosis.

GI

With inflammation and ulceration of GI mucosa, inspection of the mouth may reveal gum ulceration and bleeding and, possibly, parotitis. The patient may complain of hiccups, a metallic taste in the mouth, anorexia, nausea, and vomiting caused by esophageal, stomach, or bowel involvement. You may note a uremic fetor (ammonia smell) to the breath. Abdominal palpation and percussion may elicit pain.

Skin

Inspection of the skin typically reveals a pallid, yellowish bronze color. The skin is dry and scaly with purpura, ecchymoses, petechiae, uremic frost (most often in critically ill or terminal patients), and thin, brittle fingernails with characteristic lines. The hair is dry and brittle and may change color and fall out easily. The patient usually complains of severe itching.

Neurologic

You may note that the patient has alterations in level of consciousness that may progress from mild behavior changes, shortened memory and attention span, apathy, drowsiness, and irritability to confusion, coma, and seizures. Headache and blurred vision indicate uremia. The patient may complain of hiccups, muscle cramps, fasciculations, and twitching, which are caused by muscle irritability. He may also complain of restless leg syndrome. One of the first signs of peripheral neuropathy, restless leg syndrome causes pain, burning, and itching in the legs and feet that may be relieved by voluntarily shaking, moving, or rocking them. This condition eventually progresses to paresthesia, motor nerve dysfunction (usually bilateral footdrop) and, unless dialysis is initiated, flaccid paralysis.

Endocrine

Adults with chronic renal failure may have a history of infertility, decreased libido, amenorrhea in women, and impotence in men.

Hematologic

Inspection may reveal purpura, GI bleeding and hemorrhage from body orifices, easy bruising, ecchymoses, and petechiae caused by thrombocytopenia and platelet defects.

Musculoskeletal

The patient may have a history of pathologic fractures and complain of bone and muscle pain caused by calcium-phosphorus imbalance and consequent parathyroid hormone imbalances. You may note gait abnormalities or, possibly, an inability to ambulate.

Complications

- Anemia
- Peripheral neuropathy
- Cardiopulmonary and GI complications
- Sexual dysfunction
- Skeletal defects

TREATMENT

The goal of conservative treatment is to correct specific symptoms. The specific diet depends on the patient's signs and symptoms. A low-protein diet reduces the production of end products of protein metabolism that the kidneys can't excrete. (A patient receiving continuous peritoneal dialysis should have a high-protein diet.) A high-calorie diet prevents ketoacidosis and the negative nitrogen balance that results in catabolism and tissue atrophy. The diet should restrict sodium, phosphorus, and potassium.

Maintaining fluid balance requires careful monitoring of vital signs, weight changes, and urine volume (if not anuric). Fluid retention can be reduced with loop diuretics such as furosemide (if some renal function remains) and with fluid restriction. Digitalis glycosides in small doses may be used to mobilize the fluids causing the edema; antihypertensives may be used to control blood pressure and associated edema.

Antiemetics taken before meals may relieve nausea and vomiting, and cimetidine, omeprazole, or ranitidine may decrease gastric irritation. Methylcellulose or docusate can help prevent constipation.

Anemia necessitates iron and folate supplements; severe anemia requires the infusion of fresh frozen packed cells or washed packed cells. Transfusions relieve anemia only temporarily. Synthetic erythropoietin (epoetin alfa) stimulates the division and differentiation of cells within the bone marrow to produce red blood cells.

Drug therapy commonly relieves associated symptoms. An antipruritic, such as trimeprazine or diphenhydramine, can relieve itching, and aluminum hydroxide gel can lower serum phosphate levels. The patient may also benefit from supplementary vitamins (particularly vitamins B and D) and essential amino acids.

Careful monitoring of serum potassium levels is necessary to detect hyperkalemia. Emergency treatment for severe hyperkalemia includes dialysis therapy and administration of 50% hypertonic glucose I.V., regular insulin, calcium gluconate I.V., sodium bicarbonate I.V., and cation exchange resins such as sodium polystyrene sulfonate. Cardiac tamponade resulting from pericardial effusion may require emergency pericardial tap or surgery.

Calcium and phosphorus imbalances may be treated with phosphate-binding agents, calcium supplements, and reduction of phosphorus in the diet. If hyperparathyroidism develops secondary to low serum calcium levels, a parathyroidectomy may be performed.

Intensive dialysis and thoracentesis can relieve pulmonary edema and pleural effusion.

Hemodialysis or peritoneal dialysis (particularly the newer techniques, such as continuous ambulatory peritoneal dialysis and continuous cyclic peritoneal dialysis) can help control most manifestations of end-stage renal disease. Altering the dialysate can correct fluid and electrolyte disturbances. However, maintenance dialysis itself may produce complications, including protein wasting, refractory ascites, and dialysis dementia. A kidney transplant may eventually be the treatment of choice for some patients with end-stage renal disease.

NURSING CONSIDERATIONS

The widespread clinical effects of chronic renal failure require meticulous and carefully coordinated supportive care.

- Provide good skin care. Bathe the patient daily, using superfatted soaps, oatmeal baths, and skin lotion to ease pruritus. Give good perineal care, using mild soap and water. Pad the bed rails to guard against ecchymoses. Turn the patient often, and use a convoluted foam or low-pressure mattress to prevent skin breakdown.

- Provide good oral hygiene. Brush the patient's teeth often with a soft brush or sponge tip to reduce breath odor. Hard candy and mouthwash minimize metallic taste in the mouth and alleviate thirst.

- Offer small, palatable, nutritious meals. Try to provide favorite foods within dietary restrictions, and encourage intake of high-calorie foods. Consult with a dietician as needed.

- Monitor the patient for hyperkalemia. Watch for cramping of the legs and abdomen and for diarrhea. As potassium levels increase, watch for muscle irritability and a weak pulse rate. Monitor the electrocardiogram for tall, peaked T waves; widening QRS complex; prolonged PR interval; and disappearance of P waves, indicating hyperkalemia.

- Carefully assess the patient's hydration status. Check for jugular vein distention, and auscultate the lungs for crackles. Carefully measure daily intake and output, including all drainage, emesis, diarrhea, and blood loss. Record daily weight, presence or absence of thirst, axillary sweat, tongue dryness, hypertension, and peripheral edema.

- Monitor for bone or joint complications. Prevent pathologic fractures by turning the patient carefully and ensuring his safety. Perform passive range-of-motion exercises for the bedridden patient.

- Encourage the patient to perform deep-breathing and coughing exercises to prevent pulmonary congestion. Auscultate for crackles, rhonchi, and decreased breath sounds. Be alert for clinical signs of pulmonary edema (such as dyspnea and restlessness). Administer diuretics and other medications as ordered.

- Maintain aseptic technique. Use a micropore filter during I.V. therapy, watch for signs of infection (listlessness, high fever, and leukocytosis), and warn the patient to avoid contact with infected people during the cold and flu season.

- Carefully observe and document seizure activity. Infuse sodium bicarbonate for acidosis and sedatives or anticonvulsants for seizures as ordered. Pad the bed rails, and keep an oral airway and suction setup at the bedside. Periodically assess neurologic status, and check for Chvostek's and Trousseau's signs, indicators of low serum calcium levels.

- Observe for signs of bleeding. Watch for prolonged bleeding at puncture sites and at the vascular access site used for hemodialysis. Monitor hematocrit and hemoglobin levels, and check stool, urine, and vomitus for blood.

- Report signs and symptoms of pericarditis, such as a pericardial friction rub and chest pain. Also watch for the disappearance of friction rub, with a decrease of 15 to 20 mm Hg in blood pressure during inspiration (paradoxical pulse), an early sign of pericardial tamponade.

- Schedule medication administration carefully. Give iron before meals, aluminum hydroxide gels after meals, and antiemetics (as necessary) a half hour before meals. Administer antihypertensives at appropriate intervals. If the patient requires a rectal infusion of sodium polystyrene sulfonate for dangerously high potassium levels, apply an emollient to soothe the perianal area. Make sure the sodium polystyrene sulfonate enema

is expelled; otherwise, it causes constipation and doesn't lower potassium levels. Suggest antacid wafers as an alternative to the aluminum hydroxide gels needed to bind GI phosphate. Don't give magnesium products because poor renal excretion can lead to toxic levels.

- If the patient requires dialysis, check the vascular access site every 2 hours for patency and the arm used for adequate blood supply and intact nerve function (check temperature, pulse rate, capillary refill, and sensation). If a fistula is present, feel for a thrill and listen for a bruit. Use a gentle touch to avoid occluding the fistula. Report signs of possible clotting. Don't use the arm with the vascular access site to take blood pressure readings, insert I.V. lines, draw blood, or give injections because these procedures may rupture the fistula or occlude blood flow.

- Withhold the morning dose of antihypertensive on the day of dialysis, and instruct the patient to do the same.

- After dialysis, check for disequilibrium syndrome, a result of sudden correction of blood chemistry abnormalities. Symptoms range from a headache to seizures. Also check for excessive bleeding from the dialysis site, and apply a pressure dressing or an absorbable gelatin sponge as indicated. Monitor blood pressure carefully.

- Teach the patient how to take his medications and what adverse effects to watch for. Suggest taking diuretics in the morning so that sleep isn't disturbed. If the patient requires dialysis, instruct him on how to adjust his medication schedule as needed in relation to dialysis.

- Instruct the anemic patient to conserve energy by resting frequently.

- Tell the patient to report leg cramps or excessive muscle twitching. Stress the importance of keeping follow-up appointments to have his electrolyte levels monitored.
- Tell the patient to avoid high-sodium and high-potassium foods. Encourage adherence to fluid and protein restrictions. To prevent constipation, stress the need for exercise and sufficient dietary fiber.
- If the patient requires dialysis, remember that he and family members are under extreme stress. The facility probably offers a course on dialysis; if not, you need to teach the patient and family members. Topics to cover include reasons for the procedure; complications; signs and symptoms of the related disease; how to check for bleeding, electrolyte imbalance, and changes in blood pressure; diet; exercise; and the use of equipment.
- Refer the patient and family members for counseling if they need help coping with chronic renal failure.
- Demonstrate how to care for the shunt, fistula, or other vascular access device and how to perform meticulous skin care. Discourage activity that might cause the patient to bump or irritate the access site.
- Suggest that the patient wear a medical identification bracelet or carry pertinent information with him.

Endometrial cancer

Endometrial, or uterine, cancer involves cancerous growth of the endometrial lining. The 5-year survival rate is 75% to 95% for stage I cancers; as the stages progress, the survival rate diminishes. For stage II, there's a 50% survival rate; stage III, 30%; and there's less than a 5% survival rate for stage IV.

CAUSES AND INCIDENCE

Endometrial cancer seems linked to several predisposing factors including:

- abnormal uterine bleeding
- diabetes
- familial tendency
- history of uterine polyps or endometrial hyperplasia
- hypertension
- low fertility index and anovulation
- nulliparity
- obesity
- uninterrupted estrogen stimulation.

Endometrial cancer usually affects postmenopausal women between ages 50 and 60; it's uncommon between ages 30 and 40 and extremely rare before age 30. Most premenopausal women who develop endometrial cancer have a history of anovulatory menstrual cycles or other hormonal imbalance. About 33,000 new cases of endometrial cancer are reported annually, with about 5,500 deaths occurring annually.

PATHOPHYSIOLOGY

In most cases, endometrial cancer is an adenocarcinoma that metastasizes late, usually from the endometrium to the cervix, ovaries, fallopian tubes, and other peritoneal structures. It may spread to distant organs, such as the lungs and the brain, through the blood or the lymphatic system. Lymph node involvement can also occur. Less common are adenoacanthoma, endometrial stromal sarcoma, lymphosarcoma, mixed mesodermal tumors (including carcinosarcoma), and leiomyosarcoma. (See *Progression of endometrial cancer*, page 286.)

ASSESSMENT FINDINGS

Uterine enlargement, persistent and unusual premenopausal bleeding, and any postmenopausal bleeding are the most common

PROGRESSION OF ENDOMETRIAL CANCER

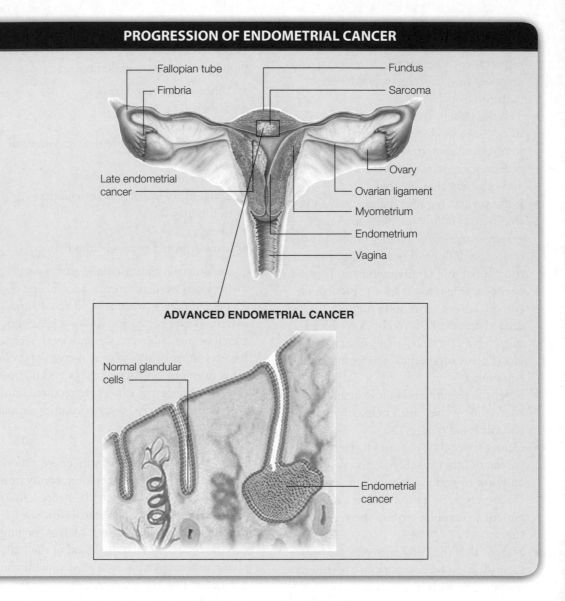

Fallopian tube

Fimbria

Fundus

Sarcoma

Late endometrial cancer

Ovary

Ovarian ligament

Myometrium

Endometrium

Vagina

ADVANCED ENDOMETRIAL CANCER

Normal glandular cells

Endometrial cancer

indications of endometrial cancer. The discharge may at first be watery and blood-streaked, but it gradually becomes bloodier. Other signs and symptoms, such as pain and weight loss, don't appear until the cancer is well advanced.

COMPLICATIONS

- Intestinal obstruction
- Ascites
- Hemorrhage

TREATMENT

Treatment varies, depending on the extent of the disease:

- Rarely curative, surgery generally involves total abdominal hysterectomy, bilateral salpingo-oophorectomy, or possibly omentectomy with or without pelvic or para-aortic lymphadenectomy. Total exenteration involves removal of all pelvic organs, including the vagina, and is done only when the disease is sufficiently contained to allow surgical removal of diseased parts.

- When the tumor isn't well differentiated, intracavitary or external radiation (or both), given 6 weeks before surgery, may inhibit recurrence and lengthen survival time.
- Hormonal therapy with synthetic progesterones, such as medroxyprogesterone or megestrol, may be administered for systemic disease. Tamoxifen (which produces a 20% to 40% response rate) may be given as a second-line treatment for advanced stage disease.
- Chemotherapy, which typically involves varying combinations of cisplatin, doxorubicin, carboplatin, topotecan, paclitaxel, and gemcitabine, is usually tried when other treatments have failed.

NURSING CONSIDERATIONS

Patients with endometrial cancer require patient teaching to help them cope with surgery, radiation, and chemotherapy. Also provide good postoperative care and psychological support.

Before surgery, take the following steps:

- Reinforce what the practitioner told the patient about the surgery, and explain the routine tests (for example, repeated blood tests the morning after surgery) and postoperative care.
- If the patient is to have a lymphadenectomy and a total hysterectomy, explain that she'll probably have a wound drainage system for about 5 days after surgery. Also explain indwelling urinary catheter care.
- Fit the patient with antiembolism stockings for use during and after surgery.
- Make sure the patient's blood has been typed and cross-matched.
- If the patient is premenopausal, inform her that removal of her ovaries will induce menopause.

After surgery, take the following steps:

- Measure fluid contents of the wound drainage system every shift. Notify the practitioner immediately if drainage exceeds 400 ml.
- If the patient has received subcutaneous heparin, continue administration as ordered until the patient is fully ambulatory again. Give prophylactic antibiotics as ordered, and provide good indwelling urinary catheter care.
- Check vital signs every 4 hours. Watch for and immediately report any sign or symptom of complications, such as bleeding, abdominal distention, severe pain, wheezing, or other breathing difficulties. Provide analgesics as ordered.
- Regularly encourage the patient to breathe deeply and cough to help prevent complications. Promote the use of an incentive spirometer several times every waking hour to help keep lungs expanded.

For the patient undergoing radiation therapy, take the following steps:

- Find out if the patient is to have internal or external radiation or both. Usually, internal radiation therapy is done first.
- Explain the internal radiation procedure, answer the patient's questions, and encourage her to express her fears and concerns.
- Explain that internal radiation usually requires a 2- to 3-day hospital stay, bowel preparation, a povidone-iodine vaginal douche, a clear liquid diet, and nothing taken by mouth the night before the implantation.
- Mention that internal radiation also requires an indwelling urinary catheter.
- Tell the patient that, if the procedure is performed in the operating room, she'll receive a general anesthetic. She'll be placed in a dorsal position, with her knees and hips flexed and her heels resting in footrests.

- Inform her that the physician may implant the radioactive source in the vagina, or a member of the radiation team may implant the radioactive source while the patient is in her room.
- Remember that safety precautions, including time, distance, and shielding, must be imposed immediately after the patient's radioactive source has been implanted.
- Tell the patient that she'll require a private room.
- Encourage the patient to limit movement while the source is in place. If she prefers, elevate the head of the bed slightly. Make sure the patient can reach everything she needs (call bell, telephone, water) without stretching or straining. Assist her with range-of-motion arm exercises (leg exercises and other body movements could dislodge the source). If ordered, administer a tranquilizer to help the patient relax and remain still. Organize the time you spend with the patient to minimize your exposure to radiation.
- Check the patient's vital signs every 4 hours; watch for skin reaction, vaginal bleeding, abdominal discomfort, or evidence of dehydration.
- Inform visitors of safety precautions, and hang a sign listing these precautions on the patient's door.

For the patient receiving external radiation, take the following steps:

- Teach the patient and her family about the therapy before it begins. Tell the patient that treatment is usually given 5 days a week for 6 weeks. Warn her not to scrub body areas marked with indelible ink for treatment because it's important to direct treatment to exactly the same area each time.
- Instruct the patient to maintain a high-protein, high-carbohydrate, low-residue diet to reduce bulk and yet maintain calories.

Administer diphenoxylate with atropine as ordered to minimize diarrhea, a possible adverse effect of pelvic radiation.

- To minimize skin breakdown and reduce the risk of skin infection, tell the patient to keep the treatment area dry, to avoid wearing clothes that rub against the area, and to avoid using heating pads, alcohol rubs, or any skin creams.
- Teach the patient how to use a vaginal dilator to prevent vaginal stenosis and to facilitate vaginal examinations and sexual intercourse.
- Remember, a patient with endometrial cancer needs special counseling and psychological support to help her cope with this disease and the necessary treatments. Fearful about her survival, she may also be concerned that treatment will alter her lifestyle and prevent sexual intimacy. Explain that except in total pelvic exenteration, the vagina remains intact and that after she recovers, sexual intercourse is possible. Your presence and interest will help the patient, even if you can't answer every question she may ask.

Ovarian cancer

Ovarian cancer is the fifth most common cancer in women and the leading cause of gynecologic deaths in the United States. In women with previously treated breast cancer, metastatic ovarian cancer is more common than cancer at any other site and may be linked to mutations in the BRCA1 or BRCA2 gene.

The prognosis varies with the histologic type and stage of the disease but is generally poor because ovarian tumors produce few early signs and are usually advanced at diagnosis. With early detection, about 90% of women with ovarian cancer at the localized stage survive for 5 years. The overall survival rate is about 45%.

More than half of all deaths from ovarian cancer occur in women between ages 65 and 84, and more than a quarter of ovarian cancer deaths occur between ages 45 and 64.

CAUSES AND INCIDENCE

Exactly what causes ovarian cancer isn't known, but the greatest number of cases occurs in women in their 40s. Other contributing factors include infertility, nulliparity, familial tendency, ovarian dysfunction, irregular menses, hormone-replacement therapy, and possible exposure to asbestos, talc, and industrial pollutants.

PATHOPHYSIOLOGY

Primary epithelial tumors—which account for 90% of ovarian cancers—arise in the Müllerian epithelium; germ cell tumors, in the ovum itself; and sex cord tumors, in the ovarian stroma. Ovarian tumors spread rapidly intraperitoneally by local extension or surface seeding and, occasionally, through the lymphatics and the bloodstream. Generally, extraperitoneal spread is through the diaphragm into the chest cavity, which may cause pleural effusions. Other metastasis is rare. (See *Looking at ovarian cancer* and *Common metastatic sites for ovarian cancer*, page 290.)

ASSESSMENT FINDINGS

Typically, signs and symptoms vary with the size of the tumor. An ovary may grow to considerable size before it produces overt symptoms. Occasionally, in the early stages, ovarian cancer causes vague abdominal discomfort, dyspepsia, and other mild GI disturbances. As it progresses, it causes urinary frequency, constipation, pelvic discomfort, distention, and weight loss. Tumor rupture, torsion, or infection may cause pain, which, in young patients, may mimic appendicitis. Granulosa cell tumors have feminizing effects (such as bleeding between periods in

LOOKING AT OVARIAN CANCER

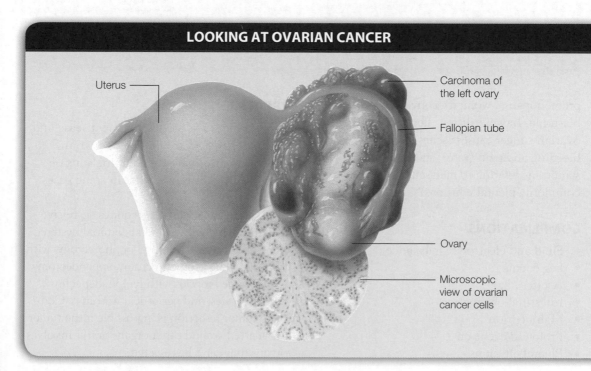

Uterus

Carcinoma of the left ovary

Fallopian tube

Ovary

Microscopic view of ovarian cancer cells

COMMON METASTATIC SITES FOR OVARIAN CANCER

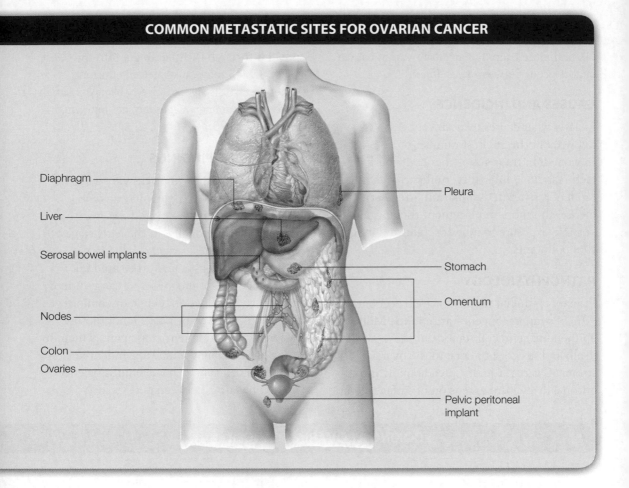

Diaphragm

Pleura

Liver

Serosal bowel implants

Stomach

Omentum

Nodes

Colon

Ovaries

Pelvic peritoneal implant

premenopausal women); conversely, arrheno-blastomas have virilizing effects. Advanced ovarian cancer causes ascites, postmenopausal bleeding and pain (rare), and signs and symptoms relating to metastatic sites (most commonly pleural effusions).

COMPLICATIONS

- Fluid and electrolyte imbalance
- Leg edema
- Ascites
- Intestinal obstruction
- Malnutrition
- Profound cachexia
- Pleural effusions

TREATMENT

According to the staging of the disease and the patient's age, treatment of ovarian cancer requires varying combinations of surgery, chemotherapy and, in some cases, radiation.

Ovarian cancer usually requires aggressive treatment, including total abdominal hysterectomy and bilateral salpingo-oophorectomy with tumor resection, omentectomy, appendectomy, lymph node biopsies with lymphadenectomy, tissue biopsies, and peritoneal washings. Complete tumor resection is impossible if the tumor has matted around other organs or if it involves organs that can't be resected.

Chemotherapy extends survival time in most ovarian cancer patients, but it's largely palliative in advanced disease. However, prolonged remissions have been achieved in some patients. Chemotherapeutic drugs useful in ovarian cancer include carboplatin, docetaxel, cyclophosphamide, doxorubicin, paclitaxel, cisplatin, and topotecan. These drugs are usually given in combination and they may be administered intraperitoneally.

Radiation therapy generally isn't used for ovarian cancer because the resulting myelosuppression would limit the effectiveness of chemotherapy. Radioisotopes have been used as adjuvant therapy, but they cause small-bowel obstructions and stenosis.

NURSING CONSIDERATIONS

The specific treatment and care plans for ovarian cancer vary widely, depending on the nature of the cancer and other factors such as patient age and overall health. However, certain nursing steps apply to all patients.

Before surgery, take the following steps:

- Thoroughly explain all preoperative tests, the expected course of treatment, and surgical and postoperative procedures.
- Reinforce what the surgeon has told the patient about the surgical procedures listed in the surgical consent form. Explain that this form lists multiple procedures because the extent of the surgery can only be determined after the surgery itself has begun.

After surgery, take the following steps:

- Monitor vital signs frequently, and check I.V. fluids often. Monitor intake and output, while maintaining good catheter care. Check the dressing regularly for excessive drainage or bleeding, and watch for signs of infection.
- Provide abdominal support, and watch for abdominal distention. Encourage coughing and deep breathing. Reposition the patient often, and encourage her to walk shortly after surgery.
- Monitor and treat adverse effects of radiation and chemotherapy.
- Provide psychological support for the patient and her family. Encourage open communication, while discouraging overcompensation or "smothering" of the patient by her family.

Prostate cancer

Prostate cancer is the most common cancer in men older than age 50. Adenocarcinoma is its most common form; sarcoma occurs only rarely. Most prostatic cancers originate in the posterior prostate gland; the rest originate near the urethra. Malignant prostatic tumors seldom result from the benign hyperplastic enlargement that commonly develops around the prostatic urethra in older men. Prostate cancer seldom produces symptoms until it's advanced.

CAUSES AND INCIDENCE

Four factors have been suspected in the development of prostate cancer: family or racial predisposition, exposure to environmental elements, co-existing sexually transmitted diseases, and endogenous hormonal influence. Eating fat-containing animal products has also been implicated. Although androgens regulate prostate growth and function and may also speed tumor growth, no definite link between increased androgen levels and prostate cancer has been found. When primary prostatic lesions metastasize, they typically invade the prostatic capsule and spread along the ejaculatory ducts in the space between the seminal vesicles or perivesicular fascia.

Incidence is highest in African-Americans and lowest in Asians. In fact, African-Americans have the highest prostate cancer incidence in the world and are considered at high risk for the disease. Incidence also increases with age more rapidly than any other cancer and is the most common cause of cancer death in men older than age 75.

PATHOPHYSIOLOGY

Typically, when a primary prostate lesion spreads beyond the prostate gland, it invades the prostatic capsule and spreads along ejaculatory ducts in the space between the seminal vesicles or the perivesicular fascia. Endocrine factors may play a role, leading researchers to suspect that androgens speed tumor growth. (See *Looking at prostate cancer* and *Pathway for metastasis of prostate cancer*.)

ASSESSMENT FINDINGS

Signs and symptoms of prostate cancer appear only in the advanced stages and include difficulty initiating a urine stream, dribbling,

urine retention, unexplained cystitis and, rarely, hematuria. The patient may feel pain in the lower back with urination, ejaculation, and bowel movement.

COMPLICATIONS

- Spinal cord compression
- Deep vein thrombosis
- Pulmonary emboli
- Myelophthisis

TREATMENT

Management of prostate cancer depends on clinical assessment, tolerance of therapy, expected life span, and the stage of the disease. Treatment must be chosen carefully, because prostate cancer usually affects older men, who commonly have coexisting disorders, such as hypertension, diabetes, or cardiac disease.

LOOKING AT PROSTATE CANCER

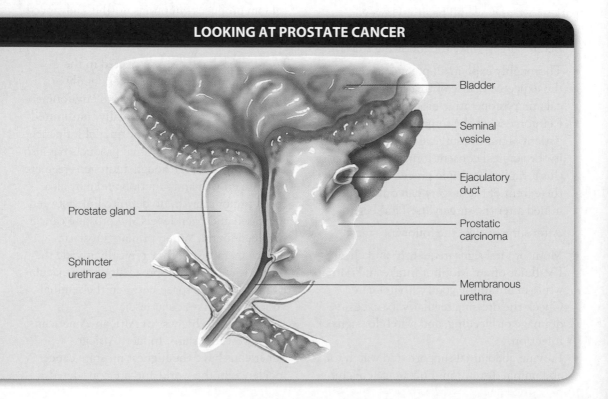

Bladder

Seminal vesicle

Ejaculatory duct

Prostate gland

Prostatic carcinoma

Sphincter urethrae

Membranous urethra

PATHWAY FOR METASTASIS OF PROSTATE CANCER

When primary prostatic lesions metastasize, they typically invade the prostatic capsule, spreading along the ejaculatory ducts in the space between the seminal vesicles of perivesicular fascia.

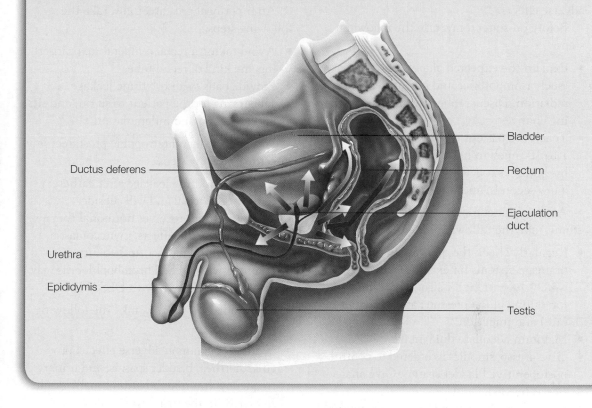

Ductus deferens

Urethra

Epididymis

Bladder

Rectum

Ejaculation duct

Testis

Therapy varies with each stage of the disease and generally includes radiation, prostatectomy, orchiectomy to reduce androgen production, and hormone therapy with synthetic estrogen (diethylstilbestrol [DES]) and antiandrogens, such as cyproterone, megestrol, and flutamide. Radical prostatectomy is usually effective for localized lesions.

External beam radiation therapy is used to cure some locally invasive lesions and to relieve pain from metastatic bone involvement. Internal radiation therapy, also known as brachytherapy, involves placing internally radioactive seeds directly in or near the

tumor. This method reduces damage to surrounding tissue. The seeds are left in place either temporarily or permanently. A single injection of the radionuclide strontium 89 is also used to treat pain caused by bone metastasis.

If hormone therapy, surgery, and radiation therapy aren't feasible or successful, chemotherapy (using combinations of mitoxantrone with prednisone, estramustine, docetaxel, goserelin, leuprolide, and paclitaxel) may be tried. However, current drug therapy offers limited benefit. Combining several treatment methods may be most effective.

NURSING CONSIDERATIONS

The care plan for the patient with prostate cancer should emphasize psychological support, postoperative care, and treatment of radiation adverse effects.

Before prostatectomy, take the following steps:

- Explain the expected aftereffects of surgery (such as impotence and incontinence) and radiation. Discuss tube placement and dressing changes.
- Teach the patient to do perineal exercises 1 to 10 times an hour. Have him squeeze his buttocks together, hold this position for a few seconds, and then relax.

After prostatectomy or suprapubic prostatectomy, take the following steps:

- Regularly check the dressing, incision, and drainage systems for excessive bleeding; watch the patient for signs of bleeding (pallor, falling blood pressure, and rising pulse rate) and infection.
- Maintain adequate fluid intake.
- Give antispasmodics as ordered to control postoperative bladder spasms. Give analgesics as needed.
- Urinary incontinence is common after surgery; keep the patient's skin clean, dry, and free from drainage and urine.
- Encourage perineal exercises 24 to 48 hours after surgery.
- Provide meticulous catheter care—especially if a three-way catheter with a continuous irrigation system is in place. Check the tubing for kinks and blockages, especially if the patient reports pain. Warn him not to pull on the catheter.

After transurethral prostatic resection, take the following steps:

- Watch for signs of urethral stricture (dysuria, decreased force and caliber of the urine stream, and straining to urinate) and for abdominal distention (from urethral stricture or catheter blockage).
- Irrigate the catheter as ordered.

After perineal prostatectomy, take the following steps:

- Avoid taking a rectal temperature or inserting any kind of rectal tube.
- Provide pads to absorb urine leakage, a rubber ring for the patient to sit on, and sitz baths for pain and inflammation.

After perineal and retropubic prostatectomy, take the following steps:

- Explain that urine leakage after catheter removal is normal and will subside.
- When a patient receives hormonal therapy, watch for adverse effects. Gynecomastia, fluid retention, nausea, and vomiting are common with DES. Thrombophlebitis may also occur, especially with DES.

After radiation therapy, take the following steps:

- Watch for common adverse effects: proctitis, diarrhea, bladder spasms, and urinary frequency. Internal radiation usually results in cystitis in the first 2 to 3 weeks.
- Urge the patient to drink at least eight 8-oz glasses (2 liters) or fluid daily.
- Provide analgesics and antispasmodics as ordered.

Sensory System

As a person ages, sensory capabilities—hearing, vision, touch, taste, and smell—deteriorate. Hearing and vision losses are usually the most upsetting, because they directly affect the ability to perform activities of daily living, threaten independence and bodily safety, and distort communication.

The major forms of hearing loss are classified as conductive loss (interrupted passage of sound from the external ear to the junction of the stapes and oval windows) and sensorineural loss (impaired cochlear or acoustic [eighth cranial] nerve dysfunction, causing failure of sound impulse transmission within the inner ear or brain).

The two most common age-related conductive losses are cerumen (wax) impaction, which results in a blockage of sound, and otosclerosis, a slow stiffening of the tiny bones (ossicles) in the inner ear. The most common sensorineural loss, presbycusis, affects the inner ear and retrocochlear area. It begins with the loss of high-frequency sounds and may progress to middle and low frequencies; degeneration of vestibular structures and atrophy of the cochlea and organ of Corti also occur.

Age-related vision changes are first noticed in the fifth decade of life. During the early to mid-40s, presbyopia, the inability to focus properly, causes most middle-aged adults to need corrective eyeglasses. The visual field narrows, reducing peripheral vision. The iris loses elasticity and responds less efficiently to light and dark; it also fades or develops irregular pigmentation. The pupil becomes smaller, reducing the amount of light that reaches the retina. The lens yellows, making it difficult to distinguish low tones of blue, green, and violet.

The vitreous can also degenerate with age, revealing opacities and floating debris, and can also detach from the retina. Floaters (bits of debris or condensation) accumulate in the vitreous humor and float across the visual field. Intraocular fluid reabsorption loses efficiency, increasing intraocular pressure and the risk of glaucoma. The cornea loses its luster and flattens. A white circle (arcus senilus) may develop around the periphery of the cornea. The sclera becomes thick and rigid, and fat deposits cause yellowing. Increased formation of connective tissue may cause sclerosis of the sphincter muscles. Reabsorption of intraocular fluid can diminish, predisposing a patient to glaucoma. The lens enlarges and loses transparency. Impaired lens elasticity (presbyopia) can decrease accommodation.

Common vision problems older patients may experience include cataracts, opacities that develop in the lens and further cloud the vision; dry eyes, which result from diminished lacrimal gland secretions; entropion and ectropion, or inversion and eversion of the eyelids, which cause irritation and poor drainage of tears through the nasolacrimal system; glaucoma, marked by high intraocular pressure that damages the optic nerve; macular degeneration, which results from hardening of retinal arteries; and retinal detachment, a separation of retinal layers.

Because hearing and vision loss can interfere significantly with individual pursuits and social interactions, periodically assess each of your older patients thoroughly to rule out conditions that can be treated by surgery or medication.

Age-related macular degeneration

At least 10% of older Americans have irreversible central vision loss from age-related macular degeneration. Two primary forms include the atrophic (also called the involutional or dry) form, which accounts for about 70% of cases, and the exudative (also called the hemorrhagic or wet) form of macular degeneration. The disorder commonly affects both eyes and is a leading cause of blindness in the United States in people over age 60.

CAUSES AND INCIDENCE

Although it's not known what causes macular degeneration, possible causes include aging,

RETINAL CHANGES IN MACULAR DEGENERATION

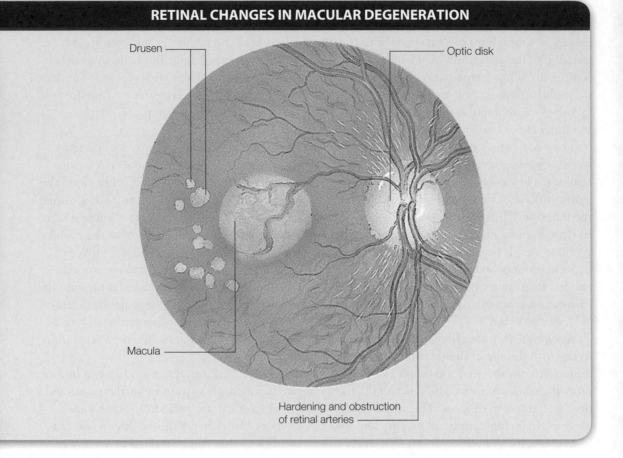

Drusen

Optic disk

Macula

Hardening and obstruction
of retinal arteries

infection, inflammation, and injury; genetics may also play a role. Cigarette smoking and a lack of antioxidants, such as vitamins C and E, may enhance occurrence.

PATHOPHYSIOLOGY

Age-related macular degeneration results from hardening and obstruction of the retinal arteries, usually associated with age-related degenerative changes. As a result, new blood vessels form (neovascularization) in the macular area and totally obscure central vision. Underlying pathologic changes occur primarily in the retinal pigment epithelium, Bruch's membrane, and choriocapillaries in the macular system.

The dry form develops as yellow extracellular deposits—tiny yellow spots called drusen—accumulate beneath the pigment epithelium of the retina; they may be prominent in the macula. Drusen are common in older adults. Over time, drusen grow and increase in number. Vision loss occurs as retinal pigment epithelium detaches and becomes atrophic.

Exudate macular degeneration develops as new blood vessels in the choroid project through abnormalities in Bruch's membrane and invade potential space underneath the retinal pigment epithelium. As these vessels leak, fluid in the retinal pigment epithelium increases, resulting in blurry vision. (See *Retinal changes in macular degeneration.*)

ASSESSMENT FINDINGS

The patient may complain of seeing a blank spot in the center of a page (scotoma) while reading. He may tell you that his central vision blurs intermittently and has gradually worsened. He may also report that straight lines appear distorted.

In the patient with dry macular degeneration, you may see drusen beneath the retina. If they're outside the macular area, the patient won't have symptoms. If they're within the macula, the patient will likely report a gradual blurring of vision that's most noticeable when he tries to read. With wet macular degeneration, signs and symptoms develop rapidly, with the patient reporting that straight lines appear crooked and letters appear broken up.

COMPLICATIONS

- Blindness
- Nystagmus

TREATMENT

Laser photocoagulation reduces the incidence of severe visual loss in patients with subretinal neovascularization. Photodynamic therapy with verteporfin, a newer form of laser therapy, is effective in selected patients.

NURSING CONSIDERATIONS

- Help the patient obtain optical aids, such as magnifiers and special lamps, for poor vision. Suggest an appointment with a low-vision specialist.
- Offer emotional support, and encourage the patient to express fears and concerns.
- Point out ways to modify the patient's home environment for safety.
- Explain that macular degeneration usually doesn't affect peripheral vision, which should be adequate for performing routine activities.

- If the patient likes to read, refer him to an agency such as the American Foundation for the Blind or Associated Services for the Blind. Agencies like these offer classes in braille and reading alternatives, such as books and other materials on audiocassettes.

Blepharitis

Blepharitis is a common inflammation of eyelash follicles and meibomian glands of the upper or lower eyelids. It gives a red-rimmed appearance to the eyelid margins. The disorder, which may affect both eyes (and both upper and lower eyelids), tends to recur and may become chronic.

CAUSES AND INCIDENCE

Seborrheic (nonulcerative) blepharitis generally results from seborrhea of the scalp, eyebrows, and ears. Ulcerative (staphylococcal) blepharitis results from a *Staphylococcus aureus* infection. (Chalazia and styes are likely to develop with this infection.)

Seborrheic blepharitis is more common in older people but also may affect people with red hair. Ulcerative blepharitis may coexist with seborrheic blepharitis. Both types can be controlled if treatment begins before the onset of ocular involvement.

PATHOPHYSIOLOGY

The pathophysiology of blepharitis usually involves bacterial colonization of the eyelids resulting from microbial invasion of tissues, immune system–mediated damage, or damage caused by the production of bacterial toxins, waste products, and enzymes.

ASSESSMENT FINDINGS

The patient typically complains that his eyelids itch, burn, or feel as if they have a foreign body in them. He may also complain that his eyelids are crusty and stick together when he awakens in the morning.

Inspection may reveal that the patient unknowingly rubs his eyes (causing the red rims) or continually blinks. You may also note waxy scales along the eyelids, indicating seborrheic blepharitis. Flaky scales on the eyelashes, missing eyelashes, or ulcerations on eyelid margins suggest ulcerative blepharitis.

COMPLICATIONS

- Keratitis

TREATMENT

Early treatment is essential to prevent recurrence or complications. For patients with seborrheic blepharitis, treatment includes daily shampooing (using a mild shampoo on a cotton-tipped applicator or a washcloth) to remove scales from the eyelid margins. Patients should also shampoo the scalp and eyebrows and follow up with warm eye compresses.

A patient with ulcerative blepharitis requires the same treatment, in addition to a sulfonamide or an appropriate antibiotic eye ointment at bedtime. A combination antibiotic and steroid such as prednisolone (Vasocidin or Blephamide) may be used.

Treatment for a patient with blepharitis resulting from pediculosis involves removing the nits with forceps or applying ophthalmic physostigmine or other insecticidal ointment. **Rx** *Medication Alert* Application of ophthalmic physostigmine or other insecticidal ointment can cause pupil constriction, headache, conjunctival irritation, or blurred vision from the film of ointment on the cornea.

NURSING CONSIDERATIONS

- Provide eyelid care at least twice daily. To do so, dip a cotton-tipped applicator in baby shampoo, and then shake the applicator to remove any excess shampoo. Using a downward motion from the eyelid margin to the tips of the eyelashes, gently clean the upper eyelid margin. Repeat on the lower eyelid margin. Use a warm, wet washcloth to rinse the shampoo away.
- Encourage the patient to participate in eyelid care.
- Show him how to use a cotton-tipped applicator or a clean washcloth to remove the scales from his eyelids. Instruct him to do this daily.
- Demonstrate how to apply warm compresses: First, run warm water into a clean bowl. Then immerse a clean cloth in the water and wring the water from the cloth. Next, place the warm cloth against the closed eyelid. (Be careful not to use hot water, which could burn the skin.) Hold the compress in place until it cools. Continue this procedure for 15 minutes.
- Instruct the patient to apply antibiotic ophthalmic ointment after a 15-minute application of warm compresses.

Cataract

Cataract—a common cause of gradual vision loss—is opacity of the lens or the lens capsule of the eye. The clouded lens blocks light shining through the cornea. This, in turn, blurs the image cast onto the retina. As a result, the brain interprets a hazy image.

Cataracts commonly affect both eyes, but each cataract progresses independently. Exceptions are traumatic cataracts, which are usually unilateral, and congenital cataracts, which may remain stationary.

CAUSES AND INCIDENCE

Cataracts are classified by their causes:

- Senile cataracts develop in older people, probably because of chemical changes in lens proteins.
- Traumatic cataracts develop after a foreign body injures the lens with sufficient force to allow aqueous or vitreous humor to enter the lens capsule.

- Complicated cataracts occur secondary to uveitis, glaucoma, retinitis pigmentosa, or retinal detachment. They can also occur with systemic disease, such as diabetes, hypoparathyroidism, or atopic dermatitis or from ionizing radiation or infrared rays.
- Toxic cataracts result from drug or chemical toxicity with prednisone, ergot alkaloids, naphthalene, and phenothiazines.

Cataracts are most prevalent in people over age 70. Surgery restores vision in about 95% of patients.

PATHOPHYSIOLOGY

Pathophysiology may vary with each form of cataract. Senile cataracts show evidence of protein aggregation, oxidative injury, and increased pigmentation in the center of the lens. In traumatic cataracts, phagocytosis of the lens or inflammation may occur when a lens ruptures. The mechanism of a complicated cataract varies with the disease process—for example, in diabetes, increased glucose in the lens causes it to absorb water.

Typically cataract development progresses through stages:

- During the immature phase, the lens isn't totally opaque.
- In the mature phase, the lens is completely opaque and vision loss is significant.
- During the tumescent phase, the lens is filled with water, which may lead to glaucoma.
- In the hypermature phase, the lens proteins deteriorate, causing peptides to leak through the lens capsule; glaucoma may develop if intraocular fluid outflow is obstructed.

ASSESSMENT FINDINGS

Typically, the patient complains of painless, gradual vision loss. He may also report a blinding glare from headlights when he drives at night, poor reading vision, and an annoying glare and poor vision in bright sunlight. If he has a central opacity, the patient may report seeing better in dim light than in bright light. This is because this cataract is nuclear and, as the pupil dilates, the patient can see around the opacity.

Inspection with a penlight may reveal a milky white pupil and, with an advanced cataract, a grayish white area behind the pupil. As the cataract matures, the red reflex is lost.

COMPLICATIONS

- Complete vision loss

TREATMENT

Surgical lens extraction and implantation of an intraocular lens (IOL) to correct the visual deficit is the treatment for cataracts. The surgery is usually performed as a same-day, or outpatient, procedure. Extracapsular cataract extraction, the most common procedure, involves removing the anterior lens capsule and cortex and leaving the posterior capsule intact. Typically, this is performed with phacoemulsification equipment, which fragments the lens with ultrasound. The fragments are then removed by irrigation and aspiration. In this procedure, the surgeon implants a posterior chamber IOL where the patient's own lens used to be. This procedure is used for patients of all ages.

Intracapsular cataract extraction involves removing the entire lens within the intact capsule by cryoextraction (the moist lens sticks to an extremely cold metal probe for easy and safe removal with gentle traction). After the surgeon removes the lens, he implants an IOL in either the anterior or posterior chamber. If the patient doesn't receive an IOL, he'll use contact lenses or aphakic glasses to correct vision.

Possible complications of surgery include loss of vitreous (during surgery), wound dehiscence from loosening of sutures and flat anterior chamber or iris prolapse into the wound, hyphema, pupillary block glaucoma, retinal detachment, and infection.

A patient with an IOL implant may experience improved vision almost immediately; however, the IOL corrects distance vision only. The patient also needs either corrective reading glasses or a corrective contact lens, which can be fitted 4 to 8 weeks after surgery.

If the patient didn't receive an IOL, he may receive temporary aphakic cataract glasses. Then, sometime between 4 and 8 weeks after surgery, he has a refraction examination for permanent glasses.

Some patients who have an extracapsular cataract extraction develop a secondary membrane in the posterior lens capsule (which has been left intact), causing decreased visual acuity. This membrane can be removed by the Nd:YAG laser, which cuts an area from the membrane center, thus restoring vision. However, laser surgery alone can't remove a cataract.

NURSING CONSIDERATIONS

- Postoperatively, monitor the patient until he recovers from the effects of the anesthetic. Keep the side rails of the bed up, monitor vital signs, and assist him with early ambulation.
- Apply an eye shield or eye patch postoperatively as ordered.
- Because the patient will be discharged after he recovers from the anesthetic, remind him to return for a checkup the next day. Caution him to avoid activities that increase intraocular pressure, such as straining with coughing, bowel movements, or lifting.
- Advise the patient to abstain from sex until he receives his physician's approval.
- Teach the patient or family member how to instill ophthalmic ointment or drops.

- Tell the patient to notify his physician immediately if he develops increased eye discharge, sharp eye pain (unrelieved by analgesics), or deterioration in vision.

Glaucoma

Glaucoma is a group of disorders characterized by high intraocular pressure (IOP) that damages the optic nerve. Glaucoma may occur as a primary or congenital disease or secondary to other causes, such as injury, infection, surgery, or prolonged topical corticosteroid use.

Primary glaucoma has two forms: open-angle (also known as chronic, simple, or wide-angle glaucoma) and angle-closure (also known as acute or narrow-angle) glaucoma. Angle-closure glaucoma attacks suddenly and may cause permanent vision loss in 48 to 72 hours.

CAUSES AND INCIDENCE

Open-angle glaucoma results from degenerative changes in the trabecular meshwork. These changes block the flow of aqueous humor from the eye, which causes IOP to increase. The result is optic nerve damage. Open-angle glaucoma affects about 90% of all patients who have glaucoma and commonly occurs in families.

Angle-closure glaucoma results from obstruction to the outflow of aqueous humor caused by an anatomically narrow angle between the iris and the cornea. This causes IOP to increase suddenly. Angle-closure glaucoma attacks may be triggered by trauma, pupillary dilation, stress, or any ocular change that pushes the iris forward (for example, a hemorrhage or swollen lens).

Secondary glaucoma can proceed from such conditions as uveitis, trauma, drug use (such as corticosteroids), venous occlusion, or diabetes. In some instances, new blood vessels (neovascularization) form, blocking the passage of aqueous humor.

One of the leading causes of blindness, glaucoma affects about 2% of Americans aged 40 to 50 years and 8% of those over age 70. It accounts for about 12% of newly diagnosed blindness in the United States. The incidence is highest among African-Americans; it's the single most common cause of blindness in this group. In the United States, early detection and effective treatment contribute to a good prognosis for preserving vision.

PATHOPHYSIOLOGY

Chronic open-angle glaucoma results from overproduction or obstruction of the outflow of aqueous humor through the trabecular meshwork or canal of Schlemm, causing increased IOP and damage to the optic nerve. In secondary glaucoma, conditions such as trauma and surgery increase the risk of obstruction and intraocular fluid outflow caused by edema or other abnormal processes.

The obstruction of acute angle-closure glaucoma that blocks the outflow of aqueous humor can stem from anatomically narrow angles between the anterior iris and the posterior corneal surface, shallow anterior chambers, a thickened iris that causes angle closure on pupil dilation, or a bulging iris that presses on the trabeculae, closing the angel (peripheral anterior synechiae). Any of these may cause IOP to increase suddenly. (See *Optical disk changes in glaucoma*, page 302.)

ASSESSMENT FINDINGS

Because open-angle glaucoma begins insidiously and progresses slowly, the patient may have no symptoms. Later, he may complain of a dull, morning headache; mild aching in the eyes; loss of peripheral vision; seeing halos around lights; and reduced visual acuity (especially at night) that's uncorrected by glasses.

Angle-closure glaucoma typically has a rapid onset and is an emergency. The patient may complain of pain and pressure over the eye, blurred vision, decreased visual acuity, seeing halos around lights, and nausea and vomiting (from increased IOP).

Inspection may reveal unilateral eye inflammation, a cloudy cornea, and a moderately dilated pupil that's nonreactive to light. Palpation may also disclose increased IOP, discovered by applying gentle fingertip pressure to the patient's closed eyelids. With angle-closure glaucoma, one eye may feel harder than the other.

COMPLICATIONS

• Total blindness

TREATMENT

For a patient with open-angle glaucoma, the initial goal of treatment is to reduce pressure by decreasing aqueous humor production with medications. These include beta-adrenergic blockers, such as timolol (used cautiously in asthmatics or patients with bradycardia) or betaxolol; alpha agonists such as brimonidine to lower IOP; and topical carbonic anhydrase inhibitors such as dorzolamide. Other drug treatments include epinephrine to dilate the pupil (contraindicated in angle-closure glaucoma) and miotic eyedrops such as pilocarpine to promote aqueous humor outflow.

Patients who don't respond to drug therapy may benefit from argon laser trabeculoplasty or from a surgical filtering procedure called trabeculectomy. This procedure involves creating an opening for out flowing aqueous humor.

To perform argon laser trabeculoplasty, the ophthalmologist focuses an argon laser beam on the trabecular meshwork of an open angle.

OPTIC DISK CHANGES IN GLAUCOMA

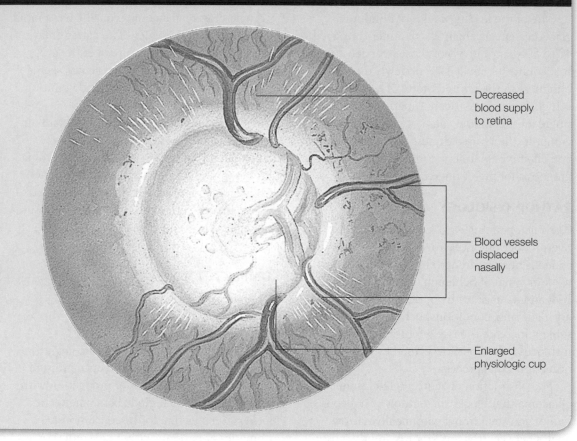

Decreased blood supply to retina

Blood vessels displaced nasally

Enlarged physiologic cup

This produces a thermal burn that changes the meshwork surface and facilitates the outflow of aqueous humor.

To perform a trabeculectomy, the surgeon dissects a flap of sclera to expose the trabecular meshwork. The surgeon removes a small tissue block and performs a peripheral iridectomy, which produces an opening for aqueous outflow under the conjunctiva and creates a filtering bleb. Postoperatively, the patient may receive subconjunctival injections of fluorouracil to maintain the fistula's patency.

Angle-closure glaucoma is an emergency that requires immediate treatment to reduce high IOP. Initial preoperative drug therapy lowers IOP with acetazolamide, timolol, pilocarpine (which constricts the pupil, forces the iris away from the trabeculae, and allows fluid to escape), and I.V. mannitol or oral glycerin (which forces fluid from the eye by making the blood hypertonic). If these medications fail to decrease the pressure, laser iridotomy or surgical peripheral iridectomy must be performed promptly to save the patient's vision.

An iridectomy is used to relieve pressure by excising part of the iris to reestablish the outflow of aqueous humor. A few days later, the surgeon performs a prophylactic iridectomy on the other eye to prevent an episode of acute glaucoma in the normal eye.

If the patient has severe pain, treatment may include opioid analgesics. After peripheral iridectomy, treatment includes cycloplegic eyedrops to relax the ciliary muscle and to decrease inflammation and thereby prevent adhesions. The end stage of glaucoma may require a tube shunt or valve to keep IOP down.

NURSING CONSIDERATIONS

- For the patient with angle-closure glaucoma, give medications as ordered and prepare him physically and psychologically for laser iridotomy or surgery.
- Remember to administer cycloplegic eyedrops in the affected eye only. In the unaffected eye, these drops may precipitate an attack of angle-closure glaucoma and threaten the patient's residual vision.
- After trabeculectomy, give medications as ordered to dilate the pupil. Also apply topical corticosteroids as ordered to rest the pupil.
- After surgery, protect the affected eye by applying an eye patch and shield, positioning the patient on his back or unaffected side and following general safety measures.
- Administer pain medication as ordered.
- Encourage ambulation immediately after surgery.
- Encourage the patient to express concerns related to having a chronic condition.
- Stress the importance of meticulous compliance with prescribed drug therapy to maintain low IOP and prevent optic disk changes that cause vision loss.
- Explain all procedures and treatments, especially surgery, to help reduce the patient's anxiety.
- Inform the patient that lost vision can't be restored but that treatment can usually prevent further loss.
- Instruct the patient's family how to modify the patient's environment for safety.

For example, suggest keeping pathways clear and reorienting the patient to room layouts, if necessary.
- Teach the patient signs and symptoms that require immediate medical attention, such as a sudden vision change or eye pain.
- Discuss the importance of glaucoma screening for early detection and prevention. Point out that all people over age 35, especially those with a family history of glaucoma, should have an annual tonometric examination.

Hearing loss

Hearing impairment is the most common disability in the United States and the third most prevalent in those over age 65. Mechanical or nervous impediment to the transmission of sound waves can produce hearing loss. The major forms are classified as conductive, sensorineural, and mixed.

In conductive hearing loss, sound is interrupted as it travels from the external canal to the inner ear (the junction of the stapes and the oval window). In sensorineural hearing loss, sound wave transmission is interrupted between the inner ear and the brain. Presbycusis, the most common type of sensorineural hearing loss, is prevalent in adults over age 50 and can't be reversed or corrected. Mixed hearing loss combines dysfunction of conduction and sensorineural transmission.

Sudden hearing loss, which can occur in a patient with no previous hearing loss, can be conductive, sensorineural, or mixed and usually affects only one ear. Depending on the cause, prompt treatment (within 48 hours) may restore hearing.

Noise-induced hearing loss may be transient or permanent. Such hearing loss is common in workers subjected to constant industrial noise and in military personnel, hunters, and rock musicians.

Hearing loss may be partial or total and is calculated using the American Medical Association formula: Hearing is 1.5% impaired for every decibel (dB) that the pure tone average exceeds 25 dB.

CAUSES AND INCIDENCE

The most common cause of conductive hearing loss is cerumen (earwax) impaction, which occurs in patients with small or hairy ear canals. Conductive loss may be caused by anything that blocks the external ear (foreign body, edema, or drainage from infection) or by thickening, retraction, scarring, or perforation of the tympanic membrane. Other causes include otitis media; otitis externa, which results from a gram-negative bacterial infection of the external ear canal; and otosclerosis, which produces ossification of the stapediovestibular joint.

Sensorineural hearing loss is caused by impairment of the cochlea or acoustic nerve (eighth cranial). Presbycusis results from loss of hair cells and nerve fibers in the cochlea or from drug toxicity. Other causes of nerve deafness include infectious diseases (such as measles, mumps, and meningitis), arteriosclerosis, otospongiosis, injury to the head or ear, and degeneration of the organ of Corti. Sensorineural hearing loss may also follow prolonged exposure to loud noise (85 to 90 dB) or brief exposure to extremely loud noise (greater than 90 dB). Occasionally, sensorineural hearing loss results from an acoustic neuroma (a benign tumor that can be life-threatening).

The cause of sudden hearing loss is unknown. However, the possibilities include occlusion of the internal auditory artery by spasm or thrombosis, subclinical mumps and other bacterial and viral infections, acoustic neuroma, or a single episode of Ménière's disease.

Sudden hearing loss also may be caused by metabolic disorders, such as hypothyroidism, diabetes mellitus, and hyperlipoproteinemia; vascular disorders such as hypertensive arteriosclerosis; neurologic disorders, such as multiple sclerosis and neurosyphilis; blood dyscrasias, such as leukemia and hypercoagulation; and ototoxic drugs, such as tobramycin, streptomycin, quinine, gentamicin, furosemide, and ethacrynic acid.

PATHOPHYSIOLOGY

In conductive hearing loss, the passage of sound from the external ear to the junction of the stapedes and oval window is interrupted. In sensorineural loss, hearing loss stems from impaired cochlear or acoustic (eighth cranial) nerve dysfunction, which causes a failure of transmission of sound impulses within the inner ear or brain. Mixed loss results from a combination of dysfunction of conduction and sensorineural transmission.

ASSESSMENT FINDINGS

For a patient with conductive hearing loss, the history may uncover a recent upper respiratory tract infection. The patient has a positive Weber's test and possibly a positive Rinne test (a positive Rinne test also may indicate sensorineural hearing loss).

A patient with sudden deafness may report recent exposure to loud noise or brief exposure to an extremely loud noise. The patient may complain of persistent tinnitus and transient vertigo. Audiometric tests indicate that the patient has a loss of perception of certain frequencies (around 4,000 Hz) or, if he's experienced lengthy exposure, loss of perception of all frequencies. Weber's and Rinne tests may indicate conductive or sensorineural hearing loss.

In sensorineural hearing loss from presbycusis, the patient history is probably the most valuable assessment tool because the patient may not have noticed the hearing loss or may deny it. The history also may expose the use of ototoxic substances. Hearing tests typically reveal a loss in the high-frequency tones. The patient may report a history of tinnitus. A positive Rinne test may indicate sensorineural hearing loss.

COMPLICATIONS

• Difficulty communicating

TREATMENT

Treatment for patients with hearing loss varies with the type and cause of impairment and may include medication to treat infections and dissolve cerumen, surgery (stapedectomy, tympanoplasty, cochlear implant, and myringotomy), hearing aids or other effective means of aiding communication, and antibiotics and decongestants for hearing loss from otitis media. Analgesics may be given for pain and antipyretics for fever. Treatment for sudden deafness requires prompt identification of the underlying cause.

For noise-induced hearing loss, overnight rest usually restores normal hearing in the patient exposed to noise levels greater than 90 dB but who hasn't been exposed to such noise repeatedly. As hearing deteriorates, treatment should include speech and hearing rehabilitation because hearing aids rarely help.

A cochlear implant may be an option for a profoundly deaf patient or one who's very hard of hearing. The device, which is surgically placed in the skin behind the ear, can provide a sense of sound to help the patient understand both auditory stimuli in his environment and speech. Unlike hearing aids, which simply amplify sound, a cochlear implant processes sounds from the environment, converting them to electrical impulses that are then transmitted to the brain for interpretation. In the United States, about 13,000 adults and 10,000 children have already received such implants.

Presbycusis may necessitate a hearing aid.

Dietary measures can help to prevent further hearing loss. Studies suggest that people with high cholesterol levels have greater hearing loss as they age than people with low cholesterol levels.

NURSING CONSIDERATIONS

• Answer the patient's questions, encourage him to discuss his concerns about hearing loss, and offer reassurance when appropriate.
• If the patient has difficulty understanding procedures because of hearing loss, give clear, concise explanations of treatments and procedures. Face him when speaking; enunciate words clearly, slowly, and in a normal tone; and allow adequate time for him to grasp what is expected. Provide a pencil and paper to aid communication, and alert staff members about his communication problem.
• To speak to a patient who can read lips, approach within his visual range and attract his attention by raising your arm or waving. (Touching him may be unnecessarily startling.) Then, stand directly in front of him in a well-lit area and speak slowly and distinctly.
• Place the patient with hearing loss in a place where he can observe activities and approach people because such a patient depends heavily or totally on visual clues.
• Encourage the patient who's learning to use a hearing aid because he may experience periods of self-doubt and apprehension about wearing the aid.
• Provide the patient and family members with opportunities to express their concerns and expectations about the hearing loss. Help them determine an alternate method of communication.

- Teach the patient and his family about hearing loss, its causes, and treatments.
- Explain all tests and procedures. For the patient who requires surgery, give preoperative and postoperative instructions.
- For the patient receiving a hearing aid, demonstrate how to operate and maintain the device and suggest carrying extra batteries at all times. Remind him that the hearing aid won't restore hearing to a normal level and that it makes speech louder but not necessarily clearer. Encourage him to experiment with the controls for best results. Advise him that lessons in lip reading may increase the effectiveness of the aid. Tell him that if the hearing aid requires repair, he may be able to borrow an aid from the repair agency.
- For the patient with temporary hearing loss, emphasize the danger of excessive exposure to noise and encourage the use of protective devices in a noisy environment.
- If the patient's hearing loss stems from cerumen buildup and the physician has advised ear cleaning or irrigation, demonstrate the proper technique for this and for instilling medication.
- If the patient has hearing loss from otitis media, discuss the antibiotics and decongestants ordered and tell him to report any adverse effects.
- Review the ordered medication, including its proper dosage, administration, and possible adverse effects.
- Encourage the patient to tell the physician about any significant earache.

Retinal detachment

In retinal detachment, separation of the retinal layers creates a subretinal space that fills with fluid. It may be primary or secondary.

The disorder usually involves only one eye but may occur in the other eye later. A detached retina rarely heals spontaneously; it can usually be reattached successfully with surgery. The prognosis for good vision depends on the area of the retina affected.

CAUSES AND INCIDENCE

A retinal detachment may be primary or secondary. A primary detachment occurs spontaneously because of a change in the retina or the vitreous; a secondary detachment results from another problem, such as intraocular inflammation or trauma.

The most common cause of retinal detachment is a hole or tear in the retina. This hole allows the liquid vitreous to seep between the retinal layers and separate the sensory retinal layer from its choroidal blood supply. In adults, retinal detachment usually results from degenerative changes related to aging (which cause a spontaneous tear). Predisposing factors include myopia, cataract surgery, and trauma.

Retinal detachment may also result from fluid seeping into the subretinal space as an effect of inflammation, tumors, or systemic disease. Or detachment may result from traction placed on the retina by vitreous bands or membranes (resulting from proliferative diabetic retinopathy, posterior uveitis, or a traumatic intraocular foreign body, for example).

The disorder is as common in men as in women. It may occasionally develop in a child from retinopathy of prematurity, tumors (retinoblastomas), or trauma. Retinal detachment can also be inherited, usually in association with myopia.

PATHOPHYSIOLOGY

Traumatic injury or degenerative changes cause retinal detachment by allowing the retina's sensory tissue layers to separate from the retinal pigment epithelium. This separation permits fluid—from example, from the vitre-ous—to seep into the space between the retinal pigment epithelium and the rods and cones of the tissue layers.

The pressure, which results from the fluid entering the space, balloons the retina into the vitreous cavity away from choroidal circula-tion. Separated from its blood supply, the retina can't function. Without prompt repair, the detached retina can cause permanent vision loss.

ASSESSMENT FINDINGS

Initially, the patient may complain that he sees floating spots and recurrent light flashes. As detachment progresses, he may report gradual, painless vision loss described as looking through a veil, curtain, or cobweb. He may relate that the veil obscures objects in a particular visual field.

COMPLICATIONS

- Severe vision impairment
- Possible blindness
- Risk of future retinal detachment in the other eye (with spontaneous detachment)

TREATMENT

Depending on the location and severity of the detachment, treatment may include restricting eye movements to prevent further separation until surgical repair can take place. The patient's head is positioned to allow gravity to pull the detached retina into closer contact with the choroid.

A patient with a hole in the peripheral retina may be treated with cryotherapy. A hole in the posterior retina may respond to laser therapy.

To reattach the retina, scleral buckling may be performed. In this procedure, the surgeon places a silicone plate or sponge over the reattachment site and secures it in place with an encircling band. The pressure exerted gently pushes the choroid and retina together. Scleral buckling may be followed by replacement of the vitreous with silicone, oil, air, or gas.

NURSING CONSIDERATIONS

- Provide encouragement and emotional sup-port to decrease anxiety caused by vision loss.
- Prepare the patient for surgery by cleaning the face with a mild (no-tears) shampoo. Give antibiotics and cycloplegic or mydri-atic eyedrops as ordered.
- In macular involvement, keep the patient on bed rest (with or without bathroom privileges) to prevent further retinal detachment.
- Postoperatively, position the patient as directed (the position varies according to the surgical procedure). To prevent increas-ing intraocular pressure (IOP), administer antiemetics as indicated. Discourage any activities that could increase IOP.
- Observe for slight localized corneal edema and peri-limbal congestion, which may follow laser therapy. To reduce edema and discomfort, apply ice packs and administer acetaminophen as ordered for headache.
- If the patient receives a retrobulbar injec-tion, apply a protective eye patch because the eyelid remains partially open.
- After removing the protective patch, give cycloplegic and steroidal or antibiotic eyedrops as ordered. Apply cold compresses to decrease swelling and pain, but avoid putting pressure on the eye.
- Give analgesics as needed, and report persistent pain.
- Encourage leg and deep-breathing exercises to prevent complications of immobility.
- Explain to the patient undergoing laser therapy that the procedure may be done in same-day surgery. Forewarn him that he

may have blurred vision for several days afterward.

- Instruct the patient to rest and to avoid driving, bending, heavy lifting, and any other activities that affect IOP for several days after eye surgery. Discourage activities that could cause the patient to bump the eye.

- Show the patient undergoing scleral buckling surgery how to instill eyedrops properly. After surgery, remind him to lie in the position recommended by the physician. Provide him with illustrations if necessary.

- Advise the patient to wear sunglasses if photosensitivity occurs.

- Instruct the patient to take acetaminophen as needed for headaches and to apply ice packs to the eye to reduce swelling and alleviate discomfort.

- Review the signs of increasing IOP and infection, emphasizing those that require immediate attention.

- Review early signs and symptoms of retinal detachment, and emphasize the need for immediate treatment.

Common Disorders, Uncommon Care

One of the difficulties of growing older is coping with a range of disorders, sometimes more than one at a time, and often chronic disorders—and all with a body that's steadily becoming less able to fight off the effects of disease. Such patients will need the best from you: compassion for what they're undergoing, knowledge of how disease affects older adults, and skill in providing the kind care older patients need. With your understanding of the disorders they face and how these disorders can affect them, you'll be able to offer all your older patients that uncommon care.

7

Sexuality:
Not Just for the Young

> *"Some things are better than sex, and some are worse, but there's nothing exactly like it."*
>
> —W.C. FIELDS

W hen we think about growing older, we don't usually think about sexuality. In fact, many people seem to think that sex pretty much fades into the background as we age, that the physical and psychological changes of aging prevent older people from wanting or being able to have satisfying sexual relationships. Our society still holds on to the stereotype that old people are unattractive, aren't interested in sex, and can't perform anyway.

We're slowly shedding this stereotype as more and more older adults make it clear that they *are* interested in sex, thank you very much, and that older is beautiful. And research backs that up, confirming that men and women maintain sexual interest and activity well into their 80s, enjoying the intimacy, pleasure, and tenderness that sexual expression provides. In fact, satisfying sexual expression helps keep older adults healthy in mind and body.

⌛ Timeline *One Hundred Years of Sex*

Older adults can well attest that sex is as old as the hills. Here's a quick look at how America's attitudes toward and tolerance of all things sexy have changed over the past century.

1943 Betty Grable becomes most celebrated pin-up girl of World War II

1946 Bikinis introduced

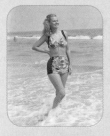

1939 Nylon stockings go on sale

1923 Charleston dance craze

1913 Mary Phelps Jacob invents modern bra

1929 D.H Lawrence's *Lady Chatterley's Lover* banned in U.S. for being obscene; ruling overturned in 1959

1917 Exotic dancer Mata Hari executed for being a spy

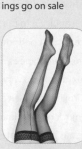

1948 Alfred Kinsey's *Sexual Behavior in the Human Male* is published to rave reviews; followed by *Sexual Behavior in the Human Female* in 1953

1900   10   20   30   40

1965 Miniskirts debut

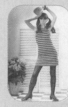

1965 "Make Love, Not War" buttons distributed at Mother's Day Peace March in Chicago; slogan adopted by countercultural factions during the 60s

1965 New York City's Great Blackout occurs on 11/9; credited with dramatic surge in births at area hospitals exactly 9 months later

1966 Masters & Johnson's *Human Sexual Response* published

1969 Gay rights movement born out of Stonewall riots in New York

1953 Marilyn Monroe poses for first issue of *Playboy*

1956 Elvis "the Pelvis" gyrates on Ed Sullivan Show

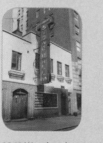

1969 Woodstock concert

1972 The Joy of Sex published

1972 *Last Tango in Paris* stars Marlon Brando; receives X rating by MPAA

1973 Abortion legalized in U.S.

1973 American Psychiatric Association eliminates "homosexuality" from official list of mental disorders

1980 Dr. Ruth Westheimer hosts radio talk show "Sexually Speaking"; premiers on TV in 1982

1989 Sean Connery (59) graces cover of *People* magazine as "Sexiest Man Alive"

1998 FDA approves Viagra as first oral treatment for impotence

1998 President Clinton impeached for perjury, obstruction of justice, and abuse of power stemming from Monica Lewinsky affair and Paula Jones lawsuit

2004 Same-sex marriages legalized in Massachusetts

Sex After 65, and Counting...

According to the Administration on Aging, almost 22 million women and 16 million men were age 65 or older as of 2008. That's 12.6% of the population, or more than one in every eight Americans—and that number is expected to grow. By 2010, 20.1% of the country's population will be 65 or older, and by 2020, a whopping 23.6.% of the population will have reached or passed age 65. At the same time, the country's birth rate continues to decline.

This shift in demographics calls for us as nurses to become more comfortable meeting the health care needs of older adults. We need to gain the necessary expertise to address issues of sexuality in older adults with sensitivity and tact. By doing so, we can help our older patients not only to improve their quality of life, but even to increase their quantity of life.

Myths and misinformation

The first step in understanding sexuality in older adults is recognizing myths for what they are. In our society, we see countless sexual images in advertising and programming on T.V., in magazines, and on the Internet. Almost all of these involve young, thin, beautiful men and women, or occasionally, very attractive middle-aged adults. Rarely are older adults portrayed as sexy. Instead, we're more likely to see images of an older adult as a grandmother knitting by the fire or a retiree reading his paper in his recliner—with not a hint of sexuality.

Here are some common myths:

- Only the young are sexually attractive.
- Sexuality in later life isn't dignified.
- Older men and women lose their ability to perform sexually after a certain age.
- People become bored with sex as they age.

MYTHBUSTING

The truth is quite different. A 1999 American Association of Retired People (AARP) survey found that adults age 45 and older actually considered their partners more physically attractive as they aged, busting the myth about sexuality waning with age. As people live longer, healthier lives and receive the health care they need, they're able to enjoy sex later into life.

A 2007 research study published in *The New England Journal of Medicine* supports the finding that older adults remain sexually active. The study examined 3,005 adults aged 57 to 85 and found that most had an active sex life with a partner or spouse. Of adults age 57 to 64, 73% reported recent sexual activity.

The percentage does decline with age. Only 53% of those aged 65 to 74 years and 26% of those aged 75 to 85 years reported recent sexual activity. Nevertheless, the study confirms that, although the percentage of sexually active older adults declines with age, most older adults still view sexuality as an important part of life. Unfortunately, the study also reports that sexual problems occur frequently among older adults, but that these adults rarely discuss such problems with their health care providers.

THE BOOMERS STEP UP

One very large group helping to dispel myths about older people and sexuality is the baby boomers. The older boomers—those just beginning to turn 65—view sex in a whole different light from previous generations. As young adults, they enjoyed sexual expression, and that hasn't changed as they've aged. Like adults from earlier generations, most boomers value the warmth, caring, and security of a loving, stable relationship. But the boomers grew into adulthood with birth control pills readily available and in a society that held a much more liberal outlook on sex. This group also helped open the door for gays, lesbians, and transsexuals to "come out" instead being forced to hide their sexual preferences from public view.

Separating myth from truth about older adult sexuality lays the groundwork for giving sexually active older adult patients good health care. The next step calls for an understanding of how physical aging and other factors affect older adults' sexuality.

Body Changes and Other Issues: Sidelining Sex?

As adults age, they experience sex-specific changes. Men take longer to achieve erections and have them for shorter periods, and women have diminished vaginal lubrication. In several landmark studies from the 1970s and 1980s, researchers found that male and female sexual responses didn't decrease significantly with age, nor did the capacity to experience orgasm. However, studies found that prolonged abstinence from sexual activity increased the risk of genital atrophy from disuse. (See *Physiologic changes that occur with aging.*)

Besides physiologic changes, other issues—including cultural taboos, rigid morality, and negative self-images—can also inhibit sexual activity. Later in this section, we'll examine how the different life spans of men and women, chronic illness, and medications can impact sexuality.

The body: Not what it once was

Although physiologic changes in sexual function are a normal part of aging, they trouble many older adults. Helping your patients understand that such changes as a slowed sexual response time are normal and reminding them that the ability to have an orgasm remains throughout life can help them cope with these changes.

CHANGES IN WOMEN...

In women, obvious changes may include wrinkles, sagging breasts, and less-erect posture. Such changes can harm a woman's sexual self-image, making her feel less desirable. Society generally portrays sexually attractive women as having no wrinkles and firm breasts, which can compound an older woman's self-image problem.

Besides these more visible changes, other, subtler changes can also affect an older woman's sexual health. Changes in the urinary tract, for instance, can have a profound impact. A roughly 50% loss of bladder capacity along with a decreased sensation of bladder

---

PHYSIOLOGIC CHANGES THAT OCCUR WITH AGING

The chart below highlights some of the key physiologic changes that occur as men and women age that can affect sexuality and sexual function.

Physiologic changes in men	Physiologic changes in women
● Slowed arousal	● Vaginal wall drying and atrophy
● Less pre-ejaculatory fluid	● Shortening and narrowing of vagina
● Decreased ejaculatory force	● Decreased acidic vaginal secretions
● Less firm erection	● Possible reduction in size of clitoris
● Shorter-lasting erection	
● Longer time to achieve another erection	
● Continued fertility	

fullness can lead to urinary incontinence, or a cystocele can lead to urinary dribbling. The fear of smelling like urine, despite frequent adult pad changes and showers, may cause an older woman to feel less desirable. But because many view incontinence as a taboo subject, the patient may have trouble discussing the problem, even with a health care professional. The impact of urinary incontinence on sexuality can make the subject even harder for the patient to discuss.

Teaching the patient Kegel exercises can help. If that doesn't help, certain medications, surgery, or other procedures can lessen the problem.

Another less-visible change, menopause decreases a woman's sexual drive, or libido. Taking a little extra time for stimulation before intercourse can help. The vaginal thinning and dryness that typically occur may also make intercourse uncomfortable; if the woman hasn't had much sexual stimulation for some time, the vaginal tissue may have atrophied, compounding the problem. Using water-based lubricants during intercourse can help improve the woman's comfort.

If the patient develops a prolapsed uterus, penile penetration can become difficult and uncomfortable. She can use a pessary during waking hours to manage the condition, or she may undergo surgical correction if necessary and if she's a good candidate for this procedure.

After menopause, a woman typically needs more time to become sexually stimulated, and she'll feel less intense stimulation than she used to. Lack of interest, loss of physical stamina, or a decrease in the ability to perform because of an underlying condition can compound the problem.

Hysterectomy, which is the second most frequent surgery (after cesarean section) performed on adult American women, can also change a woman's sexual response. About a third of women have had the surgery by the time they reach age 60. Such women may experience several effects. For instance, altering the nerve supply can lead to a change in lubrication and orgasm. Removal of the cervix and its mucous-producing glands may diminish vaginal lubrication, leading to dyspareunia. Or removal or alteration of the upper vaginal area—a highly sensitive area that expands during arousal—may result in decreased sensation and arousal. However, most women experience few adverse sexual effects from hysterectomy. Just like younger patients, an older patient facing one or more of these challenges to expressing sexuality still needs love, warmth, sharing, closeness, intimacy, sensuality, and touching. Offer support as appropriate to such a patient, including advising her about resources available to help her cope with the situation.

...AND IN MEN

Older men face many of the same challenges. They, too, experience visible physical changes—sagging skin, wrinkles, gray, thinning hair—that threaten their self-esteem and feelings of physical attractiveness. Most older men do maintain their regular interest in sex, although chronic illness may lessen stamina and interest level.

For men, the sexual act may require more time and effort just as it does for women. Older men take longer to achieve full penile erection and have less firm erections than younger men; such chronic illness as diabetes and certain medications, such as antihypertensives and antidepressants, can make an erection less firm still. Keep an eye out for the older male patient who stops taking such medications. Doing so not only puts his health at risk by may signal an underlying sexual problem.

Men may also have weaker ejaculations and less intense orgasms with age and need more time to recover between sexual acts.

Male-enhancement drugs can help with this problem, and many men do use them. *The New England Journal of Medicine* study from 2007 found that 14% of men interviewed used a drug or supplement to improve sexual function.

If your patient tells you he's having difficulty performing, recommend a full physical evaluation, including an assessment of medications and sexual difficulties, to help determine what steps can be taken and if a male-enhancement drug might be appropriate. If the patient has a cardiac condition, warn him against getting these drugs from a disreputable supplier, such as one who sells through certain Internet sites or through the mail. Also, make sure he understands the importance of thoroughly discussing these drugs and their possible effects with his cardiologist before taking anything.

Other issues: Dampening desire

Other factors can also interfere with an older adult's sexuality, everything from the availability of partners to the effects of illnesses, surgeries, and medications. The good news: For many of these situations, there are remedies.

THE PARTNER PROBLEM

One of the hard facts of aging is that women generally outlive men, with the ratio of women to men steadily increasing with advancing age. As a result, older women tend to have more difficulty finding partners, and those men who live longer may actually have multiple female partners. *The New England Journal of Medicine* study found that almost 80% of men aged 75 to 85 had a spousal or intimate relationship, compared with around 40% of women in the same age-group.

This disparity can lead to some risky behaviors. For instance, in an independent living facility where older women greatly outnumber older men, a man may have sex with several of the women, increasing the

possibility of spreading sexually transmitted infections (STIs).

A widowed or divorced older woman also has a much smaller chance of remarrying than a man in the same circumstances. Concerns over inheritance or conflicts with grown children can also interfere with remarriage for either sex, and the need to care for a chronically ill or disabled spouse can severely limit an older person's sexual choices.

CHRONIC ILLNESS...

Chronic illness can not only reduce an older adult's stamina, but some of the physical changes that can occur with certain illnesses can interfere with sex. Medication and surgery can sometimes lessen the impact of chronic illness. (See *Illness and sexuality*, page 316.)

MAJOR SURGERY...

Surgery can also affect sexual function. As mentioned earlier, hormonal and structural changes from a hysterectomy can impact a woman's sexuality, although the surgery itself doesn't typically lead to sexual dysfunction. In fact, studies indicate that not only do most women suffer few adverse sexual effects from the surgery, but some symptoms women had experienced before surgery actually stopped after surgery.

Mastectomy can also interfere with a woman's sexuality. A woman who has lost a breast may feel less feminine or fear that she's less attractive to her partner; these feeling can dampen her sexual desire.

For men, a prostatectomy may affect potency. After a transurethral resection of the prostate, men may lose potency or become impotent; they may also experience retrograde ejaculation.

...AND CREATIVE RESPONSES

Different methods—including some surprisingly simple solutions—can help many older

ILLNESS AND SEXUALITY

Illness can profoundly affect an older adult's sexuality, whether from physical or psychological effects. Several disorders that commonly occur in older adults can make sexual activity more challenging.

Heart Disease

Although older adults with heart disease may avoid sexual activity because they fear having a heart attack during sex, studies show that cardiac death rarely occurs during or after sexual activity. In fact, sexual activity provides mild exercise and tension release.

However, after an event such as myocardial infarction (MI), heart failure, or bypass surgery, it's recommended that an older patient wait for a period before resuming sexual activity. After an MI, an adult should typically wait 8 to 14 weeks before resuming sexual activity. The exact duration depends on the patient's desires, general fitness, and conditioning.

After heart failure with an episode of pulmonary edema, a patient should wait 2 to 3 weeks, or until normal exertion—such as climbing two flights of stairs—doesn't produce any symptoms. If managed effectively, sexual activity may actually help improve the patient's condition.

Older patients with angina should engage in sexual activity in a relaxed atmosphere, possibly in the late morning after a full night's sleep. The supine position may help reduce energy expenditure (equivalent to climbing a single flight of stairs or walking a city block); taking nitroglycerin before sex can prevent or treat angina. Remind your patient who takes nitroglycerin that he can't use sildenafil (Viagra) to treat erectile dysfunction because it may cause a severe, even fatal, drop in blood pressure.

Hypertension

The older patient with mild to moderate hypertension doesn't need to restrict sexual activity. Men with uncontrolled hypertension and those taking antihypertensives may experience erectile dysfunction.

Diabetes Mellitus

Older men with diabetes mellitus may experience erectile dysfunction; the rate is two to five times higher than in the general population. The disease doesn't affect sexual desire.

Stroke

Stroke may affect sexual functioning, but it doesn't typically affect sexual desire unless the patient suffered severe brain damage. Some men who have had a stroke may experience erectile dysfunction. If the stroke caused a motor dysfunction, the older adult can use pillows, headboards, or overhead grips to support the area during sexual activity.

Hypothyroidism

This disorder can reduce potency.

Arthritis

Pain from osteoarthritis or rheumatoid arthritis can decrease sexual desire and performance. Such comfort measures as exercise, rest, and heat may help reduce pain, which can in turn promote sexual activity.

Planning sexual activity for times of the day when the patient has less pain can help. For some patients, sexual activity can even decrease pain for 4 to 8 hours, possibly because of the release of endorphins, hormone production, or the physical activity.

Chronic or Recurrent Prostatitis

Pain from the disorder can diminish interest in sexual activity. Warm baths, Kegel exercises, and sitz baths may decrease discomfort.

Cystitis or Urethritis

Mucosal changes that occur during sexual activity can exacerbate these conditions.

Peyronie's Disease

For about half of men with this disorder, intercourse is uncomfortable. If the patient's penis is angled too sharply, he may not be able to achieve penetration. Medical and surgical interventions aren't considered effective, although symptoms sometimes resolve spontaneously after a few years.

Chronic Renal Disease

In chronic renal disease, both older men and women may have reduced serum testosterone levels. Many patients experience reduced libido, and men may experience erectile dysfunction. Men with this chronic condition may also experience anxiety and depression, which can affect sexual functioning.

Parkinson's Disease

With advanced neurologic involvement, older men may develop erectile dysfunction. This chronic illness also typically causes depression, which can lead to erectile dysfunction in men and lack of sexual desire in both sexes.

Chronic Emphysema and Bronchitis

Shortness of breath interferes with all physical exercise, including sexual activity. Resting during sexual activity, finding less strenuous ways to approach a partner, and using oxygen or an inhaler before engaging in sex may help.

R℞ *Medication Alert*   Medications and Sexuality

Several types of medications can affect sexual function.

Antidepressants

- Tricyclic antidepressants such as amitriptyline (Elavil), doxepin (Sinequan), imipramine (Tofranil) and nortriptyline (Aventyl, Pamelor)
- Monoamine oxidase inhibitors (MAOIs) such as phenelzine (Nardil) and tranylcypromine (Parnate)
- Anti-psychotic medications such as thioridazine (Mellaril), thiothixene (Navane) and haloperidol (Haldol)
- Anti-mania medications such as lithium carbonate (Eskalith, Lithobid)
- Selective serotonin reuptake inhibitors (SSRIs) such as fluoxetine (Prozac), sertraline (Zoloft) and paroxetine (Paxil).

Antihypertensives

- Diuretics, including spironolactone (Aldactone) and the thiazides (Diuril, Naturetin, and others)
- Centrally acting agents, including methyldopa (Aldomet) and reserpine (Serpasil, Raudixin)
- Alpha-Adrenergic blockers, including prazosin (Minipress) and terazosin (Hytrin)
- Beta-adrenergic (beta) blockers, including propranolol (Inderal) and metoprolol (Lopressor)

Hormones

- Lupron
- Zoladex

adults regain sexual enjoyment. For example, having sex in the morning, when both partners are better rested, can improve stamina. Switching to the morning can also help a patient with osteoarthritis because symptoms are typically less severe in the morning. An older adult who has a respiratory condition can use an inhaler before intercourse to improve respiratory status, which will in turn improve stamina. Taking pain medications before sex can help to reduce discomfort during intercourse.

Different positions can also make the sexual act much more comfortable. Several guides, including online sources and printed material, can help older adults decide what positions would be most comfortable for them and can save them from the embarrassment of discussing it with health care providers; make sure you steer the patient towards reputable sources.

Other suggestions include mutual masturbation as a means to maintain sexual gratification of both partners if intercourse isn't possible, or use of a vibrator when the arthritis interferes with manual stimulation.

ADDING MEDICATIONS TO THE MIX

Older adults typically take several medications, including both over-the-counter and prescription drugs. Many of these can adversely affect sexuality and sexual function. Be prepared to answer questions the patient may have about the effects of these drugs. (See *Medications and sexuality*.)

The Sexual Assessment: A Tactful Approach

A sexual assessment of an older adult calls for you to appraise and manage both the normal and pathologic aging changes that can affect the patient's sexual health. To perform the assessment and gather the necessary information, you'll need to be comfortable with the questions such an assessment requires you to ask. You may sometimes find it challenging to balance your own beliefs about sexuality and sexual functioning with the need to be open and nonjudgmental with your patients. But remember that your tactful, supportive approach goes a long way toward helping your older patients cope with their own discomfort in talking about such a private, personal topic with a health care professional.

Before beginning your assessment, select a quiet, relaxed area that ensures the patient's privacy. Maintain eye contact and demonstrate respect throughout the assessment.

Spelling it out: The PLISSIT model

One guide that can help you assess an older adult's sexuality is the PLISSIT model. This model provides an easy, step-by-step guide you can follow to make the assessment go more smoothly. (See *The PLISSIT model.*)

The PLISSIT model consists of four simple steps that can guide you through the conversation. At first, both you and the patient may feel uncomfortable with this process, but make sure you follow the steps. It's also okay to acknowledge that you both may feel a little uncomfortable with the process; your acknowledgement shows your honesty, promotes trust, helps the patient relax, and demonstrates the

importance of this part of the health history. Ask questions that guide the patient to provide enough information to give a clear picture of problems and risks.

PERMISSION

First, ask the patient for permission to ask questions about his sexual health. Doing so actively involves the patient and fosters a sense of autonomy and control over the situation. For instance, you can ask, "Would it be okay with you if I asked you some questions about your sexual health and function?"

Alternatively, you can couple the question with a lead-in statement, such as the following: "Many of my older adult patients have some trouble with their sexual health. Would it be all right if I ask you some questions about this part of your life?" Such a statement followed by a request for permission lets the patient know that he's not the only older adult experiencing sexual problems and acknowledges the importance of sexual health for older adults.

Once you've broached the topic of sexual health, you can ask questions that will garner information about important health issues and where the patient may need further guidance and education. But how much useful information you gather depends on *how* you ask questions. Don't pose yes-or-no questions or questions the patient can answer with one or two words. Try a more open-ended approach. For instance, "Do you have any concerns about your sexuality now?" may get you a simple "no" as a response. But a question such as "What concerns do you have now about your sexuality?" allows the older patient to voice concerns he may have had for a while but wasn't sure how to share, perhaps out of fear of rejection or of shocking the health care professional. Asking "How has your sexuality changed in the recent months?" can open the door to important information about health-related changes.

THE PLISSIT MODEL

Use the acronym PLISSIT to help you assess an older adult's sexuality:

- **P**: Obtain **P**ermission from the patient to initiate sexual discussion.
- **LI**: Provide the **L**imited **I**nformation necessary to dispel any misinformation the patient may have and to help the patient function sexually.
- **SS**: Offer **S**pecific **S**uggestions to address the sexual issues the patient.
- **IT**: If necessary, arrange for **I**ntensive **T**herapy to help the patient deal with specific sexual issues.

Adapted with permission from Springer Science + Business Media: Esmail, S., et al. "Sexuality and Disability: The Role of Health Care Professionals in Providing Options and Alternatives for Couples," *Sexuality and Disability* 19(4):267-82, Winter 2001.

You can often rephrase the patient's answers to such questions to gradually focus on more sensitive areas, such as methods to improve the quality of the patient's sexual life. And you can gather answers that can lead you to more focused questions to pinpoint the exact problem.

LIMITED INFORMATION

Once you've gathered the information you need, you can offer the patient information appropriate to his concerns, including an explanation of normal age-related changes and changes specifically related to any underlying condition he has or medication he uses. Be aware that your own knowledge level and how much the patient is willing to take in limit this information.

SPECIFIC SUGGESTIONS

Next, move on to specific suggestions. For instance, you may need to talk to the patient's physician about possibly changing a medication that's causing a problem. Or you may need to ask the patient how he handled a similar situation in the past to see if the same method might help now.

INTENSIVE THERAPY

You may also discover that the patient needs intensive therapy for a particular issue. If so, you'll need to make appropriate referrals. (See the *Case Study* below.)

Completing the picture

Several specific questions can lead to a more complete picture of the older adult's sexual situation and help you determine what to explore further. They include the following:

- Can you tell me how you express your sexuality?
- What concerns or questions do you have about fulfilling your continuing sexual needs?
- How has your sexual relationship with your partner changed as you've aged?
- What interventions or information can I offer you to help you to fulfill your sexuality?

As mentioned earlier, answers you receive to your questions can lead you to more focused questions. If the patient mentions using a medication—an antihypertensive, for instance—you can ask more specific questions about it to determine if a correlation exists between using the drug and a reported sexual issue. If the patient brings up a chronic health condition, you can ask specific questions to determine if the condition is affecting his sexual well-being. Then you can help the patient understand how his medication use or chronic illness is affecting his sexual health.

Throughout the assessment, demonstrate total interest and let the patient explain with minimal interruptions. As you listen, note any misunderstandings or lack of complete information, and offer suggestions as appropriate that can improve the patient's sexual health.

Case Study

A patient who has recently been diagnosed with diabetes mellitus comes to the facility where you work to discuss erectile problems he's having when he and his wife want to engage in sexual activity. Although it's clear to you that he wants help with the situation, he seems nervous and hesitant to talk with you about the situation.

Critical thinking questions

1. How would you effectively use the PLISSIT model to gather the information you need for a thorough sexual history?
2. What are two open-ended questions that would help the patient express the problem he's having with sexual functioning?

If the patient mentions anything that may put his sexual or overall health at risk, explain the risks to the patient, and discuss ways to reduce the risk if possible.

Dealing with your own discomfort

Despite your best efforts to maintain a sensitive, nonjudgmental attitude, you may find yourself becoming uncomfortable. Nursing education programs don't typically focus on sexuality, particularly in older adults. Plus, you're surrounded by the same stereotypes and myths as everyone else. You can help improve your comfort level by becoming more self-aware and more comfortable with your own sexuality. The following self-teaching methods can help you decrease your anxiety and improve your understanding of sexuality in older adults.

MAKE YOURSELF COMFORTABLE...

One way to you can become more comfortable with the PLISSIT model and other assessment questions and improve the outcome of your conversations with your older patients is to practice these questions with a colleague. Role-play interviewing different types of patients—including patients in nontraditional sexual relationships—who have different sexual health problems. Keep in mind as you role play that many older adults can be very reluctant to talk about sexuality, making this kind of practice even more important.

Caught on tape

Try videotaping the practice sessions so that you can learn from both your verbal and nonverbal responses. Watch your nonverbal responses in particular; you may be surprised at how much they reveal about your true anxiety level.

Not-so-trivial pursuit

One surprisingly effective way to learn more about older adult sexuality and lessen anxiety

in the process is the Sexual Dysfunction Trivia game. Designed to teach nurses how to identify sexual dysfunction in older adults, this game has been tested on staff nurses in a pilot project, although it's not yet available. Compared with their knowledge before playing, the nurses who played the game showed a significant improvement in knowledge about sexual dysfunctions in older adults. The tool needs more research to measure its effectiveness, but it looks promising.

The name game

Another game can help decrease your anxiety by desensitizing you to some of the sexual terms you may hear used. In this game, a group of health care professionals state alternate names for genitalia they've heard from older patients and from the general public. You'll find this game typically results in a couple of embarrassing moments—and lots of healthy laughter. By the end of the game, the participants have not only set aside much of their nervousness, but have become more aware of what people may call different body parts. Many health departments use this tool to help train health care professionals for work in STI clinics.

Outside the Norm: Alternative Lifestyles

When you begin the sexual assessment, don't be surprised if your older patient doesn't fit society's stereotype of the happily married, heterosexual couple. For instance, an older adult may be having sex outside of marriage and may be too embarrassed to share that information, especially with a younger health care professional. A patient may be gay, lesbian, or transgendered and may be afraid to discuss the issue with you. You may even find that you have a married patient who's having an affair outside of marriage with a member of the same sex. Keep in mind that your role is never to judge, but to keep communication open and to remain unbiased.

Although sex is typically thought of as an act between a man and a woman and most of the general health literature addresses it as such, the Centers for Disease Control and Prevention (CDC), the National Institutes of Health, and several other reputable Web sites offer information on gay, lesbian, and transgender people. The 2000 Census also provides some interesting statistics about older adult sexuality in the United States. For instance, at least one senior citizen in a same-sex partnership lives in 97% of U.S. counties, and in more than 1 out of every 10 same-sex partnerships, one partner is aged 65 or older.

If your patient has an alternative sexual lifestyle, keep in mind that any sexual problems he may have as a result of aging can be compounded by health risks associated with his particular lifestyle. As with all of your older patients, your compassionate listening and careful assessment play a key role in detecting risks to the patient's sexual and overall health and providing him with the help he needs.

Gay men

The public's exposure to same-sex relationships has steadily increased with the portrayal of such relationships on television in shows such as *Will and Grace* and *The L Word* and movies such as *Brokeback Mountain*. Although many people still don't accept homosexuality as "normal," homosexuals have made significant progress in being accepted by society, including winning the right to legally marry in some states. This increasing acceptance can make it easier for you to broach the subject of homosexuality with an older gay patient.

Men who engage in sex with other men (MSM) can come from any ethnicity or class. About 5% to 7% of men classify themselves as MSM, although the number is likely higher.

RISKY BUSINESS

If your older male patient engages in sex with other men, he may be at higher risk for contracting an STI, especially human immunodeficiency virus (HIV) infection, the virus that causes acquired immunodeficiency syndrome (AIDS). As of 2005, 71% of all HIV infections in men occurred in the MSM group, highlighting the risk to this population and emphasizing the need for providing reliable health care education to such patients. Gay men in stable, monogamous relationships are at much lower risk for contracting STIs.

By the numbers

Consider these statistics from a survey conducted on a community of 1,900 gay men living in British Columbia. More than 15% had used crystal methamphetamine with sex. Many had never been tested for HIV. Those that were HIV positive were more likely to use this drug than those who hadn't yet contracted the disease. Of those diagnosed with HIV, 53% expected their partners to let them know they had HIV, whereas 74% of those who were HIV negative had that expectation. Such statistics highlight the STI risk for members of the MSM group who engage in risky sexual behaviors, with those having multiple partners at greatest risk.

The danger of drugs

Use of other recreational drugs can also put this group at risk. Using alcohol alone reduces a person's inhibitions enough to risk not using protection. Using other "party" drugs, such as ecstasy, ketamine, and gamma hydroxybutyrate—sometime along with nitrate inhalants, commonly called poppers—reduce inhibitions further, increasing the risk of engaging in dangerous sexual behavior.

Using methamphetamines during anal sex also increases the risk of STI transmission. The rectum has many blood vessels very close to the surface; methamphetamine causes these vessels to engorge, creating a ready conduit for HIV, syphilis, and other STIs to pass into the bloodstream. To help prevent the spread of STIs, public health advocates recommend using condoms for anal sex, although many people ignore this recommendation.

AN UNACCEPTABLE SITUATION

Unfortunately, many in our society still stigmatize homosexuality. As recently as 1973, the American Psychiatric Association (APA) listed homosexuality as an official diagnosis in the Diagnostic and Statistical Manual of Mental Disorders, although the APA issued a statement in 1992 that homosexuality was not a mental disorder.

Despite society's increased acceptance of homosexuality, many gay men say that they don't seek health care education because homophobia continues to make it difficult. Many are still afraid to come out publicly, resulting in too many gay men—including older gay men—afraid to reach out to health care professionals for education that can improve their sexual health and decrease their risks.

Lesbian women

Like gay men, lesbians face significant health risks. The American College of Obstetricians and Gynecologists (ACOG) discusses these risks in a 2008 news release. The news release urges testing of lesbian and bisexual patients for STIs. It also states that, because most lesbians have had a male partner at some point, they're at higher risk for catching an STI, reminding health care providers that STIs pose a health risk even to women in a same-sex relationship.

The news release also discusses oral sex, anal sex, and other noncoital sexual activity, pointing out that both same-sex and heterosexual couples don't routinely use a condom or dental dam during oral sex. Unprotected noncoital sex increases the risk of passing on several STIs, including gonorrhea, chlamydia, herpes simplex virus (HSV), and syphilis, with HSV the greatest risk from oral sex.

According to ACOG, you should ask your patients, including older lesbian patients, direct, personal questions to obtain an accurate sexual health history. It's as important as checking a patient's temperature or blood glucose level and can reveal risks to both her sexual and overall health.

WHAT YOU DON'T KNOW...

It's crucial to the health of your older lesbian patients to know what questions to ask to obtain an accurate sexual history. But many lesbians, particularly older lesbians, are reluctant to openly discuss their sexual history out of fear of rejection or prejudice, and you may have a difficult time gathering an accurate, useful sexual health history. What's worse, fear of prejudice prevents many lesbians from seeking out health care at all, even when an acute situation may endanger their health. And lesbians are less likely than heterosexual women to seek preventative health care, so many lesbians lose out on the benefits of regular breast exams, Papanicolaou (Pap) tests, mammograms, cancer screenings, and other types of early detection.

If you're unsure of some of the health risks facing your lesbian patients, you can turn to a Web site maintained by the U.S. Department of Health and Human Services that answers frequently asked questions about lesbian health. You can use this excellent resource

HEALTH RISKS FOR OLDER LESBIAN WOMEN

The Lesbian Health page (http://www.womenshealth.gov/FAQ/lesbian-health.cfm), maintained by the U.S. Department of Health and Human Services, provides useful answers to frequently asked questions about lesbian health issues. It reminds us that lesbians face particular challenges when dealing with the health care system and are at higher risk for certain disorders, including those listed here:

- Heart disease
- Obesity
- Alcohol and drug abuse
- Cancer
  - Uterine
  - Breast
  - Cervical
  - Endometrial
  - Ovarian

- Domestic violence
- Polycystic ovarian syndrome
- Osteoporosis
- Sexually transmitted infections
  - Bacterial vaginosis
  - Human papilloma virus
  - Trichomoniasis
  - Genital herpes
  - Syphilis
  - Chlamydia
  - Gonorrhea
  - Hepatitis B
  - Human immunodeficiency virus
  - Acquired immunodeficiency syndrome
  - Pubic lice

when caring for an older lesbian patient to answer many of your own questions and to help you focus on what questions to ask your patient. (See *Health risks for older lesbian women.*)

DOUBLE JEOPARDY

Heart disease is the overall number one killer of women in the United States, and lesbians are anything but exempt from this killer. If anything, they may be at higher risk than the general female population, for this and other dangerous health conditions.

The risk factors for heart disease for all women include smoking, obesity, and high stress, factors that are prevalent in lesbians. An older lesbian is at even higher risk as a result of advancing age and because she's postmenopausal. If your older lesbian patient is at high risk, make sure she understands the importance of stopping smoking, limiting high cholesterol, and exercising.

Lesbian women also typically have a higher body mass than heterosexual women, with more body fat stored around the abdomen. This higher body mass increases their risk not only for heart disease, but also for cancer of the breast, ovaries, uterus, and colon.

A FEW DRINKS TOO MANY

As a whole, nontraditional populations are at increased risk from drug and alcohol abuse. And, although alcohol abuse has dropped over the past 20 years in lesbians as a group, older lesbians haven't shown a drop in alcohol consumption. Make sure you assess older lesbian patients for indications of alcohol abuse.

THE HOME FRONT

Don't overlook the possibility of domestic violence in your sexual health assessment. Lesbians may be less likely to report such violence out of fear of discrimination and misunderstanding. If a couple has children, an abused partner may be even less likely to report such violence for fear of a custody battle.

THE DANGERS OF DISEASE

Several diseases threaten the sexual health of older lesbians. Polycystic ovarian syndrome (PCOS), for instance, affects roughly 5% to 10% of all women aged 20 to 40, but evidence suggests it affects a much greater percentage of lesbians. A woman with PCOS may experience altered or absent menstruation, infertility, increased androgen levels, altered insulin production, the appearance of cysts on her ovaries, and changes to her heart, blood vessels, and general appearance. Although older lesbian patients may not be at risk for developing this disease because of their advanced age, keep in mind that they may have suffered from it earlier in life. The risks for heart attack, stroke, and diabetes from PCOS increase with age, putting an older lesbian patient with the disease at increased risk. PCOS may be one reason some older lesbians have an increased body mass index, waist circumference, and abdominal adiposity.

Older lesbians aren't immune to the risks of STIs, and the risk increases with multiple partners. STIs can pass from one person to another through menstrual blood, vaginal fluids, and other body fluids; mucosal contact; and skin-to-skin contact. Sharing sex toys can also increase the risk. Although not an STI itself, bacterial vaginosis—relatively common in women who engage in unprotected sex with partners of either sex—increases the risk for contracting an STI.

Human papillomavirus (HPV), the cause of genital warts, can also spread through sexual contact and can increase a woman's risk for cervical cancer. Because so many lesbian patients forgo such preventive care as regular Pap tests, HPV infection can remain undetected in older lesbians.

Other types of STIs include trichomoniasis, a parasite that's transmitted from one partner to another during sexual contact through vaginal secretions, and HSV, a virus transmitted by direct genital contact that can lead to painful lesions requiring medication to decrease the number and vigor of outbreaks. These lesions continue to shed the virus even when the infected partner takes medication and lesions aren't visible on the skin surface, putting the uninfected partner at risk if the two continue to have sex. Although syphilis rarely passes between female partners, if your older lesbian patient has genital lesions that aren't healing, she should be tested for syphilis.

REDUCING THE RISKS

You'll offer many of the same recommendations for maintaining or improving sexual and overall health to your older lesbian patients as you would to your other patients. Recommend regular health exams, with an emphasis on the risks that stem from being in a relationship with a person of the same sex. If the patient has multiple partners, explain that she should be regularly tested for STIs and practice safe sex.

If she's overweight or smokes, steer her toward a healthier diet, help her develop an exercise program, and suggest joining a smoking cessation program. If she abuses drugs or alcohol, help her with coping skills to reduce her stress, and recommend such programs as Alcoholics Anonymous if appropriate. If you suspect she's the victim of domestic violence, talk to her about the possibility, and provide her with information on seeking help.

Transgender adults

As people who have completed the transformation from one sex to another grow older, you're more likely to find yourself caring for transgender older adults. Although a person doesn't typically complete such a transformation until midlife, surgery to transform sex has been growing in popularity for the past 50 years, meaning that more transgender people are entering their later years.

10 THINGS...

Many health care providers don't know all that they should about transgender patients. Dr. Rebecca A. Allison, a member of the Board of Directors for the Gay and Lesbian Medical Association (GLMA), has published a list that can help. "Ten Things Transgender Persons Should Discuss with Their Health Care Providers" lists the health issues that GLMA health care providers consider the most common concern for transgender people. They are:

- access to health care
- health history
- hormones
- cardiovascular health
- cancer
- STIs and safe sex
- alcohol and tobacco
- depression and anxiety
- injectable silicone
- fitness.

Dr. Allison explains that, in the past, transgender people have been turned away and shunned by health care providers. Insurance doesn't always cover the treatments needed to change a person's sex or the possible problems that can arise, resulting in a group of people who may become very ill before seeking health care. Transgender patients may also hide their real health history from health care providers, fearing being turned away. She asks that health care professionals treat transgender patients as they would any other patient.

RATCHETING UP THE RISK

Older transgender patients face unique health risks because of the hormone therapy they received as part of their treatment. The estrogen used by men to become women can increase the risk of blood clots, hypertension, hyperglycemia, and water retention, and antiandrogens can produce dehydration, hypotension, and electrolyte imbalances. Women taking testosterone to become men can suffer liver damage. The risk increases when a patient has taken hormones from someone other than a reputable health care professional and without medical supervision.

Transgender patients also have a higher cardiovascular risk, with an increased chance of heart attack and stroke, because of factors such as hormone therapy and the overall stress from the sex-change procedure. Many also smoke, adding to the risk. And because they fear being found out, many don't seek out health care, even when they have noticeable signs and symptoms of a heart attack or stroke.

Hormone therapy increases the cancer risk for both sexes. Transgender women have an increased risk for breast cancer, and transgender men are more likely to develop liver cancer—risks that grow as the patient ages.

If a transgender man hasn't had his female reproductive organs removed, he's at risk for cancer in these organs. If the patient doesn't reveal that he still has female reproductive organs to his health care provider, it will complicate early detection of cancer. A transgender woman who still has a prostate is at risk for prostate cancer, a risk that increases if she doesn't share this information with her health care provider. In fact, not knowing such crucial facts about these patients' health histories may be the biggest cancer risk of all for transgender patients because it delays early detection, when cancer is most treatable.

THE ISOLATION ISSUE

Social isolation also poses health risks to older transgender patients, health threats that further complicate an already complicated set of health issues. Transgender people are at risk for alcohol abuse, drug use, and unsafe sex. Many also smoke and are overweight, perhaps as a result of social isolation and resultant depression and anxiety.

A specific risk to transgender women comes from the silicone injections they use to give them a more feminine appearance. Many participate in "pumping parties," where, without proper medical training, they inject silicone into each other's bodies. These transgender women are at risk for hepatitis and other disease from sharing needles, long-term problems from silicone traveling to other parts of the body, even disfigurement.

Although older transgender people compose only a small percentage of the overall population, their numbers continue to grow as more people seek to change their sex and as the current group of transgender people age. Understanding the particular health issues of older transgender people will allow you to more fully explore their health histories so that you can gain a complete and accurate picture and offer these patients the best health care.

Your role

Whenever you care for an older patient, listen carefully for clues that he may fall outside a traditional sexual relationship. If you suspect a patient is gay, lesbian, or transgender, understanding the particular health risks and concerns of these groups will allow you to offer care tailored to the patient's specific needs. You'll also be better prepared to gather a complete health history, which can sometimes be more difficult with such patients, who may have had to cope with prejudice and as a result are less forthcoming. Using tact and patience

and remaining nonjudgmental and compassionate can help you give these often-ignored patients the excellent health care everyone deserves.

Close Quarters: Long-term Care Facilities

The need for affection, closeness, and sexual expression doesn't vanish when an older adult moves to a long-term care facility. An adult who no longer has a spouse, partner, or other family members to meet such needs and may turn to another resident. Nursing staff members working in such facilities confirm that outward displays of affection commonly occur between residents.

These displays of affection can sometimes escalate into something more intimate, leaving staff members wondering how to diplomatically and equitably handle such situations and respect the needs of all parties. Things can grow more complicated if one partner has a spouse who doesn't live in the facility. Such a situation calls for open discussion with all parties, including adult children if appropriate, to define the parameters of an acceptable relationship.

Studies have shown that staff members have a variety of reactions to residents expressing their need for closeness and intimacy, ranging from confusion, embarrassment, and helplessness to humor and ridicule. Some staff members view resident's displays of affection and intimacy as a behavior problem rather than the expression of a legitimate need.

Both staff members and residents' family members need to understand that residents who have the mental capacity have the right to choose relationships that meet their sexual needs. Plus, the long-term care facility is the residents' home; residents should have the opportunity to form relationships with each other, as they would in their own homes. If two older adults both have the mental capacity to decide to engage in a relationship—whether just cuddling and touching or sexual intercourse—staff members should try to provide them with the privacy they need.

PRIVATE NEEDS, NOT-SO-PRIVATE SETTING

A couple that has one resident living in a long-term care facility and the other living at home faces a different problem: finding some privacy, especially if the resident has a roommate. The couple may be embarrassed to openly discuss the problem with staff members, fearing the stereotype that older adults don't have sex anymore. In some cases, the resident may leave the facility and move back home so that the couple can have an intimate relationship, leaving the spouse to resume caregiver duties. The burden of caregiving may end up jeopardizing the caregiver's health, resulting in a worse situation for both of them—and all because the couple needed some privacy.

Obtaining an honest, complete sexual history on admission to a long-term care facility can help avoid such a problem. Understanding a couple's need for privacy from the beginning allows staff members to look for ways to adapt the setting to accommodate the couple's need for privacy, making it less likely that the couple will want to move the resident out of the facility.

Because of cost, most residents share rooms, making it more difficult to find a private place for the couple. Some larger facilities have a cohabitation room, but smaller facilities don't typically have such a resource. Working together with trust and respect, however, staff members and couples can try to work out a solution. For instance, staff members can help

the couple find a time when a roommate is off-campus or scheduled for another activity.

THE DEMENTIA DILEMMA

The situation in a long-term care facility can become much more complicated when a resident has dementia. Although less than 10% of the population has dementia, the percentage of older adults developing dementia such as Alzheimer's disease is on the rise, particularly as baby boomers reach retirement age.

As dementia progresses, patients not only lose the capacity to make decisions but also typically lose their sexual inhibitions. Such residents can demonstrate sexually inappropriate behavior toward fellow residents, staff members, and even visitors. Dementia also makes these patients less able to provide an accurate sexual history, making it harder to know what sexual health risks they may pose.

The sexual advances of a resident with dementia towards another resident who is physically or mentally unable to resist is considered rape. This risk calls for staff members to be on the watch for such behavior and to protect vulnerable patients. To decrease the risk, a patient with dementia who has made inappropriate sexual advances may receive hormone treatment, although he's more likely to be transferred to another long-term care facility. In certain cases, the patient may undergo intensive therapy, a form of behavior modification therapy; such therapy isn't available at all facilities and its effectiveness depends on the patient's response.

Even with a willing and mentally and physically capable partner, the patient with dementia—even if he's the aggressor—isn't mentally capable of making such a decision. Plus, dementia can result in changeable behavior, potentially placing the sexual partner at risk for verbal, mental, or physical abuse. The situation places stress on all parties involved, from staff members, to other residents, to family members and other visitors. And throughout, both the rights and safety of residents and others may be at risk.

Many larger facilities have ethics committees to handle such complicated problems. Even so, such situations call for tact and careful decision-making from all parties.

Your role

If you work at a long-term care facility, understanding older adults' need for sexual expression and the importance of sexuality in later life will help you give your older patients better care. Using the PLISSIT model and open-ended question discussed earlier can help you gather a more complete sexual health history for such patients.

If necessary, staff members can receive further education and training to increase their understanding and awareness. Although state regulatory agencies require in-service training on such matters as dementia and use of restraints, such training rarely focuses on older adult sexuality. But education about how to respond to residents' sexual behavior and

giving staff members the opportunity to openly discuss their own concerns, feelings, and beliefs about older adult sexuality can help them deal with any confusion or anxiety they may feel. The result: Staff members who can respond to difficult situations with professionalism and sensitivity. (See the *Case Study* below.)

STIs: A Hidden Threat

With all the other issues surrounding older adult sexuality, it's easy to overlook the danger of STIs. But older adults are just as susceptible to STIs as younger adults. Many older adults may be at even greater risk because they're reluctant to share their sexual health history with health care providers. Older adult patients also typically have more complex health problems and chronic illnesses related to aging. As a result, signs and symptoms of an STI may be mistaken for another illness, or symptoms from a chronic illness may mask STI symptoms, delaying diagnosis and treatment of an STI.

When obtaining an older patient's sexual history, keep alert for possible signs and

Case Study

As the nursing director of a local long-term care facility, you receive a disturbing report from the night shift nursing staff: A patient diagnosed with moderate-stage Alzheimer's disease was found in bed with the very frail, bedridden woman in the next room. Staff members reported that they thought the two were just cuddling, but you're very concerned.

Critical thinking questions

1. What general concerns as well as specific concerns about lack of consent does this situation raise?
2. What risks does a resident with moderate-stage Alzheimer's disease pose to himself, other residents, visitors, and staff members?
3. What should be your immediate response this situation?
4. How can you educate staff about this type of problem? Create a brief outline for a nursing staff education program that would prepare staff members to successfully handle such situations in the future.

symptoms of STIs. If you suspect an STI, ask follow-up questions that can help identify a particular STI and request appropriate testing. If the patient is reluctant to provide details because of embarrassment, gently help him to understand the importance proper diagnosis and treatment for his and any partner's health.

If he has a bacterial STI, he most likely has acute signs and symptoms; a current partner may be the source or may have been infected by the patient. If the patient has a viral STI, he may have had the disease for a long time before any symptoms emerged, and the source of infection—as well as others the patient may have infected—may be hard to pin down. Plus, the infection may have progressed to the point where it's difficult to treat.

HIV and AIDS

One of the deadliest of the viral STIs, HIV can lie dormant for up to 10 years, delaying treatment for the patient and putting any of his partners at risk. Older patients who contract HIV also have a much higher mortality rate than younger patients, with patients aged 80 or older having a 37% chance of dying within 1 month of diagnosis.

COPYCAT SYMPTOMS

The signs and symptoms of HIV closely mimic those of common chronic illnesses in older patients. They include fatigue, flulike symptoms, respiratory problems, weight loss, chronic pain, and neurologic symptoms. As a result, they're less likely to raise your suspicion that the patient may have a more serious underlying illness, delaying an accurate diagnosis.

THE DEMENTIA DILEMMA, TAKE TWO

If the patient has dementia, gathering an accurate sexual health history—and thus moving toward an accurate diagnosis—becomes much more difficult. Because

dementia can sexually disinhibit a patient, he may have either contracted or passed on the infection more recently. Such encounters may be especially difficult to track down in a patient who lives at home rather than in a long-term care facility, where patients are more closely supervised.

If the patient contracted HIV years earlier, he may not have been aware of his exposure. Even if he knew of his exposure at the time, he may have forgotten about it because of dementia-related memory loss or he may be too embarrassed to share that information with you.

WHEN PROTECTION CAN ENDANGER

The health insurance portability and accountability act (HIPAA) rules of privacy and special rules about disclosing mental illness and HIV can make it difficult to obtain accurate information about an older adult patient. Designed to protect people against discrimination from employers, the military, and insurance companies, these rules can complicate the situation when you discover that your older patient is infected with HIV. How can you inform the spouse, family members, caregivers, and others who may be closely involved with the patient? You'll need to juggle ethical and legal responsibilities, balancing the patient's right to decline exposure of his illness with not endangering the health of others.

DRUGS: THE STRAIGHT DOPE

Antiretroviral medications approved by the Food and Drug Administration (FDA) can control or slow the HIV disease process. Unfortunately, older adults have less effective immune systems than younger adults. To work effectively, antiretroviral drugs require a healthy CD4 cell response, a response that's blunted by an older patient's less effective immune system. As a result, the virus tends to spread more quickly.

Antiretroviral drugs also have a number of adverse effects, which can complicate chronic conditions commonly found in older patients. Not only that, but there's a high risk of these potent drugs adversely interacting with medications an older adult already takes for chronic illnesses—a significant problem since 60% to 70% of older HIV patients also have another chronic illness. Given all these factors, some older adults with HIV and other chronic conditions may not receive much improvement in quality and length of life from these drugs.

BY THE NUMBERS

How prevalent is HIV infection in older adults? In 1996, the CDC reports that 7,459 people aged 50 and older were diagnosed with AIDS. Between 2000 and 2003, the CDC estimates that about 30,000 men and women aged 45 and older contracted HIV. The number of cases continues to rise, although current statistics are more complicated because people who contracted HIV as younger adults and take antiretroviral drugs are now passing age 50 and more patients over age 50 are contracting the virus.

With so many older adults infected, how much do older adults know about the disease and how it's transmitted? A 2005 Emory University surveyed 514 women aged 50 and older to try and answer this question. The nine-question survey revealed that:

- only 13% stated that condoms were effective in prevention of the transmission of HIV.
- 63% thought that kissing was the method of transmission.
- almost 50% thought that vasectomies would prevent HIV transmission.
- 44% thought abstinence wasn't effective or only partially effective in preventing HIV transmission.

Clearly, many older adults need better education about how HIV is transmitted and the steps they can take to protect themselves and their partners.

RISKS ON THE RISE?

This lack of knowledge can contribute to the spread of HIV infection among older adults. Older adults who divorce or become widowed and enter into new relationships can contract or spread the disease if they don't know the facts about HIV and the importance of testing. Studies confirm this risk: One study shows that 60% of older women who had engaged in sex during the previous 10 years hadn't used condoms.

Physiologic changes can also contribute to the risk. For instance, in older women, thinning and drying of the vaginal walls can result in tears that allow the HIV virus to enter the bloodstream. And, just as in other age groups, drug and alcohol abuse can lead to risky sexual behavior in older adults.

Older gay men in particular continue to be at high risk, with more AIDS cases occurring in this group than in any other group of older adults. Prevention education rarely focuses on this group, leaving them at risk. You can help with sensitive questioning to determine an older adult's sexual history and orientation. If you find that an older patient is gay, you can teach him the steps he can take to protect himself and any partners from HIV infection, and you can emphasize the importance of HIV testing.

TEST TIME

Although testing can help identify HIV infection in older adults, many older adults still aren't tested. If an older adult does choose to be tested, most states require such a test to be private and don't require the patient to provide his real name. Some older adults may instead choose to use an FDA-approved home testing kit. Although these kits aren't guaranteed to

Healthy living — Preventing the Spread of HIV

Many older patients don't think they're at risk for human immunodeficiency virus (HIV). But as people live longer, healthier lives and take part in sexual activity well past age 50, they remain at risk for contracting HIV. You can give your older patients these guidelines from the Centers for Disease Control and Prevention to help them decrease their risk of contracting or spreading HIV.

What People Age 50 and Older Can Do

- Abstain from sex (oral, anal, and vaginal) until you're in a relationship with only one person, you're both having sex with only each other, and you know each other's HIV status.
- Even if you think you have a low risk for HIV infection, if you're having sex or injecting drugs, get tested whenever you have a regular medical checkup.
- Talk about HIV and other sexually transmitted diseases (STDs) with each partner before you have sex. Learn about your partner's past behavior with sex and drugs.
- Ask your partner if he or she has recently been tested for HIV, and encourage your partner to be tested.
- Use a latex condom and lubricant every time you have sex.
- If you have or plan to have more than one sex partner, you should get tested for HIV.
  - If you're a man who has sex with other men, get tested at least once a year.
  - If you're a woman, you should get tested whenever you have a new sex partner.
- If you think you may have been exposed to another STD, get treatment. These diseases can increase your risk of contracting HIV.

- Don't inject illicit drugs. You can contract HIV through needles and syringes if they've been contaminated with the blood of someone who has HIV. Drugs also cloud your judgment, which may result in riskier sex.
- If you do inject drugs, do the following:
  - Use only clean needles and syringes.
  - Never share needles and syringes.
  - Don't expose yourself to another person's blood.
  - Get tested for HIV at least once a year.
  - Consider getting counseling and treatment for your drug use.
  - Get vaccinated against hepatitis A and B viruses.
- Don't have sex when you're taking drugs or drinking alcohol because being high or drunk can make you more likely to take risks.
- Because of better treatments, people with HIV can live longer, healthier lives than was possible in previous years—well past age 50. As a result, as you grow older, you'll need to continue to practice safe behaviors to remain healthy:
  - If both you and your partner have HIV, use condoms to prevent other STDs and possible infection from a different strain of HIV.
  - If only one of you has HIV, use a latex condom and lubricant every time you have sex.
  - To protect yourself, remember these ABCs:
    - A = Abstinence
    - B = Be Faithful
    - C = Condoms

The Centers for Disease Control and Prevention (February 12, 2008). "What Persons Aged 50 and Older Can Do" [Online]. Available: http://www.cdc.gov/hiv/topics/over50/print/protection.htm [July 24, 2009].

provide the same accuracy as testing performed in a lab, they can offer the patient some information about his HIV status.

The CDC now recommends HIV testing routinely for all adults up to age 64. And you can teach all your older patients—including those over age 64— about the risk factors for HIV and encourage them to receive testing. (See *Preventing the spread of HIV*.)

Other STIs: Less famous, still dangerous

HIV may be the most well known STI, but several other STIs pose a serious threat to the health of any older adult who isn't celibate or in a long-term monogamous relationship. One difficulty with detecting an STI in an older adult is that a failing immune system can mask many of the outward signs of both bacterial and viral STIs. Medications such as prednisone can also mask signs and symptoms, making diagnosis difficult. The chronic illnesses typical in many older patients can compound the situation.

THE ABCs OF STIs

Several STIs were covered earlier in the section on older adults with alternative lifestyles, but these diseases can threaten any older adult, no matter what the adult's sexual orientation is. Some STIs to be on the lookout for in your older patients include hepatitis B and C and HPV.

The viruses hepatitis B and C are sexually transmitted in the same way as the HIV virus, with similar precautions to reduce their transmission. Treatment for hepatitis is long-term and expensive. Among older adults, older gay men are more likely than other groups to contract hepatitis.

Although young women can now be vaccinated against HPV to decrease the risk of developing cervical cancer, today's older adult women don't have this protection. Men are also at risk for multiple strains of this virus, which can cause warts that typically appear in the genital area. In about 90% of the cases, the body clears itself of the disease within 2 years, but while the virus is in the body, it's easily transmitted to another sexual partner.

Your role

The first step in combatting STIs in older patients is recognizing that older patients are at risk. By asking the right questions with patience and tact during a sexual health history, you can help bring an older patient's risk to light, which can lead to diagnosis and treatment earlier on in the course of the disease, when treatment can be more effective.

The Older Adult: Still a Sexual Being

Some health care providers who work with older patients daily—particularly some who work in long-term care facilities—can struggle under the burden of caring for patients with so many health issues, health issues that can multiply as a patient ages. In such circumstances, it can be easy to forget that older people can still very much have sexual feelings and needs.

It helps to understand that sexual activity in older adults isn't all that different from sexual activity in younger adults and can include such activities as hugging, kissing, touching, caressing, anal and vaginal intercourse, oral sex, and masturbation. In 1999, the AARP conducted a survey on sexuality and followed this up with another study in 2004. Here are some of the findings:

- Increasing numbers of older adults are seeking out information about sexuality and treatment for sexual problems.
- Older men continue to increase their use of sex-enhancing drugs; use almost doubled between 1999 and 2004.
- About two-thirds of older men and half of older women state that they view a satisfying sex life as an important factor in their overall quality of life.
- Both sexes—90% of men and 85% of women—state that a good sexual relationship with a spouse or partner plays a key role in happiness.
- Almost half of older adults with partners have had intercourse once a week or more within the previous 6 months.
- Older men think about sex and feel sexual desire more frequently than older women.

The study also identified factors affecting sexual satisfaction. Not surprisingly, the study found that the availability of a sexual partner is one of the most important factors in determining an older adult's level of sexual satisfaction. A person's overall health also greatly affects their interest in sex and their ability and willingness to participate in sexual activity. The study also found that more men than women seek treatment for their sexual difficulties, with men reporting that they use male-enhancement drugs such as Viagra and women reporting that they use female hormones for treatment of sexual problems.

Because it's so easy to overlook the sexual needs and health issues of older adults, understanding older adult sexuality becomes even more important. Once you accept the reality of older adults as sexual beings, you're on your way to offering all your older patients the excellent—and complete—health care they deserve.

Caregiving: A Family Affair

When caring for older patients, remember that behind every patient is a larger family system. An older patient who needs assistance typically depends on a spouse, a child, a neighbor, sometimes a whole network of people to help him manage his illness and day-to-day functions. Any change in that family—whether to the patient or someone else—sends ripples through the family system. If the patient's condition worsens, for instance, caregivers may need to step up care, which affects not only the patient and caregiver, but the caregiver's family. An aging spouse who provides care may reach the point where she needs care herself. Or a son or daughter who serves as the main caregiver may move away, leaving the patient in need of new caregivers and affecting both the patient and any family members who have to step into the role of caregiver.

Looking beyond the patient to the family allows you to monitor the changes that inevitably happen within families, especially as the aging patient needs more care, and offer support to the entire family system. In fact, as an older patient's needs increase, the caregivers may need as much support as the patient himself.

Timeline   *Everybody Cares for Creature Comforts*

An abundance of modern appliances, home goods, and in-home services help ease the strain of caring for patients at home. Here are some examples of modern-day conveniences that were introduced over the past century.

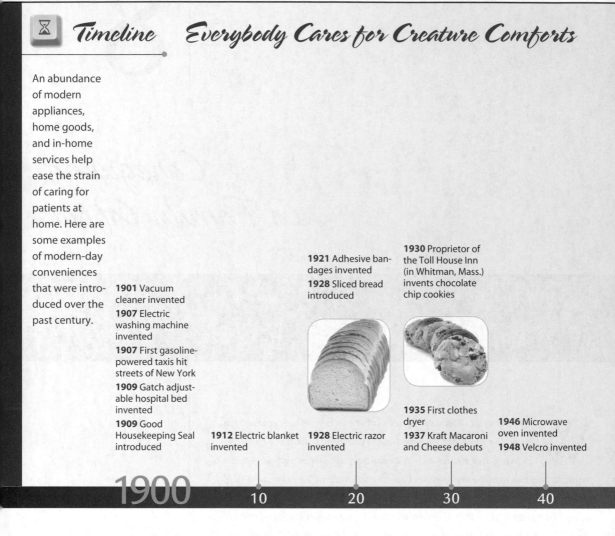

1901 Vacuum cleaner invented

1907 Electric washing machine invented

1907 First gasoline-powered taxis hit streets of New York

1909 Gatch adjustable hospital bed invented

1909 Good Housekeeping Seal introduced

1912 Electric blanket invented

1921 Adhesive bandages invented

1928 Sliced bread introduced

1928 Electric razor invented

1930 Proprietor of the Toll House Inn (in Whitman, Mass.) invents chocolate chip cookies

1935 First clothes dryer

1937 Kraft Macaroni and Cheese debuts

1946 Microwave oven invented

1948 Velcro invented

1900   10   20   30   40

What is Family Caregiving?

To offer caregivers the assistance they need, it helps to fully understand what family caregiving is. The National Family Caregivers Association defines it as "assisting someone you care about who is chronically ill or disabled and who is no longer able to care for themselves." The Hartford Institute for Geriatric Nursing defines it as "the wide range of unpaid care provided in response to illness or functional impairment to a chronically ill or functionally impaired older family member, partner, friend, or neighbor that exceeds the support usually provided in family relationships." In other words, family caregiving is taking care of a family member, whatever the needs may be. Sometimes the patient isn't even aware of all the so-called "invisible activities" a caregiver may perform to ensure the patient's safety and well-being.

1952 First automatic percolator coffeepot

1952 First transistor hearing aids developed

1952 First TV remote control (Zenith's "Lazy Bones") developed

1953 TV dinners invented; sell for 98 cents

1954 First home-delivered meal program for homebound seniors in U.S.; delivered by high school students ("Platter Angels") in Philadelphia

1963 Touch-tone telephone service made available

1965 Older Americans Act signed into law

1965 Medicaire and Medicaid enacted

1966 Home milk delivery services begin to decline

1966 Computer mouse invented

1972 HBO, the nation's first pay-TV network, launches

1973 Domino's Pizza guarantees 30-minute home delivery—or it's free!

1978 Jimmy Carter proclaims first Sunday after Labor Day as National Grandparents Day

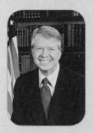

1979 Merry Maids cleaning service founded

1985 Sound-activated lamp ("The Clapper") first sold to the public

1993 Pentium processor invented

1996 Super Nintendo retails for $159

2000 Online pharmacies start to become popular

2005 YouTube introduced online

50   60   70   80   90   2010

A wide-ranging job

What kinds of tasks does caregiving involve? As patients with increasingly complicated care needs receive treatment at home, family caregiving can become very complex. The older patient's room may even begin to resemble a hospital room.

However, most caregiving is more basic than that and can include such activities as driving the patient to appointments, managing bills, and arranging for regular house cleaning and meal delivery. Specific tasks depend on the patient's needs and what the caregiver can offer, and those tasks can vary as the patient's needs change.

What caregivers need from you also varies. Some will simply need information; others will need more, including referrals, emotional support, or help with specific caregiving tasks. Whatever a patient's caregivers need, you can help them understand and manage this often-challenging role.

The times, they are a-changin'

Historically, society assumed that children would care for their parents as they aged. But times have changed significantly, for both older adults and their caregivers. For one thing, people are living longer. Older adults with chronic illnesses that affect their ability to function may need years of care; if complications develop—as they often do—the situation becomes even more challenging.

Other changes that affect family dynamics and caregiving for older adults include:

- a nationwide increase in mobility, with family members more readily moving and settling down far from each other
- a greater percentage of women entering and staying in the workforce
- a delay in childbearing, with many women waiting longer to begin having children
- changes in health care reimbursement policies and increases in health care costs, making long-term care more expensive for patients and caregivers
- improvements in technology, leading to increased treatment options and greater longevity for patients with previously difficult-to-treat or unmanageable conditions
- an increasing number of older adults as the large baby boomer generation begins to enter the ranks of older adults.

Ultimately, caregiving will be a part of every family. (See the *Case Study* below.)

By the numbers

The numbers confirm the heavy caregiving burden that rests on families. In the United States, family caregivers provide over 80% of all home care services, with 90% of all older adults who need assistance in their homes receiving at least some family caregiving. Volunteer caregivers, mostly family members, make up the largest percentage of caregivers in the country. And there are a lot of caregivers, with 21% of the U.S. population over age 18 providing unpaid care to friends or relatives aged 18 and older. More than three quarters of this group—or 16% of the U.S. populations—provide care to people aged 50 and older.

But each family situation, and every caregiver and patient, is unique. Caregivers can be adults of any age, gender, or race and live under a variety of circumstances.

WOMAN POWER

Women account for about 61% of all caregivers, with percentages varying among different ethnic groups. A typical woman caregiver is middle-aged (46 year old on average), and is likely to be employed, either as a full- or part-time worker. She spends at least 20 hours each week caring for an adult over age 50, with many caregivers spending more than

Case Study

Laura is a 40-year-old single career woman who balances caregiving with the many demands of her own life. Her mother, who has dementia, lives in the country, and Laura makes trips to her mother's home daily to make sure she's safe and has a meal. As her mother's dementia progresses, Laura worries about having to sell her mother's home and what it would be like to have her mother move in with her.

Critical thinking questions
- Would Laura fit the typical description of a family caregiver? Why or why not?
- What challenges do you think Laura faces now? What about in the future?

40 hours. She's likely to be providing care at the highest level of intensity, often helping with several ADLs.

MEN STEP UP

Men account for the other 39% of caregivers. According to a 2004 National Alliance for Caregiving/American Association of Retired People (AARP) study, more men caregivers worked full time than women caregivers. Studies have also shown that men approach caregiving somewhat differently than women, viewing caregiving more as a series of tasks to be completed, much like work. They're also more likely to seek outside help when needed.

VARIATIONS ON A THEME

The statistics vary for caregivers from different ethnic groups. About 18% of Asian-Americans and 16% of Hispanics take part in caregiving. In the Asian-American population, more than half of caregivers—54%—are men; 41% of Hispanic caregivers are men.

Caregivers from minority populations, such as African-Americans, Hispanics, and Asian-Americans, are also typically younger, usually between ages 18 and 34, whereas more caregivers 65 and older are white. Regardless of race, most caregivers are married or living with a partner, and most live near the person receiving care.

Culture Results of a national study conducted on Hispanic family caregiving in the United States revealed that more than one-third of Hispanic households have at least one family member caring for an older loved one, a percentage much higher than for total U.S. households. The study also reported that Hispanic caregivers go through major shifts in their working situations when they become family caregivers.

ON THE RECEIVING END

What's the profile of those receiving care? Like caregivers, each care receiver is unique, but the typical care recipient is over age 55, with an average age of 75. (See *The care recipient: Who is it?*)

THE CARE RECIPIENT: WHO IS IT?

According to the 2004 study by the National Alliance for Caregiving and the American Association of Retired People, the typical older care recipient is:

- female, commonly a mother
- widowed
- 75 years old
- receiving care from a relative, typically a son or daughter (if recipient is a mother)
- living either in the same household as the primary caregiver or within an hour of the caregiver's home.

Fast Facts
The study also revealed some other interesting facts about care recipients.
- African-Americans more commonly care for an aunt or uncle.
- Whites and Asian-Americans more commonly care for a father.
- Caregivers older than age 65 more commonly care for men, and caregivers younger than age 65 more commonly care for women.
- Care recipients younger than age 50 are most likely to need caregiving because of mental health disorders or emotional illnesses.
- Care recipients are most likely to require care because of old age, followed in frequency by cancer, diabetes, heart disease, and Alzheimer's disease.
- Almost all recipients aged 50 or older (92%) take prescription medications.

The "to do" list

As mentioned earlier, caregivers take part in a wide range of activities when they care for their family members. Some of these activities can be divided into instrumental activities of daily living (IADLs) and activities of daily living (ADLs).

IADLs include:

- transporting the patient, either by driving the patient (the more common approach) or by arranging for transportation such as specialized transportation services
- shopping for groceries
- helping with housework, including straightening up the house, washing dishes, or doing laundry
- preparing meals
- helping to manage the household, including paying bills, going to the bank, and completing insurance forms.

ADLs involve the patient's personal care. ADLs the caregiver typically helps the patient with include:

- getting in and out of bed or a chair
- dressing
- bathing or showering
- getting to and from the toilet
- eating.

Of these activities, more than a third of caregivers participate in helping the patient in and out of bed or a chair.

Caregivers also frequently help in a wide range of tasks related to the patient's illness. Caregivers may help the patient manage his symptoms and deal with illness-associated problems such as fatigue, weakness, and shortness of breath. Some caregivers must even perform specific procedures with specialized supplies or equipment, such as wound care or tube feedings.

Less direct but no less crucial caregiving may include managing the patient's care.

The caregiver may make sure the patient has access to necessary resources such as specialized transportation or medical equipment, for instance. Or the caregiver may be responsible for contacting the health care provider and arranging for visits or arranging for support people to help with the patient's care. The caregiver may also advocate for the patient, making sure the patient's needs and rights are met.

The costs of caregiving

No matter how you measure it—in time, in money, in the emotional toll—the cost of caregiving is high. It's especially high when a patient has a progressive disease such as Alzheimer's disease.

A LONG-TERM JOB

Family caregivers provide the bulk of care for patients with Alzheimer's disease, a disease that lasts from 3 to 20 years and averages 8 years. The caregivers, typically spouses or adult children, generally provide between 69 and 100 caregiving hours each week; half of caregivers live with the patient, providing care 24 hours a day. The estimated cost of all this "free" service? Over $350 billion a year—almost twice the amount spent on homecare and nursing home services combined. And this cost will likely grow because, as studies have shown, most families of Alzheimer's patients only turn to nursing facilities as a last resort.

STRESSED OUT

It's hard to quantify the physical, emotional, and financial impact of providing this level of care. Older adult spouses in particular experience a great deal of stress from such intensive, long-term caregiving. But any family member caring for a patient with a chronic, long-term condition such as dementia can experience effects to the immune system that last for years, even after caregiving has ended.

Other sometimes hard-to-measure costs to family members who provide hours of care each week include:

- increased rates of depression and anxiety
- job loss
- significant out-of-pocket expenses
- the need to change from full-time to part-time employment, drastically impacting the caregiver's financial status.

These individual costs ripple out to affect the larger community. By supporting these caregivers—making them part of a health care team and coaching them in caregiver roles—society in general will benefit.

Who are the Caregivers?

Every family, and each caregiver, approaches caregiving differently, with culture, age, and economics all having an effect. In many cultures, for instance, it's expected that the oldest daughter or son will carry out certain responsibilities in a particular way. As times change, however, these expectations can change. For example, a study of the Hispanic community suggests that as younger adults work to meet broader societal expectations, intergenerational living arrangements go by the wayside.

Caregivers can be almost any age, but for all, caregiving for an older adult can be a balancing act. Younger caregivers may have to put much of the energy and attention that normally would go into starting their own careers and families into caregiving. Middle-aged caregivers—the sandwich generation—often have to serve as caregivers for both children and parents. Older caregivers, including spouses and caregivers of even older parents, must juggle meeting the patient's needs with caring for themselves when their own health might be declining. (See the *Case Study* below.)

Regardless of how a family approaches caregiving, evidence confirms that family caregivers want support in providing the best care. You can help by assessing the family's situation. You can then use that information to work with the family to support them, improving their caregiving abilities. (See *Caregiver assessment categories*, page 342.)

A mix of emotions

Caregiving can raise emotional issues, especially when the patient is physically dependent. It can be especially difficult when a caregiver undergoes a perceived role reversal, serves as the sole caregiver, or has to cope with not only the patient's needs but also his own health issues. The tasks, duration, location, and responsibilities may differ from one family to the next, but research shows that all caregivers must cope with the emotional impact of caregiving.

Case Study

Jim is in his late 20s and tries to be helpful to his mother, who has Parkinson's disease and who still lives in her own, older home. Jim's mother wants to stay active, but she has trouble managing such home maintenance projects as leaky faucets and lawn care. Jim is considering moving back home with his mother to help out.

Critical thinking questions
- What role changes do you think Jim will experience if he does decide to move back home?
- What emotional issues may arise as Jim becomes more involved in caregiving?
- Do you think that Jim is prepared for caregiving?

CAREGIVER ASSESSMENT CATEGORIES

When working with a family, it helps to understand the family's social and cultural preferences and expectations. Make sure your assessment includes:

● the caregiving context (the patient's home environment or other care setting)
● the patient's needs and caregivers' perceptions of the patient's health and functional status
● caregivers' preparedness for caregiving
● informal support systems, including a determination of the quality of family relationships
● the community environment and resources
● the family's cultural preference
● caregivers' physical and mental health status.

Adapted with permission from Messecar, D.C. "Family Caregiving," in *Evidence-Based Geriatric Nursing Protocols for Best Practice*, 3rd ed. Edited by Fulmer, T., et al. New York: Springer Publishing Company, 2008.

Several surveys conducted by the National Family Caregivers Association identify some of the emotions caregivers share, including:

● intense sadness and pain
● longing for a return to normalcy
● frustration from changing family dynamics
● a sense of isolation from living outside society norms
● stress over increased and often enormous responsibilities
● depression over all the losses that result from caregiving
● a sense of fortitude and the strength to go on and make a difference
● a feeling of resourcefulness in solving problems
● a sense of strength in knowing that they can survive.

Caregivers also share similar problems that add to the stress of caregiving. When an adult child must care for a parent—a common situation—their roles seem to reverse, although the emotional dynamics prevent a true reversal. Such a situation carries emotional challenges, with the adult child feeling he must live up to society's expectations of the dutiful child and the parent not feeling ready to play a dependent role.

To help make such a situation work successfully, both parent and child need to develop new supportive, interdependent roles. However, how to make these shifts successfully and what it means to take on the role of caregiver or to become dependent on another person still needs more study.

Even when caregiver and recipient have a situation worked out, changes in the life of either party can knock things out of balance. An acute change, such as a fracture or a cancer diagnosis, can quickly change the dynamic. Gradual changes, such as the steady progression of a chronic disorder, can also call for rethinking a situation.

As a patient's health declines, a caregiver who already feels isolated may face increasing isolation. Any intimacy and companionship with the patient may suffer, especially if the patient suffers from dementia, and the increasing demands on the caregiver can lead to less time and capacity for other close relationships. The caregiver can feel increasingly trapped, with no real relief or escape on the horizon.

Preparation: The key to success

The best way to have a successful caregiving situation is preparation. But caregivers too often aren't prepared, especially since society generally doesn't do much of a job preparing people for this demanding role. Family members may be quite willing to care for an older adult, but if they don't have the right teaching and guidance, if they don't know what resources they can tap into, then they're set up for failure. Most family caregivers receive too little information, no formal caregiving training, and little help in communicating with health care providers. And caregiving classes that do exist typically have a limited scope.

Despite the lack of preparation and despite not always receiving credit for their work, family caregivers contribute significantly to patients' health outcomes. They complete tasks ranging from the most basic, such as helping with shopping, to very advanced, such as wound care. And they do this even as they cope with the emotional burden of their family life changing and a family member growing more disabled.

You can help both caregivers and patients by helping to develop educational programs for caregivers and by advocating community-based caregiver educations opportunities.

What's the Job Description?

Unfortunately, there's no universal "job description" for a caregiver. But you can help a family develop their own job description, based on their needs and situation and the needs of the patient they must care for. Such a job description should include the types of tasks needed and how many tasks a caregiver must regularly perform. You can then plan interventions to help the family that match these needs.

That task list can be extensive. The AARP, for instance, includes more than 29 topics

on caregiving at their Web site, including "balancing work and caregiving" and "caregiving from afar." Such topic titles make it clear that caregiving can involve much more than hands-on physical care. By keeping in mind that physical care is just one part of caregiving, you can make sure to cover other aspects when creating a job description with the family and planning interventions.

The types of tasks

To understand the range of potential caregiving tasks, it helps to categorize tasks into types. Thirteen general categories of task types exist, including facilitating transportation and making medical decisions. An even more general grouping includes three broad areas:

- direct assistance tasks, in which caregivers provide hands-on care and must be readily available
- societal tasks, in which caregivers perform financial services, deal with legal issues, and interact directly on the patient's behalf with other family members and service providers
- monitoring and coordinating tasks, in which the caregiver carries out or arranges for such tasks as grocery shopping and transportation and makes other necessary service arrangements.

Even after you and the family caregivers have developed a job description for their situation and come up with a basic plan of how to carry it out, you need to help them understand that the plan can and most likely will change as the situation changes. Make sure the family understands that they face changing tasks as the patient's health deteriorates—for instance, when an older adult who needed minimal care loses the ability to drive, he'll need help from his family for a whole new range of tasks. And help the family understand that it's okay to have an emotional reaction to those changes, and to reach out for help coping with new tasks as the patient and family move through these transitions.

How Can You Help?

You can provide vital support to family caregivers shouldering the burden of caring for an older family member. Such ongoing support can help prevent the burnout that can occur when a caregiver faces the challenges of caring for an increasingly ill patient alone—burnout that can lead to two patients instead of just one.

Keep in mind that no two family situations are quite the same; because of that, no one set of detailed guidelines describes the best way to help family caregivers. You also may need more than one approach to provide the support the family and patient need.

You should, however, follow some basic nursing steps, including assessing the family situation, developing structured problem solving, adapting the patient's environment, teaching the caregiver, matching the family with appropriate resources, and helping the caregiver find a support system.

Assessing the situation

The first step is assessing the patient, the family, and the community they're each part of. Such an assessment can help match the family with the most appropriate resources.

You'll gain a more complete and accurate picture if you perform not just a health assessment but also a broad functional assessment to determine the patient's ability to carry out such diverse daily activities as doing laundry, getting groceries, fixing meals, and caring for the house and yard. Such an assessment lets you generate a list of tasks that the patient needs help with. The list can serve as a guide for determining who should perform what tasks—the patient,

family caregivers, or someone brought in to help with specific tasks—and what methods might work best for completing these tasks.

CULTURAL SENSITIVITY

Understanding the family's culture will allow you to steer your assessment more closely to the patient's and family's needs. For instance, several cultures view the oldest son as the family caregiver and decision maker; others have historically provided extended care in the home. Within the context of the family's culture, however, make sure you determine the impact of the family's unique history and preferences.

A family's culture also affects what teaching and services the family needs. Illness and health mean different things to different cultures; even language differences can affect how families understand health concepts. Remaining open-minded and listening to the family's stories will help you understand and value the family's perspective. The University of Michigan's Web site on cultural competency (http://www.med. umich.edu/Multicultural/ccp/index.htm) offers useful information on diverse cultures.

When assessing the family, use broad, open-ended questions. Such questions help guide the assessment and give the family and patient a chance to elaborate on their perspective on health. Using the set of questions developed by Arthur Kleinman, a psychiatrist and anthropologist, can help you gain an understanding of the patient's and family's underlying cultural perspective. (See *The Kleinman questions*.)

You should also use specific assessment questions and tools with all families and patients, regardless of culture. Such questions and tools can help you identify preferences, assess abilities and motivations, determine other major roles and responsibilities caregivers may have, and identify available informal support systems (family, friends, and neighbors)

THE KLEINMAN QUESTIONS

Answering these questions can give the patient and family a chance to express what they think and feel about the patient's illness.

1. What do you think caused the problem?
2. Why do you think it happened when it did?
3. What do you think your sickness does to you? How does it work?
4. How severe is your sickness? Will it have a short course?
5. What kind of treatment do you think you should receive?
6. What are the most important results you hope to receive from this treatment?
7. What are the chief problems your sickness has caused for you?
8. What do you fear most about your sickness?

From Kleinman, A., et al. "Culture, Illness, and Care: Clinical Lessons from Anthropologic and Cross-cultural Research," *Annals of Internal Medicine, 88*(2):251-258, February 1978.

and formal support systems (chore services, social services, and health agencies). The Hartford Institute for Geriatric Nursing (http://hartfordign.org/Resources/Try_This_Series) provides sample assessment tools that can help.

VALUING THE FAMILY

During the assessment, focus on the family's values and preferences. By having this discussion early on rather than waiting until problems arise and by including the family in the assessment and planning process, you can help make sure the plan meets the family's needs and wishes.

Questions you might ask:

- Which members of the family are willing to take responsibility for care?
- What money and time limits affect the care the family can provide? How much money is the family willing and able to pay for care, especially if the patient's insurance doesn't cover all aspects of care?
- What kind of care does the patient and family need now? What kind of care does the family envision needing in the future?

You may also need to ask how the patient and family feel about having an outside person provide some or all of the care; in some situations,

you may need to address the possibility of the patient receiving care outside the home, including what type of care the patient may need and how long he may need such care.

DETAIL WORK

Make sure you find out the details of the patient's routines and preferences. Ask about ADLs, such as bathing and dressing. Does the patient prefer a bath or shower? At what time of day? Would the patient be uncomfortable having a person of the opposite sex perform care—for instance, how would a father feel about having his daughter help him with bathing? What time does the patient wake up? What kinds of foods does he prefer?

Such questions can help open up communication among family members, and in particular, between the patient and caregivers. These discussions, in turn, foster patient and caregiver autonomy and enhance their decision-making skills, ultimately improving outcomes and the patient's and family's quality of life.

When problems arise

In any family caregiving situation, problems are bound to arise—sometimes very complex,

PROBLEM SOLVING: THE COPE MODEL

According to the American Geriatric Society, problem solving involves four components: creativity, optimism, planning, and expert information. Family caregivers can remember these four simple components by remembering the acronym COPE. Each component offers caregivers several ways to approach problem solving.

Creativity
- Imagine how someone else might solve the problem.
- Use something that may have worked in the past, and adapt or improve it.
- Break the task or action into smaller tasks or more reasonable goals.
- Brainstorm about unusual ideas, and then select a practical one.

Optimism
- Maintain a positive attitude.
- Give yourself a pep talk; use positive statements such as "I can do this."
- Realize that you have had past successes to help you understand that success can occur in the future.

Planning
- Gather all the facts.
- Have a clear idea of the goal and what needs to be done to reach that goal.
- Set realistic goals.
- Keep the plan in your head or, if necessary, write it down.
- Organize the plan, and check for results.
- If the plan isn't successful, make adaptations to the plan.

Expert Information
- Seek out sources of reputable information, including Web sites, health care professionals, and others who have had similar experiences.
- Talk with other family caregivers; find a family caregiver support group.

From American Geriatrics Society (www.americangeriatrics.org), "Problem solving: COPE," in *Eldercare at Home,* 2nd ed, © 2007. Used with permission from the American Geriatrics Society.

multilayered problems—requiring caregivers to make decisions and set new priorities. Putting such problems in context and teaching problem-solving strategies can help caregivers learn how to deal with problems as they arise.

Strategies to help caregivers solve problems as they arise include problem logs, problem framing, and problem-solving models. In a problem log, the family keeps track of a particular patient concern to identify patterns over time. Problem framing puts a problem into context, taking into account family values, experiences, and emotions. Structured problem-solving models can help families recognize that most problems have more than one component and fall within a cultural, economic, and even political context. The American

Geriatric Society provides an *Eldercare at Home* resource, available online, to help caregivers with problem solving. Their problem-solving model identifies four components caregivers can use to help solve problems: creativity, optimism, planning, and expert information, or COPE. (See *Problem solving: The COPE model.*)

The level of help caregivers need determines the appropriate level of intervention. Caregivers may simply lack information and need an appropriate educational handout, or they may need a hands-on demonstration of a procedure. You can also refer caregivers to specific training to help them understand common caregiving issues and learn how to make decisions and solve caregiver-related problems.

If you need to step in to help caregivers solve a problem, make sure you first understand the problem, including:

- possible causes
- when the problem is most likely to occur
- what can be done to help
- what the family's goals are.

Once you understand the problem, you can help the family figure out what they can do to manage it when it occurs, and ultimately, how to prevent it if possible. This involves planning a response to a problem, learning how to implement the response, determining if the response is helping to resolve the problem, and adjusting the plan if it isn't. You also need to help the family understand what problems call for outside, professional help.

The environment: A structured approach

One way to help prevent problems as well as make life more manageable for both the patient and caregivers is to help the family structure the patient's environment so it's safe and functional. For example, assessing an older adult's kitchen for safety might include determining the adult's ability to access cupboards easily and use the stove, toaster oven, and microwave safely, including putting pots and pans on stove burners and taking them off again. Creating a more functional kitchen might include rearranging cupboards so the older adult can easily reach commonly used items from standing level and providing tools such as lazy Susans or long-handled grabber tongs to reach some items. You can give family caregivers a checklist to help them assess the safety and function of the patient's living environment. (See *Helping caregivers promote safety and function*, page 348.)

THE TOOLS OF THE TRADE

Several assistive devices and technologies—ranging from low- to high-tech—can help promote function and safety. Several tools can help with mobility, continence, memory, and hearing deficits. New devices and technologies being developed include a "smart house" that has several automated functions, such as lights and motion detectors.

Some current assistive resources include:

- telehealth monitoring, which allows a caregiver who doesn't live near the patient to check in on and monitor the patient
- Web resources, which can provide education and information
- online support groups, which provide caregivers with a chance to support each other and share ideas
- environmental assistive devices such as medical alert systems (Lifeline), which offer assistance with patient monitoring.

Coaching the caregiver

Perhaps one of the most important ways you can help both the patient and family caregivers is to teach caregivers, helping to make them part of the health care team. For most caregivers, you'll need to do more than just provide patient-teaching handouts. And although there's literature and research on environmental and behavioral approaches to patient problems, caregivers may not have ready access to such information or they may need help interpreting it.

A crucial part of coaching caregivers is helping them communicate effectively with health care providers; problems have been reported in such interactions, which can prevent caregivers from getting the help they need. You should also determine caregivers' health literacy, making sure not only that they can read, but that they understand the concepts covered in any health care literature you

HELPING CAREGIVERS PROMOTE SAFETY AND FUNCTION

When you work with caregivers to assess a patient's environment, these guidelines can help both you and the caregivers make sure the environment is safe and functional.

The First Step: Safety Checklists
Use a safety checklist to identify environmental hazards, including:

- electrical outlets, switches, and electrical and phone cords that pose an electrical hazard
- throw rugs, runners, mats, and cords that run across the floor that pose a tripping hazard
- hard-to-reach shelves that can cause a patient to overreach and fall or knock items down onto himself
- space heaters, wood-burning stoves, or fireplaces that pose a fire risk
- improperly stored volatile or flammable liquids (most patients shouldn't have such liquids readily available)
- a cluttered basement, garage, workshop, or storage area
- improperly working kitchen appliances, appliances that the patient can't safely operate, and poorly organized, crowded, or hard-to-reach storage.

Also, make sure the patient has:

- a working telephone, with emergency contacts and phone numbers readily available
- a working doorbell
- working smoke and carbon monoxide detectors
- an emergency exit plan
- a bedroom and living room or family room that doesn't pose safety risks
- bright lighting, clear passageways, and manageable steps in all hallways, stairways, and entryways
- nonskid surfaces, grab bars, safe water temperature (not too hot), and bright lighting in all bathrooms
- safely stored and organized medications; pill dispensers may help the patient take medications more safely.

The Next Step: Meeting Specific Needs
You can also take other steps tailored to the patient's specific needs:

- Consider safety-proofing medications and the household for Alzheimer's and dementia patients to prevent medication mismanagement and wandering.
- Adapt the environment to improve function for patients with specific deficits; for instance, have grab bars installed in the bathroom for a patient with mobility deficits, and provide tongs or "grabbers" for a patient who has arthritis or another disorder that makes it hard to reach for items.
- Consider using devices to improve specific disabilities; for instance, use auditory devices—such as a sound amplifier or a screen to display the words being said—for the telephone, television, radio, and stereo for a patient with a hearing deficit.

provide. Tools such as the "Ask Me 3" guide, which suggests specific questions the patient can ask health care providers, can help improve communication, and organizations such as the Family Caregiver Alliance and American Geriatric Society offer resources for family caregivers. And don't forget your role in helping caregivers sort through the often-complex paperwork.

You can steer caregivers to several Web resources, but keep in mind that too much information can overwhelm a caregiver. With all the health care information available on the Web, that's a real risk. Try to determine if the caregiver is self-directed and Web-savvy enough to use these resources well, and provide help and education where needed. (See *Selected Web resources for caregiving*.)

Care for the caregiver: A resourceful approach

Keeping older adults in their homes as long as possible has benefits: Most older adults prefer it, and it typically places a lower cost burden on society. But to keep an older adult who needs caregiving in his own home can cost the family caregivers a great deal—in resources, in stress, and in time providing care and managing services to support the older adult's quality of life. By reaching the family caregivers at a serviceable moment—that is, when the caregivers are ready to receive help—you can better help them access both the formal and informal community-based resources they need to continue to provide home care, and you can improve their ability to deal with the challenges of the health care system.

KEEPING IT CASUAL: INFORMAL RESOURCES...

Informal resources for an older adult include family members, friends, neighbors, and community organizations. The most important informal resource, family members can provide continuity and consistent care. But other informal supports can help, too, because they usually involve little or no cost. Most importantly, people in an informal support network may know the family and the older adult and may provide more personalized care.

The drawback is that such support people may lack caregiving knowledge; they may even add stress to the family, despite their best intentions, by unintentionally interfering or offering the wrong kind of help. Make sure the main family caregivers understand that it's okay—in fact, it's very appropriate—to ask for the help they need. Suggest that they reach out beyond the immediate family circle of caregivers to such possible helpers as children,

grandchildren, church members, neighbors, and informal community service providers. Such helpers can provide continuity and consist care and may be able to take on specific care issues such as driving an older adult to church or regularly checking in on an older adult whose main caregivers don't live nearby.

...BUT DON'T DISPENSE WITH THE FORMALITIES

Family caregivers also need more formal support, and you can help them navigate formal support systems. Formal support systems include agencies designed specifically to provide health services, social services, or both in the older adult's community. They can step in when the older adult's care needs are beyond what informal caregivers can offer, either because the adult's care needs call for skills or training the caregivers don't have or require more time than the caregivers can offer. Such services can provide stability, offering care day in and day out for as long as needed. And they don't run the risk of becoming too ill, frail, or just plain tired out to provide care.

Like informal resources, formal resources have drawbacks. For one thing, they frequently require payment for services. They're also often viewed as providing more impersonal care. Knowing what services are available, understanding how to set up such services for an older adult, or meeting eligibility requirements for a particular service can also be challenging.

Accessing agencies

The Administration on Aging (part of the U.S. Department of Health and Human Services) and the National Association of Area Agencies on Aging serve as resources for families. Types of formal community-service providers include adult day care, meal services (such as Meals On Wheels), transportation services, chore services, home health care agencies, and clinical care agencies.

Some agencies provide nurse case managers or navigators; the patient's primary health care provider may also identify someone to serve informally as a case manager to help families screen for problems and identify resources. If you serve such a role for a family, it helps to be aware of the criteria for services that some agencies use, such as medical or financial need. It also helps to know when a patient may need referrals, what agencies have waiting lists, and what services the patient's community provides. A rural community with a smaller population, for instance, may have fewer supportive resources. To best help families, make sure you understand what services are available, accessible, and affordable; if a community lacks needed services, you may need to advocate for those services.

Keeping track of the situation

Both the patient and family caregivers require monitoring to make sure the patient and caregiver plans remain adequate and appropriate, with the patient receiving good care and family caregivers having the support and access to services they need. Even the best plan needs adjustment when the patient's functional level or a caregiver's abilities change. A caregiver may grow ill, for instance, or need to relocate, disrupting care and calling for a new care plan. And a patient with a progressive condition such as Alzheimer's disease will need periodic adjustments to a care plan.

A standardized functional assessment can help you monitor the continued adequacy of a nursing and service care plan and the changing needs of the patient and caregivers. The Hartford Institute for Geriatric Nursing provides such tools. You'll also need to monitor the service plan, making sure that patients and caregivers are accessing and using the appropriate services—or finding out what's preventing them from using the services.

Finding the right setting

Families provide care for older adults in various settings, and each setting has its advantages and challenges. But no matter what the setting, the basic interventions and goals remain the same: safety, optimal patient function, and adequate quality of life. Helping the family and patient find the right setting for them helps ensure that the patient receives the best care and family caregivers receive the support they need.

THE INVISIBLE FAMILY

Some of these settings don't always provide both the patient and caregivers with what they need. Society tends to think of patient care in medical terms, focusing on patient needs. In primary care clinics, for instance—typically the point of entry for patients and their families—the focus can be so much on the patient's needs that family caregivers are almost invisible. As a result, they may not get the support and access to resources that they need. You can help in such a setting by addressing the needs of both patient and family caregivers, resulting in a healthier situation for all.

THE HOME FRONT

If the patient is receiving some care at home from one or more caregiver assistants, you can help family caregivers understand the importance of clarifying the job description for each assistant. Agency guidelines may specify that a caregiver in a particular position may only help buy groceries, another may only prepare meals, and another may just help with physical caregiving.

HOME AWAY FROM HOME

When family caregivers can no longer provide adequate care at the patient's home or their own home, they may face the difficult task of placing the patient in a long-term care facility. You can help with this transition, teaching caregivers about changes in their role and promoting as much continuity as possible for the patient and family. If a patient is moving from a hospital setting to a long-term care facility, discharge planners and navigators or case managers can help family caregivers with decisions. (See *When care settings change: Questions to ask*.)

Once a patient moves from his home—whether to a retirement community, an assisted-living facility, or a more acute care setting—the role of family caregivers is likely to change.

Family caregivers can use your help to determine what services the older adult will receive in the new setting and what the family's new role should be. For instance, family caregivers may need to monitor the patient fairly closely in a setting that doesn't provide extensive services, or they may need to clarify with facility personnel who should supervise a patient's medications.

When the end draws near

As a patient with a progressive disease moves closer to death, family caregivers will likely need even more support. Patients and families must deal with the physical effects of such illnesses as end-stage cardiac or respiratory disease, which can be very difficult. But the progressive mental decline from Alzheimer's disease and other forms of dementia presents unique challenges. Providing care for such patients becomes increasingly complex for caregivers as the disease progresses. (See the *Case Study* below.)

Case Study

Mary lives at home in an urban setting with her husband, who has dementia. She tries to maintain her busy outside activities while keeping her husband safe and engaged in activities so he will sleep at night. But when she next sees you, she reports that one night he left the house unnoticed and wandered barefoot for over a mile before he was found.

Critical thinking questions
- What issues do family caregivers like Mary face in creating a safe and functional environment?
- Would a dementia patient in a long-term care facility face similar issues? What would be the similarities and differences?
- What specific safety issues should you discuss with Mary?

Described as an at-risk population, caregivers for Alzheimer's patients face different challenges as the patient passes through the different stages of the disease. Such caregivers need stage-specific assessment to determine their needs. The caregiver for a patient with moderate-stage Alzheimer's who's living at home, for instance, has very different needs from the caregiver of a patient with end-stage disease who's living in a long-term care facility.

A MODEL FOR FAILURE

The medical model, which focuses primarily on the disease state of the patient, doesn't fit well in such situations because it doesn't address the care setting and the various problems each caregiver faces. In fact, the issues and needs of families dealing with late-stage Alzheimer's are rarely addressed. As a result, when caregivers most need support—with few emotional, physical, and financial resources left after years of caregiving, and with the even more painful loss of the person they're caring for as dementia deepens—they may be left high and dry.

OFFERING A HELPING HAND

You can make a real difference for family caregivers as they lose a patient to any type of progressive disease by bridging the medical model and offering treatment for the patient and support for the family. By partnering with family caregivers as the disease progresses, you and the health care team can help with transitions as care needs change, help the family understand the diagnosis, identify resources and available support groups, make sure someone is available for calls and concerns, and help caregivers to take care of themselves. Make sure the family has a contact person—you or another case manager—to help form strategies to deal with disease-specific deficits as the disease progresses.

For a family dealing with Alzheimer's and other forms of dementia, you can also help them understand the patient's behaviors, help deal with behavioral problems, and make sure that acute problems receive appropriate treatment instead of just being mislabeled as a worsening of dementia. Spotting and treating such problems early on before they progress can help prevent hospitalization, saving money and preventing a decrease in the quality of life for the patient and caregivers.

You can also provide information on support groups and caregiving resources so families know they aren't alone in providing long-term care. Make sure you evaluate educational programs and support groups to determine if they address the issues particular to late-stage disease; some groups may not be appropriate, and many community education programs and resources focus on earlier stages of chronic disease.

Caregivers coping with late-stage disease may also need help with facing ethical decisions, finding sufficient and appropriate supportive care, and dealing with the inevitability of death. Keep in mind that a family's culture will likely influence such discussions. And perhaps one of the most important supports you can offer caregivers is helping them understand that palliative care is just a different type of care, one that offers compassion and support to the patient and family as the patient approaches death.

The caregiver at risk

Caregivers do so much to improve outcomes for patients and decrease the burden on our health care system. So much, in fact, that caregivers themselves are at increased risk for health problems. Caregivers generally don't receive any special training to take on the stressful role of caring for an aging parent, spouse, or other family who has become physically dependent; they're simply thrust into the situation. They must respond to the demands of caregiving but can't just ignore their other responsibilities Plus, they must cope with their own emotional distress as they watch the older adult they care for—and care about—have increasing difficulty with such seemingly simple tasks as meal preparation, dressing, even eating.

Many caregivers are so busy juggling their other responsibilities with the care they're providing that they don't focus on their own needs. But ignoring their own needs for too long can threaten caregivers' mental and physical health, leading to depression, a sense of being overburdened and, eventually, burnout.

GETTING DOWN TO SPECIFICS

Although any of these stressful situations can lead to burnout, the specific stressors vary. For example, a caregiver may not know what to expect or how best to help. Other types of

---

THE MODIFIED CAREGIVER STRAIN INDEX

This assessment tool consists of 11 broach categories that measure the level of strain a caregiver experiences. Ask the caregiver to place a check under the answer that best applies. Then score each category as follows:

- Give 2 points for "Yes, on regular basis."
- Give 1 point for "Yes, sometimes."
- Give 0 points for "No."

The higher the score, the greater the caregiver's risk for strain, and the greater the need for a more in-depth assessment to identify problems and plan appropriate interventions.

	Yes, on a regular basis	Yes, sometimes	No
My sleep is disturbed.			
I find caregiving inconvenient.			
I find caregiving physically straining.			
I find caregiving confining.			
I've had to make family adjustments.			
I've had to make changes in my personal plans.			
I have other demands on my time.			
Some of the patient's behaviors upset me.			
I find it upsetting that the person I care for has changed so much from his or her former self.			
I find caregiving a financial strain.			
I feel completely overwhelmed.			
Total score			

Thornton, M., and Travis, S.S. (2003). Analysis of the reliability of the Modified Caregiver Strain Index. *The Journal of Gerontology*, Series B., Psychological Sciences and Social Sciences, 58(2), p. S129. Copyright The Gerontological Society of America.

Adapted from Sullivan, M. "The Modified Caregiver Strain Index (CSI)," in *Try this: Best Practices in Nursing Care to Older Adults*, Issue 14, revised 2007. The Hartford Institute for Geriatric Nursing, New York University [Online]. Available: http://consultgerirn.org/uploads/File/trythis/issue14.pdf [August 27, 2009].

stressor include financial hardship, emotional stress, and physical strain.

Research shows that certain factors predict caregiver distress, including patient behavioral problems, insufficient social supports, and inadequate coping responses. Certain patient symptoms also cause more stress, including incontinence or sleep issues that prevent the caregiver from sleeping. A synthesis of studies shows that, overall, the demands of caregiving can result in both increased stress and physical and psychiatric illnesses.

THE RISK LIST

Some specific risks to caregivers include:

- long-term caregiving
- multiple losses
- social isolation
- being a sole caregiver
- depression

- caring for an older adult and children at the same time (the sandwich generation)
- being frail themselves
- not having the financial resources for professional help.

STRESS CHECK TIME

Several tools allow you to assess caregivers, including such general tools as the modified caregiver strain index as well as tools for specific patient populations such as caregivers of patients with Alzheimer's disease and other forms of dementia. It also helps to screen caregivers for depression. If caregivers are under a great deal of stress, you'll also need to be alert to the possibility of patient neglect or abuse. The goal, of course, is to help caregivers before they reach such drastic levels. (See *The modified caregiver strain index*, page 353, and *The Alzheimer's caregiver stress check*.)

THE ALZHEIMER'S CAREGIVER STRESS CHECK

You can give this assessment tool to caregivers of patients with Alzheimer's disease so that they can gauge the amount of stress they're under. The greater the number of yes responses, the greater the degree of stress.

Do you regularly....

Feel like you have to do it all yourself, and that you should be doing more?	❑ Yes	❑ No
Withdraw from family, friends, and activities that you used to enjoy?	❑ Yes	❑ No
Worry that the person you care for is safe?	❑ Yes	❑ No
Feel anxious about money and health care decisions?	❑ Yes	❑ No
Deny the impact of the disease and its effects on your family?	❑ Yes	❑ No
Feel grief or sadness that your relationship with the person isn't what it used to be?	❑ Yes	❑ No
Get frustrated and angry when the person with dementia continually repeats things and doesn't seem to listen?	❑ Yes	❑ No
Have health problems that are taking a toll on you mentally and physically?	❑ Yes	❑ No

Alzheimer's Association (October 17, 2008). "Caregiver Stress Check" [Online]. Available: http://www.alz.org/stresscheck/ [August 27, 2009].

Care for the whole family

Family caregivers are in a unique position, providing care for older adults and yet very much needing care and support themselves. When they don't get the guidance, education, resources, and support they need, the whole family—patient and caregivers alike—can suffer.

You can promote the health of the whole family by encouraging caregivers to care for themselves. Teach caregivers the basics of healthy eating, regular exercise, and adequate sleep. Encourage them to find something enjoyable to do each day; you can suggest such coping tools as reflective writing, exercise, art, and music. You might even write out a prescription to remind caregivers of the importance of caring for themselves. (See *Caring for yourself*, pages 355 and 356.)

Healthy living   Caring for Yourself

Caring for a person who needs full-time supervision and care adds a great deal of stress to a person's life, placing the caregiver at physical and emotional risk. Heed the warning signs of stress and take necessary precautions to avoid feeling overstressed.

The Warning Signs
Keep an eye out for the warning signs of stress. They include:

- having trouble getting organized
- crying for no apparent reason
- feeling short-tempered
- feeling numb and emotionless
- having increasing difficulty accomplishing everyday tasks
- feeling constantly pressed for time
- feeling like you can't do anything right
- feeling like you have no time for yourself.

What You Can Do
If you have one or more of these warning signs, you may be feeling the stress of caregiving. The following tips can help you meet your own needs so that you can give better patient care.

Get enough rest
Exhaustion magnifies pressures and reduces your ability to cope. So the first step is to get a good night's sleep every night, if possible. Here's how:

- First, decide how much sleep you usually need—say, 7 hours—and set aside that much time. Then, when you go to bed, try not to replay the day in your mind. This isn't the time to solve problems.

- To help control disturbing thoughts, practice relaxation techniques, such as deep breathing, reading, or listening to soft music. Or try dimming the bathroom lights and taking a warm bath or shower to relieve muscle tension and help you wind down before bed.
- Avoid strenuous activity near bedtime. Strenuous activity earlier in the day, however, can promote sleep by tiring you physically. It also increases your physical stamina, improves your self-image, brightens your outlook, and gets you out of the house.
- If possible, hire a relief caregiver so you can attend aerobics classes, go for a brisk walk, or get some kind of exercise for at least 1 hour, three times a week.
- Try to schedule three or four short breaks during the day. Resting for 10 minutes with your feet up and your eyes closed can rejuvenate you and counteract the cycle of frantic activity that's probably keeping you up at night.
- Use medications only as a last resort and only temporarily. These drugs have side effects that can cause more problems for you in the long run. Instead, to induce drowsiness, try drinking a glass of warm milk.

Eat well
Eating regular, well-balanced meals helps you keep up your energy and increases your resistance to illness.

- Avoid skipping meals or eating on the run because these practices can cause vitamin and mineral deficiencies such as anemia (a shortage of iron in the blood that depletes your strength and make you feel exhausted).
- Avoid alcohol.

- Choose foods from the food-guide pyramid and avoid empty calories. And, unless you're overweight and your physician advises it, don't diet. You need increased calories to fuel your increased activity.

Don't try to be superhuman

After you've been caregiving for several weeks, reappraise your earlier plans. How much can you really do? How much time do you need for yourself?

- Make a list of tasks that you need help with, and ask friends or relatives for help. Delegate tasks. If possible, hire extra caregivers or someone to help with housework and shopping.
- Contact local support agencies for help. Send your laundry out. Remember, you don't have to do it all today, or accomplish everything on your list. Do only what's absolutely necessary, and learn to set priorities.
- Remember to save some time for pleasant activities. If you have 15 minutes of free time, listen to music or take a walk. If you want to have friends over for dinner, go ahead; just ask everyone to bring a course.

Confide in someone

A family member or close friend can help you resolve conflicts, be a sounding board for your anger and frustration, and offer emotional support. A support group can accomplish this too, as well as offer practical hints for patient care.

Be social

Don't isolate yourself. You may need to do some advanced planning to accomplish this goal. However, getting out with others helps to reduce stress.

Schedule some quality time alone

Free time won't happen automatically; you have to schedule it. In fact, your patient also needs time for himself. So allow yourself and your patient some personal space and private time. If you don't, you'll become too dependent on each other.

- Try to keep your life as normal as possible. Continue to do things that you enjoy, either by yourself or with your friends. Remember: Meeting your own needs isn't selfish, even if the patient is homebound. If you continue to feel guilty about taking some time for yourself, go for counseling.
- Determine how much time you need to be alone. At the very least, you need to take the time to attend to your important personal needs, such as bathing, washing your hair, and dressing. Or you might want or need to have a part-time or full-time job. If so, arrange for a caregiver to take care of the patient while you're working away from home. Make sure this arrangement fits your needs and your relationship with the patient.

Focus on the positive

If necessary, hold a family meeting to help resolve conflicts or gather support. Feel confident about your accomplishments as a caregiver.

The goal is to provide the best quality of life for the patient *without* sacrificing your own. How you accomplish this is up to you. But if you feel content and satisfied with the arrangement and the patient seems to be reasonably content, it's working.

Particularly when caregivers must cope with a challenging situation such as dementia, you can take steps to help maintain a healthy family system, including:

- promoting health, including screening for and diagnosing potential problems
- providing anticipatory guidance about what to expect from the patient's medical condition, especially in progressive disease
- attending to caregiver self-esteem needs and helping families be self-advocates
- screening the patient and caregivers for depression
- finding outside help for the caregiver as needed
- finding support systems for caregivers to share emotions and discuss problems.

TAKING A BREAK

When long-term caregiving becomes too much despite self-care measures, respite care can help. Respite care provides temporary relief from caregiving duties, either by providing caregiving services in the patient's home or by taking a patient temporarily into an assisted-living or extended care facility.

SEEKING SUPPORT

Although caregivers can benefit from a respite from long-term caregiving, they still need ongoing support from and a chance to share feelings with others who understand their situation. Individual counseling and organized support groups can both help. Some community-based agencies, such as the Alzheimer's Association, sponsor caregiving support groups. Different groups vary in what they provide, but they all generally offer opportunities for caregivers to share feelings and discuss problems and potential solutions. Many also give members a chance to share information about updates in services and new research that may have come out. Such groups can help families deal with stress and promote emotional and psychological well-being.

Online support groups can also help. They're especially useful for allowing people from many different locations to share ideas and support as well as for those whose caregiving duties prevent them from getting to meetings.

Make sure you're familiar with all these resources so you can provide caregivers with the information they need. If a support group isn't available but would be helpful to caregivers, you can advocate for the formation of such a group.

The Silver Lining

We all know the enormous challenges caregiving presents to families. But caregiving can also offer singular gifts, to both older adults and those caring for them. Caregiving can draw families closer together, and many caregivers report that they have gained emotional rewards from the experience; the shared experience can enhance family bonds. After all, caregiving can be very much an act of love. Many older adults receiving care can also give back to their caregivers, passing on the family's history as they interact with their caregiving children on a daily basis and having a chance to be loving grandparents to grandchildren.

And such rewards don't necessarily stop with the family. When you take part in supporting such a family, you receive the rich reward of knowing that you've improved people's lives and helped make a family stronger.

Abuse: A Breach of Trust

"Among our greatest challenges as a nation today is making America a safe place to grow old."

—LISA NERENBURG

Elder abuse—mistreatment of an older adult—afflicts some of the most vulnerable people in our society. According to the National Center on Elder Abuse, more than 2 million people in the United States age 65 and older are injured, exploited, or otherwise mistreated each year. And for every case of elder abuse, neglect, financial abuse, or self-neglect that's reported, it's estimated that 5 cases go unreported. Research by the National Center on Elder Abuse indicates that only 1 in 14 cases of elder abuse that occur in the home are reported; an even smaller proportion of financial abuse cases come to light, with only 1 in 25 cases reported.

Why are these crimes so underreported? Several factors come into play. Some victims may be in denial about the abuse, and some will deny being abused if asked. Health care workers may fail to recognize or report abuse. Many victims believe their cries for help will fall on deaf ears or that an abuser will retaliate if they tell the truth, so they don't seek help. Or they may have tried to tell someone, but found that no one listened to or believed them.

When the abuser is a family member—the majority of abusers—a victim may remain silent to protect his family member from legal consequences. Or he may be too embarrassed to admit that a supposed loved one is committing the abuse. When a victim doesn't or can't report abuse, another family member, friend, or neighbor may need to go to the authorities.

⌛ Timeline   *Fighting Elder Abuse*

Elder abuse didn't begin to receive much national attention until sometime in the mid-20th century. Awareness continues to grow; unfortunately, the incidence of elder abuse also continues to grow. This timeline covers some significant events in the recognition of and response to elder abuse in the United States along with other important historical events.

1920 18th Amendment prohibits alcohol; repealed with ratification of 21st Amendment in 1933

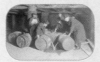

1920 19th Amendment grants women the right to vote

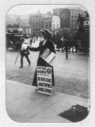

1917 Selective Service Act creates draft

1929 Stock Market crashes (Black Tuesday, October 29), heralding The Great Depression

1933 Franklin Roosevelt's first *Fireside Chat* radio broadcast

1935 Social Security Act passes

1941-1945 America's involvement in World War II

1948 Cold War begins

1900   10   20   30   40

Facts and Figures

Abuse can affect any older adult, regardless of race, ethnicity, socioeconomic level, religion, education, gender, or geographic location. (See *Elder abuse: An indiscriminate crime*, page 362.)

Statistics indicate that women are the most common victims of abuse and suffer the most severe injuries. But these statistics may somewhat distort the picture because women may be more apt to report abuse. Men may not report abuse because of the stigma of being a victim or fear of ridicule or of not being believed. Society may also be at fault, perpetuating the stereotype that abuse happens mainly to women.

The breakdown of alleged perpetrators lists adult children as the most likely abusers

1980 Prevention, Identification and Treatment of Adult Abuse Bill introduced in Congress; fails to pass

1985 Representative Claude Pepper issues report titled, "Elder Abuse: A National Disgrace"

1988 National Committee for the Prevention of Elder Abuse formed

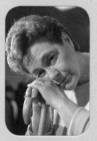

1950 President Truman initiates first National Conference on Aging

1955 In *Brown v. Board of Education,* Supreme Court orders desegregation of schools

1960-1965 Civil Rights movement

1963 National Council on Aging conducts earliest study of adult protective services (APS)

1965-1970 Demonstrations against Vietnam War

1974 Passage of Title XX of Social Security Act provides social service block grants (SSBGs) for APS

1978 Select Committee on Aging conducts first intensive investigation into elder abuse

1989 National Association of Adult Protective Services Administrators (NAAPSA) created

1992 American Association of Retired People (AARP) holds national forum on needs of older battered women

2004 First New York State Summit on Elder Abuse held

2009 Elder Abuse Victims Act introduced in Congress

50   60   70   80   90   2010

(33%), followed by family members other than spouses or children (22%), strangers (16%), and spouses or intimate partners (11%). Sadly, most reported incidents of elder abuse occur in the victim's home, although abuse has also been reported at other relatives' homes, homeless shelters, and other facilities, including adult day care centers, residential care facilities, skilled nursing facilities, and hospitals.

Home, not-so-sweet home

Several factors contribute to elder abuse. In the past, families typically lived near each other and shared responsibility for aging family members. Today, families may be scattered across the country, leaving the responsibility for caregiving to fall on the family member who lives closest to the older adult needing care. If an older adult has no family living close by, he may be alone and isolated, with no one to look after him—and particularly vulnerable to exploitation and abuse.

ONE IS THE LONELIEST NUMBER

When one family member has sole responsibility for an older adult, abuse may occur if the caregiver lacks the necessary skills to provide proper care. Conflict can also arise in the caregiver's household because of stress from caring for the older adult. A history of violent behavior within the family may also lead to elder abuse, with the abuse a continuation of what's gone on in the family for years. An adult child may take the opportunity to turn the tables on the abusive parent by physically abusing, neglecting, withholding nourishment, or overmedicating the parent. Elder abuse can also occur when someone who's dependent on an older adult—for instance, a mentally ill or developmentally challenged child—reacts inappropriately as the older adult grows increasingly frail.

MOVING IN, STRESSING OUT

When a frail or disabled older parent moves into a family member's home, the family must make sometimes-overwhelming adjustments. At the least, the house becomes more crowded. Even when the older adult is relatively independent, having another person in the household can still add responsibility and stress for the primary caregiver and other family members. An adult child—often a daughter—may find herself sandwiched between her parent and her own children, caring for both at the same time and possibly juggling all this with an outside job.

A caregiver also may not know exactly what kind of care the older adult needs or expects. If the older adult has a chronic, disabling condition, the caregiver may have even more trouble meeting the adult's needs as the older adult becomes less functional and more dependent. The caregiver may feel overwhelmed and trapped, especially if unaware of available caregiver resources that could help. Given that caregiver stress is a significant risk factor for abuse and neglect, such combined stresses may lead the caregiver to act out by mistreating the older adult.

When care facilities fail

Only about 4% of older adults live in residential and skilled nursing facilities, and most of them have their physical needs met with no abuse or neglect. When abuse or neglect does occur, direct care providers are commonly the perpetrators. They may either physically harm an older adult or fail to attend to hygiene or dietary needs. Sometimes, inadequate skills and training are to blame; for instance, abuse may occur if a caregiver doesn't have adequate training to manage difficult patients, such as those with dementia. A caregiver may also lack the skills necessary to manage resident aggression and interpersonal conflicts.

Facilities may also contribute to abuse by failing to meet older adults' physical and mental health needs or by having inadequate staffing, which can lead to neglect. Staffing shortages and mandatory overtime can also cause stress and burnout—especially in workers who need to hold more than one job to make ends meet—which can lead to abuse.

An Inventory of Abuse

Elder abuse occurs in many forms and as a single event or repeated acts that harm or increase the risk for harm. Types include domestic violence, financial abuse, neglect, and physical, psychological, or sexual abuse.

Domestic violence

Domestic violence is an increasing pattern of violence or intimidation used to exercise power and control over a partner. The abuser is typically a spouse or intimate partner, and most abusers are men. The pattern of abuse may have started when the couple was younger and persist into old age, or a previously strained relationship may escalate into abuse as the partners age. Some older adults may enter an abusive relationship later in life.

When abuse begins or worsens as the couple ages, it's commonly linked to issues surrounding medical or psychological disability, retirement, or family role changes. The frequency and severity of abuse may intensify over time, and the victim may have internal injuries, bruises, dislocations, or fractures in various stages of healing. The victim may also suffer from severe confusion and disassociation.

Financial abuse

Financial abuse—taking or misusing an older adult's money or assets for personal gain—can take many forms. The abuser may take money or property, use the victim's property or possessions without permission, or forge the older adult's signature on important documents. He may coerce the older adult to sign a deed, will, or power of attorney or may promise lifelong care in exchange for money and then refuse to provide the care. Or an abuser may use deception, scare tactics, or exaggerated claims to trick or scare an older adult into sending money or making charges on his credit card.

WHO'S CASHING IN?

The abuser may be a family member, a predator, or an unethical businessperson. But regardless of who perpetrates the crime, financial abuse can devastate an older adult, especially if the abuse depletes the victim's savings and leaves him unable to meet his financial needs.

A family member may financially abuse an older adult for several reasons. He may have gambling or financial problems or a history of substance abuse. He might be estranged from the older adult and feel entitled to the money or property, he may feel he deserves the money because of all the care he provides, or he may feel justified because he's slated to inherit the money anyway. Or he may dislike the rest of the family and want to prevent the older adult's assets from going to anyone else.

A predator deliberately seeks out vulnerable older adults with the intent to exploit them. The predator may gain access to the older adult by looking for people who live alone or by looking through newspaper death notices and then contacting a recently widowed person.

Unethical businesspeople may abuse older adults by overcharging for services and products. They may use their position to gain trust and then engage the older adult in unfair business practices. Older adults with mental or physical disabilities and those who are lonely and isolated are at greatest risk for such abuse.

THE MONEY TRAIL

Signs of financial abuse include:

- withdrawals from bank accounts
- bank transfers that the older adult can't explain
- unpaid bills
- notices about discontinuing utilities
- eviction notices
- the sudden appearance of a new close "friend"

- legal documents that the older adult has signed but doesn't understand
- unfamiliar signatures on legal documents and checks.

Neglect

Neglect occurs when a caregiver fails to provide needed care. Like financial abuse, it can take several forms, including active neglect, passive neglect, and self-neglect. In active neglect, the caregiver intentionally withholds care, food, medications, or other necessities. In passive neglect, the caregiver can't provide the necessary care because of a disability, illness, or stress. In self-neglect, the older adult refuses needed care.

Caregivers of all types may actively or passively neglect an older adult, including paid care attendants, family members, and employees of long-term care facilities. Reasons for neglect include financial gain, ill feelings toward the older adult, substance abuse or other mental health problems, and a lack of proper training or necessary skills.

TELLTALE SIGNS

Victims of all types of neglect can share common signs, including:

- dehydration
- difficulty sleeping
- emotional detachment
- emotional distress, such as depression and crying
- evidence of malnutrition
- insect or animal infestations in the home
- lack of food, water, or clothing
- lack of dentures, eyeglasses, hearing aids, wheelchairs, or walkers
- poor personal hygiene
- pressure ulcers
- regressive behavior
- skin rashes

- soiled clothing
- substandard living conditions
- sudden loss of appetite
- untreated or worsening medical conditions.

Physical abuse

Physical abuse is any act of violence, such as assault, battery, or inappropriate restraint, against a person that causes physical pain or harm. Those who physically abuse older adults are commonly unmarried, unemployed, and live with the victim. Some abusers have a history of alcohol or drug abuse.

PLAYING DETECTIVE

Because an abuser can frequently pass off an older adult's injuries as having another cause, physical abuse can be hard to detect. Look for clues; for instance, note when injury patterns don't fit the explanation. Keep in mind that patterns of injury suggest abuse more than a single injury, especially when there's no other proof of abuse. Suspect physical abuse if an older adult frequently visits the emergency department for similar injuries or if medical care for an injury is delayed.

Signs of physical abuse include:

- strap or rope marks on the arms, legs, or torso
- bilateral arm bruising
- internal injuries
- bleeding from orifices
- cigarette burns
- bilateral inner thigh bruising, which may also indicate sexual abuse
- bruises that encircle the torso, arms, or legs
- multicolored bruises, which indicate bruises in various stages of healing
- bone fractures in various stages of healing
- sprains
- dislocations.

Psychological abuse

In psychological abuse, a person verbally or nonverbally humiliates or threatens an older adult, causing mental or emotional distress. The abuser may also isolate the older adult and refuse to speak to or comfort him. The abuser of an older adult is typically a caregiver, family member, friend, or other acquaintance.

Victims of such abuse may have trouble sleeping and appear confused, anxious, depressed, agitated, withdrawn, emotionally upset, or unresponsive. They also may have low self-esteem, exhibit unusual behavior, and tremble or shy away from the abuser.

Sexual abuse

Sexual abuse is nonconsensual sexual contact, such as rape or molestation, or sexual contact with a person who's not mentally capable of giving consent. Those at greatest risk include women, isolated older adults, and those who suffer from physical or cognitive disabilities. Abusers may be caregivers, family members, spouses, or other acquaintances.

Indications of sexual abuse include unexpected sexually transmitted disease. Other signs include:

- torn or bloodstained undergarments
- difficulty sitting
- difficulty ambulating
- bruising of the inner thighs
- bruising of external genitalia
- genital injury, pain, or bleeding
- anal injury, pain, or bleeding.

Assessment: On the Alert

Health care workers—including physicians, nurses, emergency medical services personnel, dentists, and physical, occupational, and speech therapists—work in both inpatient and outpatient settings where they come in contact with older adults. Such contact places a unique responsibility on health care workers to assess older adults for the risk of abuse and detect signs of abuse. All health care workers must learn to recognize the clinical signs of elder abuse and know what actions to take if they suspect abuse.

You should assess every patient for abuse as part of the initial assessment. Unfortunately, most health care providers—including nurses—haven't had adequate training in conducting a thorough assessment for abuse. Some patients have obvious signs of abuse, but others may have subtle signs that can go unrecognized without a more thorough assessment.

The power of observation

One reason you may not readily spot signs of abuse is that they can easily appear to stem from other health problems. But if you look closely, you may note signs of abuse in the patient's physical appearance, general state of health, and the nature and extent of injuries. Listen closely, too, to both the patient and family members or other caregivers. Watch how the patient and caregiver interact with each other. Does the patient seem reluctant to speak in front of the caregiver? Do they argue with each other? Does there seem to be tension between the patient and the caregiver?

The tools you can use

Next, use a screening tool to guide your assessment and aid in the screening process. The Elder Assessment Instrument (EAI) is a useful tool that consists of a 42-item checklist broken into five major assessment categories. You can use the checklist to guide your assessment and help make sure you address specific items that may indicate abuse:

The assessment categories and items include:

- general assessment: clothing, hygiene, nutrition, and skin integrity
- possible abuse indicators: bruising, lacerations, fractures, various stages of healing of any bruises or fractures, evidence of sexual abuse, or a statement by the older adult related to abuse
- possible neglect indicators: contractures, dehydration, diarrhea, depression, impaction, malnutrition, pressure ulcers, poor hygiene, urine burns, failure to respond to warnings of obvious disease, inappropriate medications, repetitive hospital admissions, or a statement by the older adult related to neglect
- possible exploitation indicators: misuse of money, evidence of exploitation, reports of demands for goods in exchange for services, inability to account for money or property, or a statement by the older adult related to exploitation
- possible abandonment indicators: evidence that the caregiver has withdrawn care without alternate arrangements, evidence that the older adult has been left alone in an unsafe environment for extended periods without adequate support, or a statement by the older adult related to abandonment.

When using this tool, report suspected abuse if you see any physical evidence of abuse without another clinical explanation, the older adult complains of mistreatment, or you believe there's evidence of abuse, neglect, exploitation, or abandonment. The EAI requires training to use, but it's easily administered and can be used in several settings, including patients' homes, clinics, hospitals, and emergency departments.

THE BRIEF ABUSE SCREEN FOR THE ELDERLY

Commonly referred to as BASE, the brief abuse screen for the elderly is a screening tool practitioners can use to help them assess the likelihood of abuse.

1. Is the patient an older person who has a caregiver?   Yes _____ No _____

2. Is the patient a caregiver of an older person?   Yes _____ No _____

3. Do you suspect abuse?
   (See also questions #4 and #5)

   i) By a caregiver (comments) _____

1	2	3	4	5
no, not at all	only slightly, doubtful	possibly, somewhat	probably, quite likely	yes, definitely

   ii) By a care receiver or other (comments) _____

1	2	3	4	5
no, not at all	only slightly, doubtful	possibly, somewhat	probably, quite likely	yes, definitely

4. If any answer for #3 except "No, not at all," indicate what kind(s) of abuse(s) is (are) suspected.

   i) physical _____ ii) psychosocial _____ iii) financial _____
   iv) neglect _____ (includes passive and active)

5. If abuse is suspected, about how soon do you estimate that intervention is needed?

1	2	3	4	5
immediately	within 24 hours	24–72 hrs	1 week	2 or more weeks

Copyright © The Gerontological Society of America. Reprinted by permission of the publisher. Reis, M., and Nahmiash, D. "Validation of the Indicators of Abuse (IOA) Screen," Figure 2, *The Gerontologist*, 38(4):471-80, 1998.

Another screening tool, the Brief Abuse Screen for the Elderly consists of five items that focus on the caregiver. Health care providers and social workers can administer this tool. (See *The brief abuse screen for the elderly*.)

THE ELDER ABUSE SUSPICION INDEX

The Elder Abuse Suspicion Index (EASI) was designed to help health care providers decide if they should suspect elder abuse.

When you use the EASI, ask the patient the first five questions. The first question establishes that the patient relies on one or more caregivers, and the next four questions focus on potential abuse indicators. Answer the last of the six questions yourself based on your observations. If you find you have a "yes" answer to any of the last five questions, suspect abuse.

Over the Last 12 Months:

1. have you relied on other people for any of the following: bathing, dressing, shopping, banking, or meals?
   __Yes __No __Didn't answer

2. has anyone prevented you from getting food, clothes, medication, glasses, hearing aids, or medical care, or from being with people you wanted to be with?
   __Yes __No __Didn't answer

3. have you been upset because someone talked to you in a way that made you feel shamed or threatened?
   __Yes __No __Didn't answer

4. has anyone tried to force you to sign papers or to use your money against your will?
   __Yes __No __Didn't answer

5. has anyone made you afraid, touched you in ways that you did not want, or hurt you physically?
   __Yes __No __Didn't answer

Your Observations

6. Poor eye contact, acting withdrawn, sign of malnourishment, poor hygiene, cuts, bruises, inappropriate clothing, and poor medication compliance may all indicate elder abuse. Have you noticed any of these in the patient today or in the previous 12 months?
   __Yes __No

Yaffe, M.J., et al. "Development and Validation of a Tool to Improve Physician Identification of Elder Abuse: The Elder Abuse Suspicion Index (EASI)©," *Journal of Elder Abuse and Neglect* 20(3):276-300, December 6, 2008. © 2008 Routledge (Taylor & Francis).

THE RIGHT ROUTINE

Keep in mind that nurses aren't the only health care providers who should assess the patient for abuse; the patient needs a thorough interdisciplinary assessment. In fact, the American Medical Association (AMA) recommends that physicians routinely question older adult patients about abuse during regular visits. Such regular screenings help decrease the risk of attributing signs and symptoms caused by an unrelated medical problem to abuse.

Health care providers can easily use the Elder Abuse Suspicion Index (EASI), a validated, user-friendly, six-question index, in a physician's office or clinic. The EASI is designed for use with cognitively intact older adults to identify suspicion of abuse and justify a referral to an appropriate community expert in elder abuse. (See *The elder abuse suspicion index.*)

The interview: Handle with care

If you suspect abuse, you'll need to interview the older adult about the abuse. Question the older adult alone, and help him to feel at ease by letting him know that questions about abuse are routine.

Begin by asking where he lives and whether he's afraid of anyone. Make sure you give him enough time to respond to the question. If he says he's afraid, thank him for the information and ask follow-up questions, such as "Can you please give me an example of what made you feel afraid?" and "When did you last feel afraid?" If the older adult mentions physical abuse, ask questions to illicit information about the abuse. For example, ask, "Have you ever been hit or physically hurt by anyone?" Make sure you provide emotional support throughout, and address the older adult's concerns for personal safety.

DOCUMENTATION DETAILS

After you complete your assessment, carefully document your findings. Include the older adult's responses to questions you asked and any discussion held with the caregiver. Identify each speaker in your documentation and use direct quotes; doing so eliminates liability because your opinions aren't included. Keep in mind that your documentation may be invaluable evidence if the case ever goes to court. Make sure you document any discrepancies between what the patient said while alone with you and what the patient said when the caregiver was present.

Reporting: Get the Word Out

If you suspect abuse, you'll need to know your facility's policy for reporting your suspicions. In many facilities, you'll notify the case manager or social worker of suspected abuse. They'll then report the suspected abuse to adult protective services, the agency that investigates the case, intervenes, and offers protective services for the older adult. If a crime was committed, local law enforcement should also be notified. (See *Adult protective services: Protecting the rights of older adults.*)

State laws: A patchwork approach

Because of the magnitude of elder abuse, all 50 states have implemented mandatory reporting laws, special services, and training laws. However, there's no standard set of federal guidelines for reporting and managing cases of elder abuse, although both the AMA and the American Nurses' Association have developed guidelines for diagnosing and treating elder abuse. Make sure you know both your state's guidelines and your facility's policy for reporting abuse.

WHOSE JOB IS IT ANYWAY?

Because of the patchwork of laws, those legally mandated to report suspected or known abuse vary by state. For example, California mandates that physicians, clergy, all health care facility employees, and any person who assumes responsibility for the care or custody of an older adult report elder abuse. Those who fail to report elder abuse may be guilty of a crime. In Florida, state law requires that any person who knows of or suspects abuse of any vulnerable adult must report it to adult protective services.

Prevention: Stop it From Starting

Several organizations, initiatives, and other groups exist to help prevent elder abuse. Together, they offer considerable resources to help protect the elderly. (See *Combining forces to prevent abuse,* page 370.)

The power to protect

The National Center on Elder Abuse (NCEA), a national resource center, is committed to preventing elder abuse and neglect. Established by the U.S. Administration on

ADULT PROTECTIVE SERVICES: PROTECTING THE RIGHTS OF OLDER ADULTS

Adult protective services (APS) helps older adults and people with disabilities who are at risk for being mistreated or neglected, can't protect themselves, and have no one who can help them. APS receives reports of abuse, exploitation, and neglect and then investigates, monitors, and evaluates them. It also coordinates services the victim might need—including medical care, legal and economic services, and housing—contacts law enforcement when needed, and provides other protective emergency services.

APS functions under the following principles:

- Adults have the right to be safe.
- Adults retain all their civil and constitutional rights unless some of these rights have been restricted by court action.
- Adults have the right to make decisions that don't conform with societal norms as long as these decisions don't harm others.
- Adults are presumed to have decision-making capacity unless a court adjudicates otherwise.
- Adult have the right to accept or refuse services.

APS provides services by adhering to the following practice guidelines:

- The interests of the adult are the first concern of any intervention.
- Personal values shouldn't be imposed on others.
- Informed consent should be sought before providing services.
- The adult's rights to keep personal information confidential must be respected.
- Individual differences, such as cultural, historical, and personal values, should be recognized.
- The right of the adult to receive information about his or her choices and options in an understandable format should be honored.
- The adult should be involved as much as possible in formulating the service plan.
- Case planning should focus on maximizing the older adult's independence and choices according to each older adult's ability.
- Community-based services should be used first when possible, before institutionally based services.
- Family and informal support systems should be used first if it's in the best interest of the older adult.
- Clear and appropriate boundaries should be maintained.
- Casework actions should be in the older adult's best interest when the older adult is unable to express his wishes.
- Substituted judgment in case planning should be used when historical knowledge of the adult's values is available.
- Inadequate or inappropriate intervention may be worse than no intervention.

Aging in 1988, the NCEA provides information about elder abuse to both health care providers and the public as well as training for state and local agencies. The organization consists of a multidisciplinary team of experts in elder abuse, neglect, and exploitation that serves as a resource to all those working with older victims, including adult protective services, law enforcement agencies, health care workers, domestic violence networks, and national, state, and local aging networks. The NCEA also focuses on meeting the needs of disadvantaged people, including those who speak little English. The organization disseminates information to help build and strengthen elder rights networks and improve state and local elder abuse prevention and intervention programs.

The Second International Conference on Elder Abuse convened in California in 2008. At the conference, geriatric physicians, psychologists, social workers, and long-term care ombudsmen met to find ways to recognize and stop elder abuse. From this conference came the Elder PEACE movement, which hopes to inspire a national audience to join

COMBINING FORCES TO STOP ABUSE

By pooling their efforts, several groups can heighten the awareness of elder abuse, intervene when abuse occurs, and perhaps eventually stop abuse from happening. Each group plays a vital role:

- Adult protective services (APS) is designated as the primary agency in most states to receive and investigate reports of elder abuse.
- Professionals in the field of aging provide a critical link between victims of abuse and APS and may be the first to discover cases of abuse. They also help educate other professionals about the special needs of older adults.
- Health care providers may also be the first to identify suspected victims of abuse—typically in emergency departments, where physicians and nurses follow protocols designed to help identify abuse.
- Researchers provide insight about the risk factors, etiology, and incidence of elder abuse. Their research helps guide prevention efforts, interventions, and services to help elder abuse victims. A 2008 study by the National Social Life, Health, and Aging Project was the first population-based, national study to question more than 3,000 community-dwelling older adults about their recent experience with abuse. Information from this study provided valuable insight into elder abuse.
- The media can heighten awareness and educate the public about abuse as well as help shape the public's perceptions about elder abuse. Media outlets can also enlist the public's help in identifying abuse and educating policy makers about the need for improved services and public policy. Plus, they can educate victims about available services—and abusers about the consequences of their actions.
- Concerned citizens can stay alert for suspected abuse among older friends and neighbors and report incidents. The can also help raise awareness of the problem, volunteer their time, and advocate for needed services and policies.

the cause against elder abuse. PEACE stands for Protection, Education, Advocacy, Collaboration, and Eradication—the goals of the movement.

As a group, older adults are also looking out for their own rights and safety. Baby boomers—those born between 1946 and 1964—are beginning to reach retirement age, and they're concerned about elder abuse. Rebecca Guider, director of adult services and assistance programs for Orange County, California, notes that "aging boomers are already making a difference." More educated than previous generations about their rights, boomers are less likely to put up with abusive situations, and many are likely to become active in organizations that help prevent elder abuse and work to revise and enforce elder abuse laws.

Home: A safe haven?

Unfortunately, most elder abuse occurs in the home, at the hands of family members or other caregivers. To help prevent such abuse, all

people—but especially family members and other caregivers of older adults—need to be made aware of the risk factors for abuse, including caregiver stress, and the special needs of older adults. They also should have the chance to discuss their concerns and needs with a social worker, who can give them guidance about available services.

As mentioned in previous chapters, respite care can help reduce caregiver stress, a major risk factor for abuse. Respite care provides care for the older adult so that the caregiver can temporarily have some relief from the responsibility of caring for the older adult. Taking such a break can be crucial for those caring for older adults with dementia (such as Alzheimer's disease) or severe disability. Respite care doesn't have to come from an agency, though; sometimes friends or other family members can take on temporary caregiving.

Adult day care can help when a family caregiver must work outside the home and the older adult can't be left alone. Adult day care provides a safe environment for the older adult and provides peace of mind for the working caregiver. It also offers the older adult who might otherwise be isolated a chance to socialize with his peers.

Family caregivers might also benefit from a support group or other social network. Sharing similar stresses and situations can help caregivers find solutions for care issues and help relieve tensions. Sometimes group members also band together to provide respite for one another.

A family caregiver who's having trouble coping with the stress of caring for an older adult may benefit from counseling. A counselor can help the caregiver find solutions and coping mechanisms for stress.

Even with counseling, sometimes a family caregiver simply can't cope with the stress of caring for an older adult. In that case, both the older adult and the caregiver may be better off if the older adult moves into a long-term care facility.

Care facilities: Setting the standard

The Joint Commission has developed standards to help prevent abuse in long-term care facilities. The 2010 standards state that facilities must:

- have written criteria to help identify victims of abuse or neglect
- maintain a list of private and public community agencies that can assess and care for victims of abuse
- educate appropriate staff members about abuse, neglect, and exploitation and how to report it appropriately
- use criteria to assess for abuse, neglect, or exploitation on entry to the facility and on an ongoing basis
- make sure that staff members assess for abuse, neglect, or exploitation or, if they

can't do so, make an appropriate referral for the assessment process
- ensure that all cases of suspected abuse, neglect, or exploitation are reported immediately within the facility
- report all cases of suspected abuse, neglect, or exploitation to appropriate agencies according to facility policy and state laws and regulations.

The Joint Commission also has standards about the use of restraints. Specifically, a facility may not allow the use of physical or chemical restraints to discipline residents, to prevent them from wandering, or for staff convenience. A facility may only use them to support or facilitate the treatment of a medical condition, and even in these instances, the patient has the right to refuse restraints.

GOING THE EXTRA MILE

Long-term care facilities can also take further measures to help prevent abuse. All facilities should perform background checks on all staff members, as mandated by state laws, to make sure they avoid hiring anyone with a history of abusing others. They should also make sure that staff members understand what constitutes physical and psychological abuse and neglect and teach them about dementia, handling difficult resident care situations, reducing stress, and recognizing cultural differences between residents and staff members. When assigning staff members, facilities can match the needs of each resident with the capabilities of staff members. And to make sure they hire and keep excellent personnel, facilities should provide competitive salaries, maintain adequate staffing, offer opportunities for advancement and personal growth, and keep clear lines of communication open between direct care staff members and the administration.

RESOURCES FOR REPORTING ABUSE

Several agencies can help with reporting elder abuse, providing general information and referrals to protect the victim, obtaining services for victims, and investigating allegations of abuse.

Eldercare Locator

To use the Eldercare Locator (which is sponsored by the Administration on Aging), a person who suspects abuse calls the service and provides the address and zip code of the abused older adult. Eldercare Locater then uses that information to tell the caller what agency in the area to call to report the suspected abuse. Their toll-free number is 1-800-677-1116.

Area Agency on Aging

Most states have a local information and referral line, which a caller can use to locate services for victims of abuse. The local Area Agency on Aging is listed in the local telephone directory.

Medicaid Fraud Control Unit

The Medicaid Fraud Control Unit investigates and prosecutes Medicaid provider fraud and patient abuse and neglect in health care programs and home health programs that participate in Medicaid. Federal law requires each state's attorney general office to have a Medicaid Fraud Control Unit.

National Domestic Violence Hotline

The hotline, which operates 24 hours a day, 365 days a year, provides support counseling for victims of domestic violence. It provides a link to over 2,500 local support services for abused women. Their toll-free number is 1-800-799-SAFE (7233).

The Laws of the Land

Protecting older adults has been a large part of policy development in the United States for more than 30 years. In 1978, the U.S. House of Representatives Aging Subcommittee began looking at the issue of elder abuse. Between 1980 and 1986, 26 states passed laws that mandated the reporting of elder abuse. By 1997, 42 states had enacted elder abuse legislation.

A class act

The Older Americans Act illustrates the nation's commitment to protecting vulnerable older adults at risk. This act requires states to have a long-term care ombudsman program to protect the rights, health, safety, and welfare of those who live in long-term care facilities. Each facility is assigned an ombudsman, who makes regular visits to establish relationships with residents, families, staff members, and the administration. The ombudsman resolves complaints made by or for the residents, monitors long-term care laws, and helps prevent elder abuse by improving communication among residents, families, and staff members.

Bestselling titles

In 1992, Congress created and funded Title VII, Vulnerable Elder Rights Protection, to prevent abuse, neglect, and exploitation. Provisions added in 2000 encouraged states to promote greater coordination of law enforcement agencies with the court system. Congress made further amendments in 2006, adding new language to Title VII as well as to Title II, Elder Abuse Prevention and Services. The changes emphasized multidisciplinary and collaborative approaches to addressing elder abuse, especially when developing programs and long-term strategic plans. Title VII also includes a provision for a position that assists at the state level to develop programs that coordinate the provision of legal services for the elderly.

Community: Sharing the Responsibility

Despite the best laws and regulations, elder abuse won't be eradicated unless people in communities throughout the United States are willing to do their part to support and protect elders. Unfortunately, many people fear reporting suspected abuse because they may be wrong.

Community education should focus on the importance of reporting abuse, emphasizing that it's better to report suspected abuse and be wrong than allow someone to continue living in an abusive situation. Some people may think that reporting suspected abuse is meddling in other people's business; education can help them understand that a life may be at stake, that they should err on the side of caution and report the suspected abuse.

Third-party observers—not abuse victims— report at least 70% of elder abuse cases.

Remind community members that every state has a service designated to receive and investigate allegations of elder abuse and neglect. These agencies make referrals for counseling, even if they only find the potential for abuse. (See *Resources for reporting abuse*.)

Also, make sure you explain that, no matter how well meaning, a neighbor or friend should never confront a possible abuser; they should instead report the suspected abuse. If any type of confrontation were to take place, the neighbor or friend must first have the victim's permission as well as a well-thought-out plan to immediately move the victim to a safe place. (See the *Case Study* below.)

We all have a role to play in preventing abuse—legislators, health care professionals, family members, and friends and neighbors. As more of us understand the importance of recognizing abuse and taking the right steps to stop it, elder abuse may eventually become a thing of the past.

Case Study

Evelyn, an 86-year-old widow with Parkinson's disease, moved in with her 68-year-old daughter Kay because of health problems. Both of them find the situation difficult. Sometimes Kay feels as if she's at the end of her rope, caring for her mother, and worrying about her grandchildren and her husband, who also has health problems. Kay has caught herself calling her mother names and accusing her mother of ruining her life. This leaves Evelyn feeling frightened, isolated, trapped, and worthless.

Critical thinking questions
- Evelyn is a victim of which type abuse?
- How would you council Kay?
- What resources would you suggest for Kay?
- What resources would you suggest for Evelyn?

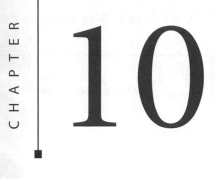

10

End-of-Life Care: Easing the Transition

> "A dying man needs to die, as a sleepy man needs to sleep, and there comes a time when it is wrong, as well as useless, to resist."
>
> —STEWART ALSOP

A s an older adult approaches death, caring for the patient doesn't stop—but the focus of that care shifts. Instead of seeking to cure or manage disease, end-of-life care seeks to relieve suffering, make the remainder of the patient's life as comfortable as possible, and help both the patient and family with the patient's transition from life to death.

Such end-of-life, or hospice, care has received more and more attention over the past several years. A number of factors have contributed to this increased attention, including the Medicare Hospice Benefit, developed in 1982 by the Centers for Medicare & Medicaid Services; Supreme Court decisions on end-of-life issues, such as the continuing controversy over *Roe v. Wade*, the Karen Quinlan case, and Kevorkian's championing of a patient's right to die; and the Patient Self-Determination Act, which increased the ability of patients to make their wishes known and direct their end-of-life care. Researchers also continue to study end-of-life care issues and point to areas for improvement, and health care organizations across the globe have implemented major initiatives to improve education on end-of-life issues for patients, families, and health care providers. This focus on end-of-life issues will likely continue as the average age of the U.S. population increases. By 2030, when the first of the baby boomers will be approaching age 85, nearly 9 million Americans will already be over age 85.

⧖ *Timeline* *Death and Dying: Issues and Trends*

This timeline traces some of the major issues and trends related to death and dying in the United States over the past century.

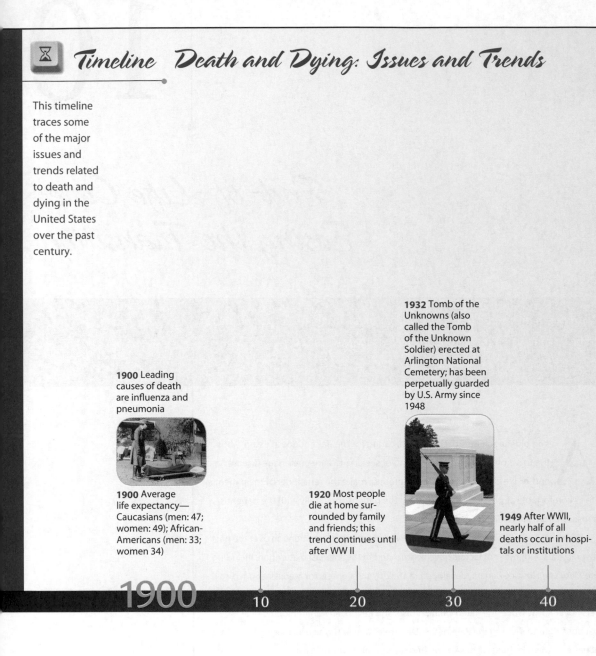

1932 Tomb of the Unknowns (also called the Tomb of the Unknown Soldier) erected at Arlington National Cemetery; has been perpetually guarded by U.S. Army since 1948

1900 Leading causes of death are influenza and pneumonia

1900 Average life expectancy—Caucasians (men: 47; women: 49); African-Americans (men: 33; women 34)

1920 Most people die at home surrounded by family and friends; this trend continues until after WW II

1949 After WWII, nearly half of all deaths occur in hospitals or institutions

1900   10   20   30   40

A "Good" Death

One of the most important specific issues health care providers and advocates must address is where people face the end of life. About 75% of those deciding where they want to die say they want to receive care and die at home, but only 18% actually do. Improvement initiatives are trying to address this discrepancy, allowing health care providers to better protect their patients' wishes.

1964 Term *brain death* coined

1967 Leading causes of death in the U.S. are heart disease and neoplasms

1967 Saunders founds first modern hospice (St. Christopher's Hospice) in residential suburb of London

1968 Uniform Anatomical Gift Act makes it legal to donate deceased individual's tissues and organs for transplantation

1969 Dr. Elisabeth Kübler-Ross publishes *On Death and Dying*, based on more than 500 interviews with dying patients

1959 Herman Feifel, a Veterans Administration psychiatrist, publishes *The Meaning of Death*, leading the way for professional discussions about trends and issues in death and dying

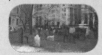

1974 The Connecticut Hospice opens as first hospice in the U.S.

1979 The Health Care Financing Administration (HCFA) initiates demonstration programs at 26 hospices across the country

1981 Uniform Determination of Death Act approved

1984 Congress prohibits selling of organs and tissues; establishes Organ Procurement and Transplantation Network to ensure fair, equitable method to allocate donated tissues and organs

1986 Congress makes the Medicare Hospice Benefit permanent; states given the option of including hospice in Medicaid programs; hospice care is made available to terminally ill nursing home residents

1991 Patient Self Determination Act passed by Congress; mandates that all Medicare/Medicaid-reimbursed hospitals must provide patients with written information about their right to execute advance directives

1993 Hospice is included as a nationally guaranteed benefit under President Clinton's health care reform proposal

2002 Three leading causes of death in people over age 65 are heart disease, malignant neoplasms, and stroke

2010 Projected average life expectancy— Caucasians (men: 77; women: 81); African-Americans (men: 70; women: 77)

50   60   70   80   90   2010

Regardless of where the patient receives end-of-life care, the overall goal remains the same: to improve the quality of the patient's life and his ability to function while minimizing symptoms. Providing successful end-of-life care can lead to what's described as a "good" death. Such care includes pain and symptom management, collaboration and communication with the patient and family, respect for the patient's wishes, and use of evidence-based clinical standards to give exceptional care. You can offer your dying older patients this kind of care if you have the most current knowledge, the appropriate skills—and, of course, compassion.

A Different Kind of Care

Geared specifically toward the needs of dying patients and their families, hospice offers a different kind of care: palliative rather than curative. Palliative care doesn't aim to cure the patient. Instead, it strives to relieve suffering and support the best possible quality of life for patients with advanced chronic or life-threatening illnesses.

Hospice programs provide this palliative care, supporting patients during the last phases of incurable disease so that they may live as fully and comfortably as possible. These programs also reach out to family members, offering help while their loved ones are dying and after they're gone. Specific types of care include treating pain, alleviating symptoms, decreasing stressors, supporting daily living tasks for the patient and family, helping the patient and family with difficult medical decisions, and ensuring that the patient's and family's wishes for care are respected and followed.

Originally, the hospice movement focused mainly on cancer patients near the end of life. Today, however, hospice services provide care to terminal patients with any serious illness, including cardiovascular and pulmonary diseases, neurodegenerative disorders, stroke, cancer, human immunodeficiency virus (HIV), and renal failure. Although some of these patients haven't yet reached old age, many hospice patients are older patients.

Hospice vs. palliative

Before getting into further detail about hospice care, it helps to understand that, even though some may use the terms "hospice" and "palliative" almost interchangeably, there are differences. Both types of care are, essentially, palliative in that they focus on relief of suffering and improvement of the quality of life—comfort care—rather than cure. However, a patient receiving palliative care can be in any stage of an illness, whereas a patient receiving hospice care typically has a life expectancy of less than 6 months (although there's a growing trend of hospice organizations offering palliative care earlier in the course of a patient's illness). Palliative care also doesn't preclude curative treatment; the patient can receive both curative or life-prolonging treatment as well as "comfort" care. Care for a hospice patient doesn't typically include more aggressive, life-prolonging treatment, instead focusing on helping the patient face the end of his life.

They're also typically administered in different settings. Hospice is typically offered in the patient's home by home health agencies or hospital systems, although hospice can take place in a variety of other settings, including hospitals, residential facilities, long-term care facilities, and even prisons. Palliative care typically takes place in acute care hospitals and outpatient settings.

Payment also differs, depending on where the care is provided. Palliative care, typically administered through a hospital or regular medical provider, is usually covered under regular medical insurance. Coverage for hospice care varies, with many hospice programs covered by Medicare (discussed in more detail later) and some hospice programs offering subsidized care for the economically disadvantaged.

Despite these differences, both palliative and hospice care provide much-needed support to regular facility staff members, family members, and the patient, who are all coping with the patient's increased and urgent medical needs as he nears death.

Medicare's role

Medicare plays a key role in the delivery of hospice care in the United States by offering the Medicare hospice benefit to pay for hospice programs that meet federal regulations. Most hospice patients and programs rely on this benefit as a payment option. The Medicare hospice benefit allows for hospice care from an interdisciplinary team that has skills in pain management, symptom control, and bereavement assistance. The benefit also covers the cost of durable medical equipment and drugs, although some drugs may require a nominal copayment fee.

To receive this benefit, the patient must meet the following conditions:

- The patient must be eligible for Medicare Part A (hospital insurance).
- The patient's physician and the hospice medical director must agree that the patient has a life expectancy of 6 months or less if the illness runs its usual course.
- The patient must elect the Medicare hospice benefit for coverage of all services related to his terminal illness.
- The patient must receive care from a Medicare-approved hospice program.

Keep in mind that receiving the Medicare hospice benefit doesn't preclude the patient from receiving benefits for a covered illness not related to the terminal illness.

An unconventional approach

End-of-life care doesn't have to be limited to conventional medicine. Many dying patients, weary of sometimes-invasive treatments and adverse effects of "modern" medicine, wish to turn to alternative therapies. The National Center for Complementary and Alternative Medicine defines those therapies that fall outside the conventional medical approach as complementary and alternative medicine (CAM) therapies. It further divides CAM therapies into four basic domains: mind-body medicine, biologically based practices, manipulative and body-based practices, and energy medicine. Specific therapies used in palliative care include massage therapy; physical, occupational, and speech therapies; pet therapy; herbal and aromatherapy; acupuncture; healing touch; imagery; magnets; and music therapy.

These therapies can play a crucial role for a dying patient, complementing conventional treatments—music therapy, for instance, may enhance pain relief for some patients—or serving as an alternative when traditional medicine no longer provides relief. Keep these therapies in mind as you care for patients approaching death so that you can offer them the fullest possible range of options. The National Center for Complementary and Alternative Medicine maintains a Web site (http://nccam.nih.gov) that offers more information about these alternative therapies.

The nursing process

As it does for all nursing care, the nursing process will help you deliver effective, consistent end-of-life care. The five steps—assessment, diagnosis, planning, implementation, and evaluation—provide a framework to help you recognize and respond to health issues as they arise.

ASSESSMENT

For your assessment, make sure you include subjective and objective data for both physiologic and psychosocial factors. Take into account input from family, friends, and caregivers, especially for a patient receiving care at home. Information from caregivers particularly helps your ongoing assessment, providing valuable data about changes in status and the effectiveness of treatments.

Use the pneumonic device OLD CART—onset, location, duration, characteristics, associated symptoms, relieving factors, and attempted treatment—during your interview of the patient and caregiver to help you remember what data you need to gather. You can use this information in conjunction with objective data to help you quickly identify a course of action and plan symptom management.

DIAGNOSIS

Use your assessment data to determine or validate an appropriate nursing diagnosis. Your working nursing diagnosis may include two or three parts and may be an actual or at-risk diagnosis. Several physiologic and psychological nursing diagnoses typically apply to patients receiving end-of-life care, including (but not limited to) *Chronic pain, Activity intolerance, Ineffective coping, Risk for injury, Anxiety, Imbalanced nutrition: Less than body requirements, Decisional conflict, Impaired skin integrity,* and *Bathing self-care deficit.*

PLANNING

When planning care and identifying outcomes, make sure you include the patient and any caregivers or family members the patient wants included. As the patient moves toward the end of life, his goals will shift from a curative intent to comfort and supportive management.

IMPLEMENTATION

When implementing the care plan, keep in mind the goal of improving quality of life by minimizing symptoms and improving functional ability. Make sure you're all clear on who's providing any hands-on care. Teach the patient, family members, and any other caregivers about the disease, strategies for care, and expected signs and symptoms; include written instructions for all medications. Encourage deep-breathing and relaxation techniques for both the patient and family members to decrease anxiety.

EVALUATION

When evaluating the effectiveness of the care plan, make sure you include feedback from the patient, family members, and caregivers as well as your own assessment of the patient's response to therapies.

Clear communication: A key to good care

Throughout care—from making your initial assessment through helping family members cope with the loss of their loved one—don't lose sight of the role of effective communication. Offer accepting, supportive listening to help the patient and family members freely discuss their wishes, concerns, and fears. Use clear, educationally appropriate language—avoiding medical jargon—to talk with them about the patient's illness, treatments, and what to expect; use a translator if necessary.

You can use such communication techniques as open-ended questions, reflection, and silence to allow the patient to voice concerns, values, cultural differences, and wishes for care. Use open body language, focus on the patient, offer empathy, eliminate distractions, and be aware of the patient's culture; all will improve communication.

Watch out for the pitfalls that can interfere with effective communication, too. Avoid clichés, false reassurances, judgmental statements, and closed-ended questions, and don't change the subject when the patient or family members need to talk, even if the subject might make you uncomfortable. Also, make sure you communicate clearly with other health care team members, making sure you include information about the patient's needs and wishes.

Palliative Care: Addressing All the Aspects

It's easy to understand the basic philosophy of relieving suffering and supporting the best quality of life for dying patients. But keeping current on the practices and guidelines for providing end-of-life care presents a greater challenge. Fortunately, three organizations have stepped in to address these issues. The American Academy of Hospice and Palliative Medicine, the Hospice and Palliative Nurses Association, and the National Hospice and Palliative Care Organization have developed end-of-life care guidelines, and they continue to work together to promote program development, establish quality control and consistency of education, set national goals, and foster continuity of care.

A framework for care

One of the most useful tools for providing consistent, quality care for dying patients is the *Clinical Practice Guidelines for Quality Palliative Care*. Developed by the National Consensus Project for Quality Palliative Care, the guidelines include eight aspects of care that serve as a framework for providing care for dying patients. These aspects range from the structure and process of care, to the physical aspects, to the ethical and legal aspects of care. They can help you understand and address the different medical priorities—including evaluating and managing symptoms and their causes—of dying patients, who aren't focused on returning to health but instead are moving through the last stages of life. (See *Aspects of palliative care*.)

Structure and processes

Caring for a dying patient calls for a comprehensive, interdisciplinary approach, from assessment to implementation of care.

The specific guidelines for the structure and processes of delivering palliative care to a dying patient focus on the importance of including not just traditional health care providers, but also those who can offer spiritual support, friends of the patient, appropriate volunteers, physical therapist, practitioners of alternative medicine, other specialists—the list can go on, and it varies for each patient, depending on the patient's and family's wishes and needs. The guidelines also recognize the importance of identifying those wishes and needs, the impact of caring for a dying patient on those who provide that care, and the importance of the environment where that care takes place. You can read the full list of guidelines at the National Consensus Project's Web site (http://www.nationalconsensusproject.org).

Physical aspects

Physical care for a dying patient focuses on controlling pain and other symptoms and mitigating adverse effects of both the underlying illness and medications. Interventions should help improve the patient's physical well-being, bringing it closer to the World Health Organization (WHO) definition of health as "a state of complete physical, mental, and social well being and not merely the absence of disease or infirmity."

A TIME FOR TEACHING

Physical aspects of care include teaching the patient and his family about disease symptoms and common adverse effects as well as preventive interventions that can help alleviate those effects. For instance, teach the patient and caregiver how to modify oral care, feeding, bathing, and other activities of daily living (ADLs) to ease symptoms. Show them techniques to prevent bedsores and contractures, including range-of-motion (ROM) exercises. Demonstrate the correct method of transferring a weak patient to prevent injury to both the patient and caregiver.

IN CASE OF EMERGENCY…

As appropriate, recommend that the at-home hospice patient have an emergency kit customized to meet his anticipated needs. Such a kit allows family members and other caregivers to provide immediate palliative care for common end-of-life symptoms, such as pain, fatigue, dyspnea, nausea, vomiting, constipation, and excessive respiratory secretions. Contents of the emergency kit may include morphine, lorazepam (Ativan), scopolamine, haloperidol (Haldol), prochlorperazine (Compazine), and diphenhydramine (Benadryl). It may also include medication compounds, such as ABHR, which includes lorazepam (Ativan), diphenhydramine (Benadryl), haloperidol (Haldol), and metoclopramide (Reglan).

FACING THE PHYSICAL PROBLEMS

Dying patients typically face a cluster of physical problems, which, depending on the disease, may include anorexia, nausea and vomiting, constipation, coughing and respiratory secretions, dyspnea, and fatigue. Unfortunately, for most patients, physical care also must include pain management.

ANOREXIA

Anorexia is the loss of appetite resulting in the inability to eat. It can result from both the underlying disease and treatment modalities. Cachexia, or wasting syndrome, is often seen in patients with cancer or HIV and may lead to anorexia.

When assessing such a patient, ask about eating patterns, mouth sores or taste changes, bowel patterns, pain level, sleep patterns, fatigue, anxiety, and the patient's ability to cook for and feed himself. Compare his current weight and body mass index to his baseline, and assess his oral cavity and throat for sores or lesions that indicate impaired mucous membrane function.

Interventions include steps to stimulate the patient's appetite to increase his food intake. Common treatments include parenteral nutrition, appetite stimulants, and nutritional supplements. Effective appetite stimulants include dronabinol (Marinol), cyproheptadine, and megestrol acetate (Megace); mirtazapine (Remeron), typically used to treat depression, also increases appetite. Nonpharmacologic interventions include preparing food at a different site to minimize odors; providing small, frequent meals; and praising the patient for any amount of food he eats. A little light exercise—such as walking, passive ROM exercises, yoga, or stretching—may also increase appetite. CAM therapies that may help stimulate the patient's appetite include omega 3 fatty acids, ginger, and fennel.

Keep in mind that the nutritional goal isn't so much the quantity the patient takes in, but nutrition to maintain his quality of life. A successful intervention may be the patient simply enjoying the taste of food and the social aspects of eating a meal. Family members who feel emotionally distressed at the decreased amount their loved one is eating may find the support of a chaplain or social worker helpful. Reassure the family that decreased thirst and hunger is normal as the physiologic demands on the patient's body decrease.

CONSTIPATION

Constipation—the decrease in the normal frequency of bowel movements with difficult passage of hard, dry stool or incomplete passage of stool—can be very uncomfortable for a patient nearing the end of life and can lead to fecal impaction. Leading causes include dehydration, medications, depression, and ascites.

During your assessment, ask about:

- nutrition and hydration status
- bowel frequency
- stool characteristics and amount
- abdominal discomfort
- flatulence
- nausea
- rectal fullness
- incomplete evacuation.

R̟ Medication Alert Provide preventive teaching and ongoing assessment for patients receiving narcotic pain medications because these medications place them at risk for constipation.

You should also auscultate bowel sounds in all four quadrants, palpate the abdomen for tenderness or masses, and perform a digital rectal examination if the patient complains of incomplete evacuation or if you suspect he's too weak to evacuate completely.

To help manage constipation, the patient should increase fluid intake and dietary fiber. Encourage physical activity to promote intestinal motility. Recommend the patient use a toilet or bedside commode, which is more comfortable and promotes more natural bowel movements, rather than a bedpan.

Many palliative care programs employ a stepped bowel regimen to handle constipation, starting with a stimulant. If that's not effective, the regimen progresses to a saline enema, then to an oral saline agent, and finally an osmotic laxative. Keep in mind that bowel stimulants may cause uncomfortable cramping in patients with neuropathies or in extremely weak patients; stool softeners and daily or every-other-day enemas may be preferable for such patients.

The patient or a family member may express concern that the patient doesn't have a bowel movement daily. If so, encourage the patient to maintain the bowel regimen, and explain that a pattern of every other day may be appropriate. Make sure the patient receives ongoing assessment to ensure adequate bowel elimination.

COUGHING AND RESPIRATORY SECRETIONS

Coughing and increased respiratory secretions are commonly seen in patients in the final stages of end-stage renal disease, heart failure, and lung diseases, such as lung cancer or chronic obstructive pulmonary disease. Coughing is a protective mechanism that clears mucous, fluids, and inhaled foreign bodies from the trachea and bronchi, but it can be uncomfortable, troublesome, and persistent at the end of life.

Assess the patient's cough for frequency, duration, and aggravating and alleviating factors. Also check the color, amount, and consistency of sputum the cough produces.

When the underlying cause of the cough can't be treated, you can help managing the cough with antitussives, such as benzonatate (Tessalon Perles) and dextromethorphan/

guaifenesin (Robitussin DM). The patient may also choose to take small doses of morphine every 3 to 4 hours if he hasn't taken opioids before. If he's already taking morphine, his dose can increase by 25%, with an additional 25% if needed. Alternatives for managing cough may include codeine and hydrocodone preparations; furosemide (Lasix) may also decrease coughing in patients with heart failure and those who have excess fluid with pitting edema.

CAM therapies may include warm elixir of honey and lemon, ventilation from an opened window, cool cloths to the patient's face, and water to help loosen sputum. You may need to remind the patient to cough and teach him to cough effectively to prevent secretions from pooling in his lungs. Also tell family members not to smoke, cook, or allow overcrowding in the patient's room.

DYSPNEA

Dyspnea—a subjective experience of difficulty breathing, an uncomfortable awareness of breathing, and shortness of breath—becomes more likely as a patient approaches death. It may result from the collection of fluid around the heart, lungs, or abdomen.

It's a frightening experience not just for the patient but also for family members and caregivers. If your patient finds it difficult to speak or eat, or if answering questions exacerbates his problem, you may need to intervene first and ask questions later.

During your physical assessment, measure the patient's respiratory rate, auscultate his lungs, monitor oxygen saturation, and assess the skin for oxygenation clues. The patient experiencing dyspnea is typically anxious, so make sure you assess him before, during, and after a dyspneic episode.

Management of dyspnea includes both pharmacologic and nonpharmacologic measures.

Drug treatment includes diuretics, opioids, anxiolytics, bronchodilators, and corticosteroids. Other treatments include positioning the patient as close to a sitting position as possible and discontinuing I.V. fluids for a time. Humidified oxygen, cooling the air in the patient's room or using a fan, and breathing techniques such as pursed-lipped breathing can also help.

Closely monitor the patient, and make sure he has a way to call for help—such as a bell or a bedside monitor—to help ease his anxiety about difficulty breathing. Family members, friends, or a caregiver may also want to remain close to the patient in case they're needed.

FATIGUE

Fatigue is a common effect of chronic illness. Descriptions vary, ranging from becoming easily tired to reacting in a more emotional way than usual. Many factors can contribute to fatigue, including medications, chemotherapy and radiation therapy, stress, depression, infection, and inadequate nutrition and hydration.

If the patient complains about fatigue, ask him about feelings of depression, causative factors, aggravating and alleviating factors, and fatigue patterns. Also assess him for signs of anemia, depression, and sedation.

Pharmacologic interventions include psychostimulants, corticosteroids, antidepressants, and blood products. To help improve fatigue, suggest balancing activity and rest, prioritizing activities, exercising regularly if possible, and participating in activities (such as playing cards or reading) that can focus attention on something other than fatigue, pain, and the underlying disease. CAM therapies include omega 3 fatty acids, meditation, and herbal preparations. Explain to the patient and his family that fatigue levels may increase as the disease progresses.

NAUSEA AND VOMITING

Unfortunately, nausea and vomiting commonly occur during end-of-life care, with 40% to 70% of advanced cancer patients reporting these symptoms. Nausea and vomiting occur more often in women, patients younger than age 65, and patients with either breast or stomach cancer.

During your assessment interview and physical examination, use the OLD CART pneumonic. Note the volume, color, consistency, and contents of emesis, determine the status of bowel movements, and consider possible interactions of prescribed medications.

The mainstay of therapy for nausea and vomiting at the end of life, antiemetic drugs include ondansetron (Zofran), metoclopramide (Reglan), transdermal scopolamine, and prochlorperazine (Compazine). Giving drugs orally before meals can help prevent nausea and vomiting; antiemetics can also be given rectally, by the transdermal route, or parenterally (I.M. or I.V.).

Nonpharmacologic interventions to control nausea and vomiting include distraction, relaxation, acupuncture, dietary changes, and celiac plexus block. Offering foods that the patient enjoys in small, frequent meals can also help increase intake. Sips of water, juice, tea, or ginger drinks with meals can help the food go down easier. CAM therapies may include peppermint and ginger, meditation, distraction, massage, and herbal preparations.

PAIN

Many dying patients need some kind of help with pain management. Pain can dramatically interfere with the patient's quality of life, affecting virtually every aspect of the patient's life. It has obvious physical effects, but it can also affect the patient's emotions, thinking, behavior, ability to interact with others, even spirituality.

When assessing the patient's pain, ask him about:
- location
- quality
- duration
- aggravating and alleviating factors
- impact on function and quality of life
- response to current and past treatment
- goals and expectations.

To assess the severity of pain, you can use the visual analog scale, which asks the patient to rate his pain intensity on a scale of 0 to 10, with 0 being no pain and 10 being the worst pain possible. Also watch the patient's gestures, posture, body movements, and facial expressions—all nonverbal indicators of pain. Assess the patient's respiratory rate, blood pressure, pulse, and skin color and condition.

Both opioid and nonopioid drugs can help control pain in dying patients. Remember to ask your patient about his pain medication preferences and past experiences. The WHO analgesic ladder provides a protocol for administering pain medications. (See *The analgesic ladder*, page 386.)

When administering morphine, keep its adverse effects in mind, including constipation, respiratory depression, itching, and urinary retention. Teach the patient and family members about the pain medications the patient is receiving, including potential adverse effects and how to contact health care providers in case of emergency. CAM therapies that can help with pain control include massage, ice or heat, and distraction.

SLEEP DISTURBANCES

Sleep disturbances in patients nearing the end of life can result from medications, diet, depression, infection, and anxiety. Evaluate these possibilities, and discuss sleep issues with the patient.

THE ANALGESIC LADDER

The World Health Organization uses an analgesic ladder to guide the treatment of pain. If the patient's pain persists or increases, move up the ladder. If it abates, you may be able to move down the ladder.

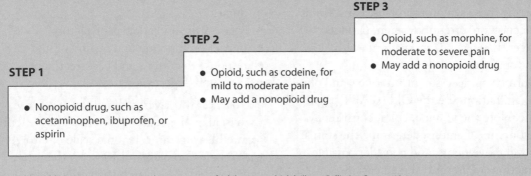

STEP 3
- Opioid, such as morphine, for moderate to severe pain
- May add a nonopioid drug

STEP 2
- Opioid, such as codeine, for mild to moderate pain
- May add a nonopioid drug

STEP 1
- Nonopioid drug, such as acetaminophen, ibuprofen, or aspirin

World Health Organization. *Integrated Management of Adolescent and Adult Illness.* Palliative Care, p. 12.

Pharmacologic treatments include benzodiazepine hypnotics, nonbenzodiazepine hypnotics, antidepressants, and pineal gland hormones. The choice of medication depends on the type of sleep problem the patient has.

Nonpharmacologic interventions include reducing noise, administering pain medications if appropriate, reducing caffeine later in the day, offering herbal tea or warm milk, improving sleep hygiene, and giving the patient a chance to express his fears and anxieties, which may be contributing to insomnia.

Psychological and psychiatric aspects

Beyond the physical effects, approaching death has profound psychological effects. Patients and family members can experience acute anxiety and depression as they cope with the reality of death. The delirium and terminal agitation that can occur shortly before death affect not only the patient but also family members, who feel increasingly helpless. Your compassionate care can help both the patient and family members coping with psychological and psychiatric aspects of care.

ANXIETY

Anxiety is the most common symptom not only of patients but also of family members, friends, and home caregivers as the patient approaches death. For the patient, anxiety may stem from the underlying disease—cardiac, endocrine, pulmonary, neurologic, and hematologic illnesses can all increase anxiety—or from nutritional deficits or adverse effects of drugs. Anxiety can also result from anger, guilt, and spiritual distress. Ask your patient about past experiences with anxiety, coping mechanisms, medications, and support systems.

Anxiety management should include the entire palliative care team. Reassure the patient that anxiety is common, and encourage him to discuss his fears to help alleviate anxiety. Medications that relieve anxiety include anxiolytics, neuroleptics, non-benzodiazepines, and antihistamines. CAM therapies that can help include imagery, massage, meditation, herbal preparations, and music.

DEPRESSION

Like anxiety, depression commonly occurs in dying patients and their family members, although the symptoms of grief that accompany the end of life may mask the depression. Symptoms from the underlying illness may also overlap with symptoms of depression.

During your assessment for depression, include questions about changes in mood, sleep patterns, diet, and fatigue. To determine if the patient is at risk for suicide, inquire about feelings of hopelessness, worthlessness, and helplessness. If he has signs and symptoms of depression, ask about suicidal thoughts.

Common medications used to treat depression include tricyclic antidepressants, selective serotonin reuptake inhibitors (SSRIs), serotonin norepinephrine reuptake inhibitors, norepinephrine dopamine reuptake inhibitors, and other antidepressants. For patients with a terminal illness, SSRIs have less of a sedative effect than other antidepressants. For severely depressed patients, psychostimulants such as methylphenidate (Ritalin) may enhance mood, increase appetite, and reduce fatigue. Psychostimulants administered with an antidepressant relieve depression more quickly. Patients with both depression and anxiety may need treatment for both conditions. CAM therapies that may alleviate some of the symptoms of depression include cognitive-behavioral, color, music, and pet therapy as well as guided imagery and aromatherapy.

DELIRIUM AND TERMINAL AGITATION

When a dying patient displays agitation, confusion, and cognitive failure—all signs and symptoms of delirium and terminal agitation—family members often feel helpless, unable to communicate with and comfort the patient. To help ease their fears, reassure them that such behavior often occurs in dying patients.

During your assessment, determine the patient's psychiatric history. Also assess medications, bowel habits, infection status, respiratory patterns, and urinary habits to see if the patient's symptoms might have another cause.

ASSESSING SOCIAL NEEDS

When assessing the social needs of a dying patient and his family, you'll need to consider several factors, including:

- access to needed equipment
- access to nutritional products
- access to prescription and over-the-counter drugs
- access to transportation
- caregiver availability
- community resources, including school and work settings
- family structure and geographic location
- finances
- legal issues
- lines of communication
- living arrangements
- medical decision making
- perceived social supports
- relationships
- sexuality and intimacy
- social and cultural networks.

Pharmacologic interventions for delirium and terminal agitation include haloperidol (Haldol), quetiapine (Seroquel), and chlorpromazine hydrochloride (Thorazine). You can also help the patient explore his concerns about death, unfinished tasks, and spirituality. Monitor the patient's safety, keep him in a familiar environment, and discuss the patient's approaching death with his family.

Social aspects

A dying patient and his family members can have a wide range of social needs, calling for a detailed social assessment. Focus on supporting the family as a unit and also on each family member in his or her unique role. A social assessment should include equipment, nutritional needs, medications, finances, relationships, and other social networks. It's often helpful to have a social worker or chaplain to help you address these needs. (See *Assessing social needs*.)

Spiritual, religious, and existential aspects

Spiritual health doesn't have a single definition; each person defines what spiritual health means to him. Studies do link regular attendance in spiritual activities to maintaining physical health and lowering the risk of death from diseases such as atherosclerosis, emphysema, cirrhosis, and suicide.

Many patients feel spiritual distress as death approaches, whether from regret over unfulfilled dreams, guilt for a misdeed, sadness for those they leave behind, or fear of dying and of death itself. Other feelings associated with spiritual distress include abandonment, anger, betrayal, despair, sorrow, remorse, and depression.

Family members may also feel spiritual distress. To help the patient and family members, listen with empathy, accept reactions of anger, and discuss their fears. If they wish, arrange for visits with a chaplain or spiritual counselor. Understand the different ways people cope with and express spiritual distress; some would rather talk about meaning in their life than speak directly about spirituality or religion.

Cultural aspects

When caring for dying patients, you'll most likely interact with people from a variety of cultures. To help these patients and their families, you'll need to offer culturally competent care and be able to work with people from several ethnicities. By providing information in a culturally sensitive manner, you'll be able to provide the best care for the patient and his family.

A cultural assessment includes language, beliefs, rituals and customs, and the role of family in cultural life. Make sure you determine the effect of the patient's culture on such issues

as diet and medication administration and understand his cultural daily practices to better plan and provide care.

The family's health care beliefs and illness philosophy can also affect care; in some cultures, for instance, discussion of illness and prognoses may be taboo. The family's role in health care decisions becomes particularly important when the course of an illness makes it difficult or impossible for the patient to make decisions. As possible, make sure the patient understands his decision-making rights and advanced directives.

Care of the imminently dying patient

As the patient approaches death, his family members are likely to grow increasingly anxious. To help them cope, teach them how to recognize the signs of impending death and reassure them that interventions are in place to make the patient as comfortable as possible. Make sure they understand that hearing is the last sense to leave a dying person and that the patient can still hear them, even if he can't communicate. Encourage them to speak to and touch their loved one, to reassure him and, if possible, to allow him to release his emotional anxieties and to die a more peaceful death.

IMPENDING DEATH

Impending death causes recognizable changes. Signs and symptoms the patient already has may grow worse. He may also report changes in appetite or his enjoyment of food, or he may begin to have trouble swallowing. It's not uncommon for the patient very near death to request a favorite dish but not be able to eat it. Family members may also ask for other means to feed the patient.

Several other changes also occur during the patient's final days. Changes in circulation may cause changes in skin temperature and the

SIGNS AND SYMPTOMS OF APPROACHING DEATH

Teaching your patient's family about the signs and symptoms of impending death can help relieve their anxiety about what to expect. Common signs and symptoms are listed here.

BODY SYSTEM	SIGNS AND SYMPTOMS
Respiratory	• Shortness of breath • Cough • Mucus production
Gastrointestinal	• Nausea and vomiting • Sore mouth • Poor appetite and weight loss • Constipation or diarrhea
Musculoskeletal	• Obvious deterioration • Weakness • Sluggishness, lethargy, lack of energy
Skin	• Irritation or dryness • Pressure areas that appear quickly • Pressure ulcers (possible) • Jaundiced, pale, or gray color • Loose skin from weight loss • Aversion to touch, including blankets
Genitourinary	• Urinary tract infections • Foul smelling, cloudy, or concentrated urine • Bladder spasms • Urine retention
Cardiac	• Edema of the limbs (possible) • Abdominal swelling (possible)
Neuropsychological	• Less engagement in family activities • Less concern with talking or hearing about family news • More focus on personal needs • Less ability to empathize with others' needs or feelings • Agitation with unclear cause, including picking at covers or clothes (possible)

appearance of what looks like bruising on the skin, which can frighten the patient and family; explain that these are expected changes. The patient's breathing may alter and may be accompanied by a gurgling sound, or "death rattle." Changing position may help, but suctioning won't decrease the sound. Incontinence may also develop, causing distress for both the patient and family members, who may feel overwhelmed and unprepared to deal with the level of care the patient needs. Cachexia, agitation, and altered senses also progress as the patient nears death.

The patient may also be aware for shorter periods of time, which the family may interpret as "giving up." As the patient becomes aware of death drawing near, he may talk about conversations with dead family members, see friends that have passed, or discuss packing a bag for a long trip; anecdotal evidence supports such occurrences in patients very near death. (See *Signs and symptoms of approaching death*.)

POSTMORTEM CARE

Once the patient has died, care differs for each situation. If the patient died at home, family caregivers may be more involved in postmortem care. Such care may offer some satisfaction for the caregivers, and making sure a strong support system is in place at this time can give family members invaluable help at a time when they're most vulnerable—help they won't soon forget.

BEREAVEMENT

During bereavement, survivors experience grief and go through mourning. The reaction to the loss of a loved one includes a mixture of feelings and observable changes in behavior. A survivor going through the grief process requires ongoing assessment and monitoring for anxiety, depression, and other emotional symptoms.

But the survivors aren't the only ones who go through bereavement. Both the patient facing death and his family can benefit from bereavement counseling, a process that maintains open communication to help the patient and family accept the patient's death. Reassure the patient and his family that grieving is an individual process without a timeframe or emotional constraints. Recognize that the patient and family members may experience the five stages of grief—denial, anger, bargaining, depression, and acceptance—or they may not experience these emotions at all, or at least not in a particular order. Help the patient and family members to be patient with themselves and to accept and experience the flow of emotions they're going through.

You can also help the patient and family through bereavement by asking the patient how he wishes to die and ensuring that his wishes are respected. A social worker can meet with the patient and family members to help them work through financial concerns, legal issues, and care and support for family members after the patient dies.

Ethical and legal aspects

As your patient faces the end of his life, he and his family face a number of legal and ethical issues—and so do you. Fortunately, several tools exist that can help you with such issues. Nursing education programs cover ethical issues in their curriculums. The ethical principles in the American Nurses Association's (ANA) *Code of Ethics for Nurses with Interpretive Statements* can also serve as a useful resource that, in the words of the ANA, can help nurses "carry out nursing responsibilities in a manner consistent with…the ethical obligations of the profession." The ANA's guidelines can help you deal with such issues as pain management, do-not-resuscitate (DNR) orders, and advanced directives. Colleen Scanlon, a palliative care nurse, has also written about the role of education and competency in end-of-life care to help nurses provide high-quality care with professional integrity to dying patients. You can learn more by reading Scanlon's *Ethical Concerns in End-of-Life Care* at http://www.aacn.nche.edu/elnec/pdf/PalliativeCareAJN5.pdf.

SOME TOOLS OF THE TRADE

Certain legal guidelines help make some ethical decision easier. For instance, advanced directives provide a way for the patient to communicate his wishes in a legal format. He may choose to outline specifics for the management of a terminal illness, allowing the family to have a clear understanding of his priorities. The patient can also choose to have a DNR order in place, refusing life-sustaining treatment if his heart and lungs stop functioning. A patient can also have some control over what happens to his body after he dies, choosing to donate his organs to help others or his body for scientific study. Your facility should have protocols in place for these issues.

A HOST OF ISSUES

Other ethical and legal issues include whether the patient can continue his day-to-day responsibilities (such as bill paying) and who should take over these responsibilities when the patient can't handle them, whether and how to tell friends or acquaintances about the patient's illness, funeral arrangements, how to distribute personal and sentimental items, and which treatments to choose or refuse. When dealing with such issues, patients and families in nontraditional situations—such as unmarried couples and same-sex couples—may face extra challenges. Such families will need your unbiased support to help them handle legal and ethical situations.

MAKING THE BEST DAY-TO-DAY CHOICES

Despite legal guidelines, you're likely to face some difficult ethical and legal situations in your day-to-day care. If the patient can make decisions, of course his wishes should guide his care as well as how involved his family is in his care. However, if the patient can't make and communicate decisions, you'll need to rely on advance directives; the patient's previously expressed wishes, values, and preferences; and appropriate surrogate decision makers. When possible, urge patients and families to finalize their advance directives, wills, guardianship agreements, and other legal documents before the patient becomes unable to express his wishes. (See *Advantages of advance directives*.)

ADVANTAGES OF ADVANCE DIRECTIVES

Advance directives offer several advantages, including:

- peace of mind for the patient that his wishes will be carried out even if he can't communicate
- clear directions for the family and significant others about the patient's wishes
- clear directions for health care providers about the patient's wishes
- prevention of family arguments and increased stress at an emotionally difficult time.

As legal and ethical concerns arise, keep in mind the principles of compassion, self-determination, confidentiality, and informed consent. Always keep patient and family care consistent with the nurse's professional codes of ethics, and include the hospice or palliative care team in such ethical issues as withholding nutrition and hydration, adopting DNR orders, and giving sedatives.

A Final Gift

Whenever you provide end-of-life care, you're caring for patients as they face their own mortality. You're with patients and families at one of the most vulnerable times in their lives. Caring for and supporting them through such a time—offering them your best nursing skills, your respect, and your compassion—can be one of the greatest gifts you'll ever offer.

Selected resources

The following list of national organizations can provide more information on aging and age-related health problems. Consult your telephone directory for state and local agencies.

Government agencies

Administration on Aging
One Massachusetts Ave. NW
Washington, DC 20201
Tel: 202-619-0724 or 800-677-1116
Fax: 202-357-3555
http://www.aoa.gov

National Association of Area Agencies
    on Aging (n4a)
1730 Rhode Island Ave. NW
Suite 1200
Washington, DC 20036
Tel: 202-872-0888
Fax: 202-872-0057
http://www.n4a.org

National Council on Aging
1901 L St NW
4th Floor
Washington, DC 20036
Tel: 202-479-1200
http://www.ncoa.org

National Institute on Aging
Building 31, Room 5C27
31 Center Dr., MSC 2292
Bethesda, MD 20892
Tel: 301-496-1752

TTY: 800-222-4225
Fax: 301-496-1072
http://www.nia.nih.gov

Health organizations

American Association for Geriatric Psychiatry
7910 Woodmont Ave
Suite 1050
Bethesda, MD 20814
Tel: 301-654-7850
Fax: 301-654-4137
http://www.aagpgpa.org

American Geriatrics Society
Empire State Building
350 Fifth Ave.
Suite 801
New York, N.Y. 10118
Tel: 212-308-1414
Fax: 212-832-8646
http://www.americangeriatrics.org

American Health Care Association
1201 L St. N.W.
Washington, DC 20005
Tel: 202-842-4444
Fax: 202-842-3860
http://www.ahcancal.org

(continued)

Selected resources *(continued)*

American Nurses Association
8515 Georgia Ave.
Suite 400
Silver Spring, MD 20910
Tel: 301-628-5000 or 800-274-4ANA
   (274-4262)
Fax: 301-628-5001
http://www.nursingworld.org

American Society of Geriatric Dentistry
(Special Care Dentistry)
401 N. Michigan Ave.
Suite 2200
Chicago, IL 60611
Tel: 312-527-6764
Fax: 312-673-6663
http://www.ada.org/ada/organizations/orgdetail.
   asp?OrganizationID=881

Gerontological Society of America
1220 L St. NW
Suite 901
Washington, DC 20005
Tel: 202-842-1275
Fax: 202-842-1150
http://www.geron.org

Health Resources and Services Administration
P.O. Box 2910
Merrifield, VA 22118
Tel: 888-ASK-HRSA (275-4772)
TTY/TTD: 1-877-4TY-HRSA (489-4772)
Fax: 1-703-821-2098
http://www.hrsa.gov

National Association for Home Care
   and Hospice
228 Seventh Street SE
Washington, DC 20003
Tel: 202-547-7424
Fax: 202-547-3540
http://www.nahc.org

National Gerontological Nursing Association
7794 Grow Dr.
Pensacola, FL 32514
Tel: 850-473-1174 or 800-723-0560
Fax: 850-484-8762
http://www.ngna.org

Social welfare organizations

American Association of Retired Persons
601 E St. NW
Washington, DC 20049
Tel: 888-OUR-AARP (687-2277)
TTY: 877-434-7598
http://www.aarp.org

American Bar Association
Commission on Legal Problems of the Elderly
321 N. Clark St.
Chicago, IL 60654
Tel: 800-285-2221
http://www.abanet.org/aging

Children of Aging Parents
P.O. Box 167
Richboro, PA 18954
Tel: 800-227-7294
http://www.caps4caregivers.org

Institute for Retired Professionals
The New School
66 West 12th Street, Room 502
New York, NY 10011
Tel: 212-229-5682
http://www.newschool.edu/irp

National Adult Day Services Association
85 S. Washington
Suite 316
Seattle WA 98104
Tel: 877-745-1440
Fax: 206-461-3218
http://www.nadsa.org

National Caucus and Center on Black Aged
1220 L St. NW
Suite 800
Washington, DC 20005
Tel: 202-637-8400
Fax: 202-347-0895
http://www.ncba-aged.org

National Gray Panthers
1612 K St. NW
Suite 300
Washington, DC 20006
Tel: 202-737-6637 or 800-280-5362
Fax: 202-737-1160
http://www.graypanthers.org

National Senior Citizens Law Center
1444 Eye St. NW
Suite 1100
Washington, DC 20005
Tel: 202-289-6976
Fax: 202-289-7224
http://www.nsclc.org

Older Women's League
1828 L St. NW
Suite 801
Washington, DC 20036
Tel: 800-825-3695
Fax: 202-332-2949
http://www.owl-national.org

Specialized organizations
ALCOHOLISM
Alcoholics Anonymous
475 Riverside Drive at West 120th St.
11th Floor
New York, NY 10115
Tel: 212- 870-3400
http://www.aa.org

Al-Anon/Alateen
1600 Corporate Landing Pkwy.
Virginia Beach, VA 23454
Tel: 757-563-1600 or 888-4AL-ANON
  (425-2666)
Fax: 75-563-1655
http://www.al-anon.alateen.org

ALZHEIMER'S DISEASE
Alzheimer's Disease Education and Referral
  Center
P.O. Box 8250
Silver Spring, MD 20907
Tel: 800-438-4380
Fax: 301-495-3334
http://www.nia.nih.gov/alzheimers

Alzheimer's Foundation of America
322 8th Ave.
7th Floor
New York, NY 10001
Tel: 866-AFA-8484 (232-8484)
Fax: 646-638-1546
http://www.alzfdn.org

ARTHRITIS
Arthritis Foundation
P.O. Box 7669
Atlanta, GA 30357
Tel: 800-283-7800
http://www.arthritis.org

CANCER
American Cancer Society
Tel: 800-ACS-2345 (227-2345)
TTY: 866-228-4327
http://www.cancer.org

National Cancer Institute
NCI Public Inquiries Office
6116 Executive Blvd.
Room 3036A

(continued)

Selected resources *(continued)*

Bethesda, MD 20892
Tel: 800-4-CANCER (422-6237)
http://www.cancer.gov

HEARING DISORDERS

Alexander Graham Bell Association for the
    Deaf and Hard of Hearing
3417 Volta Pl. NW
Washington, DC 20007
Tel: 202-337-5220
TTY: 202-337-5221
Fax: 202-337-8314
http://www.agbell.org

International Hearing Society
16880 Middlebelt Rd.
Suite 4
Livonia, MI 48154
Tel: 734-522-7200
Fax: 734-522-0200
http://www.ihsinfo.org

National Association of the Deaf
8630 Fenton St. Suite 820
Silver Spring, MD 20910-3819
TTY: 301-587-1789
Voice: 301-587-1788
Fax: 301-587-1791
http://www.nad.org

HEART DISEASE

American Heart Association
7272 Greenville Ave.
Dallas, TX 75231
Tel: 800-AHA-USA-1 (242-8721)
http://www.americanheart.org

KIDNEY DISORDERS

National Kidney Foundation
30 East 33rd St.
New York, NY 10016

Tel: 212-889-2210 or 800-622-9010
Fax: 212-689-9261
http://www.kidney.org

MENTAL HEALTH DISORDERS

National Association of Psychiatric Health
    Systems
900 17th St. NW
Suite 420
Washington, DC 20006
Tel: 202-393-6700
Fax: 202-783-6041
http://www.naphs.org

NUTRITIONAL ISSUES

American Dietetic Association
120 South Riverside Plaza
Suite 2000
Chicago, Illinois 60606
Tel: 800-877-1600
http://www.eatright.org

American Society for Parenteral and Enteral
    Nutrition
8630 Fenton St.
Suite 412
Silver Spring, MD 20910
Tel: 301-587-6315
Fax 301-587-2365
http://www.nutritioncare.org

Meals on Wheels Association of America
203 S. Union St.
Alexandria, Virginia 22314
Tel: 703-548-5558
Fax: 703-548-8024
http://www.mowaa.org

National Association of Nutrition and Aging
    Services Programs
1612 K St. NW
Suite 400
Washington, DC 20006

Tel: 202-682-6899
Fax: 202-223-2099
http://www.nanasp.org

PARKINSON'S DISEASE

American Parkinson Disease Association
135 Parkinson Ave.
Staten Island, NY 10305
Tel: 718-981-8001 or 800-223-2732
Fax: 1-718-981-4399
http://www.apdaparkinson.org

National Parkinson Foundation, Inc.
1501 NW 9th Ave. / Bob Hope Road
Miami, FL 33136
Tel: 305-243-6666 or 800-327-4545
Fax: 305-243-6073
http://www.parkinson.org

RESPIRATORY DISORDERS

American Lung Association
1301 Pennsylvania Ave. NW
Washington, DC 20004
Tel: 202-785-3355
Fax: 202-452-1805
http://www.lungusa.org

SPEECH DISORDERS

American Speech-Language-Hearing
  Association
2200 Research Blvd.
Rockville, MD 20850
Tel: 301-296-5700
http://www.asha.org

STROKE

American Stroke Association
National Center
7272 Greenville Avenue
Dallas TX 75231
Tel: 888-4-STROKE (478-7653)
http://www.strokeassociation.org

VISION DISORDERS

American Council of the Blind
2200 Wilson Blvd.
Suite 650
Arlington, VA 22201
Tel: 202-467-5081 or 800-424-8666
Fax: 703-465-5085
http://www.acb.org

American Foundation for the Blind
2 Penn Plaza
Suite 1102
New York, NY 10121
Tel: 212-502-7600
Fax: 212-502-7777
http://www.afb.org

American Printing House for the Blind
1839 Frankfort Ave.
P.O. Box 6085
Louisville, KY 40206
Tel: 502-895-2405 or 800-223-1839
Fax: 502-899-2274
http://www.aph.org

Blinded Veterans Association
477 H St. NW
Washington, DC 20001
Tel: 202-371-8880 or 800-669-7079
Fax: 202-371-8258
http://www.bva.org

Prevent Blindness America
211 West Wacker Dr.
Suite 1700
Chicago, IL 60606
Tel: 800-331-2020
http://www.preventblindness.org

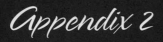

Patient-teaching aids for the older adult

Using and caring for your hearing aid

Dear Patient:

Adjusting to your hearing aid takes patience, practice, and hours of wear. Several weeks or even several months may pass before you feel completely comfortable. But don't be discouraged. Once you learn how, inserting, removing, and caring for your hearing aid will become just another daily routine, like brushing your teeth. You'll be glad that you made the effort when you notice how much your hearing improves.

These guidelines will help you learn to use and care for your hearing aid as well as ease the period of adjustment.

Inserting your hearing aid

First, wash your hands. Make sure the hearing aid is turned off and the volume is turned all the way down.

Next, examine the earmold to determine whether it's for the right or left ear. Look in the mirror and line up the parts of the earmold with the corresponding parts of your external ear. Then rotate the earmold slightly forward, and insert the canal portion.

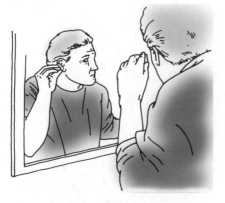

Gently push the earmold into the ear while rotating it backward. Adjust the folds of your ear over the earmold, if necessary. The earmold should fit snugly and comfortably.

After inserting the earmold, adjust other parts of the hearing aid as needed. For example, place a behind-the-ear hearing aid over your ear and clip a body aid to your shirt pocket, undergarment, or hearing aid harness carrier.

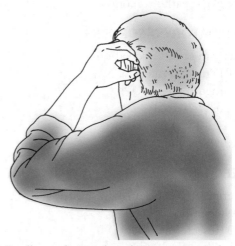

Finally, set the switch to the on position and slowly turn the volume halfway up. Adjust the volume as necessary.

Removing your hearing aid

First, set the switch to the off position and lower the volume. Then, looking in the mirror, remove the earmold by rotating it forward and pulling outward. Next, remove or unclip the hearing-aid case. After removal, store the hearing aid in a safe place. If possible, use the same place each time.

(continued)

Using and caring for your hearing aid (*continued*)

Adjusting to your hearing aid

To help ease your period of adjustment, follow these guidelines:

- Wear your hearing aid only for short periods at first. For example, wear it for 15 minutes the first 2 days; then increase your time 30 minutes each day until you feel completely comfortable. If you get nervous or tired, turn off the aid and rest for awhile.

- When you're comfortable wearing the aid, wear it as much as possible.

- Don't turn up the volume too high. This distorts sound and may also cause feedback, a whistling or squealing noise. (These sounds may also signal a loose-fitting earmold.)

- Try to block out background sounds when listening to conversations. This takes practice. If the background noise gets too annoying, turn down the volume on your hearing aid and watch the speaker's face closely.

- Talk to only one person at a time until you get used to the hearing aid. Experiment to see if you can hold a conversation in difficult situations — for example, with loud music in the background.

- When you're in a large group, sit as close to the speaker as possible.

Cleaning the earmold

- Keep the earmold of your hearing aid clean and free from excess wax to prevent infection and keep the aid working efficiently:

- To clean a body aid, first detach the earmold from the receiver. For a behind-the-ear or eyeglass aid, first detach the earmold where its tubing meets the hook of the hearing-aid case, if possible. Don't remove the earmold if glue or a small metal split ring secures the earmold tubing to the hearing aid case.

- After detaching the earmold, soak it in a mild soapy solution; then rinse and dry it well.

- Blow out excess moisture through the earmold opening.

- If the opening is clogged with wax or debris, use a pipe cleaner or toothpick to remove it, but avoid pushing debris into the opening.

- Store the dry, clean earmold in the hearing aid case.

- If you wear an in-the-ear aid with an unremovable earmold, wipe the earmold with a damp cloth.

Maintaining your hearing aid

- Your hearing aid is a delicate electronic instrument, so avoid wearing it outside for long periods in hot, humid, or cold weather.

- Never store it near a stove, heater, or on a sunny windowsill.

- Don't wear it in the rain, in the bathtub or shower, during activities that cause excessive perspiration, when using a blow-dryer or hairspray, or when using a vaporizer.

- Never clean or immerse any part except the earmold in water. Don't insert sharp objects into the microphone or receiver opening — only an audiologist or hearing aid dealer should clean these parts.

- Take care not to drop your hearing aid on a hard surface. Work over a bed or similar soft area when changing batteries or removing the aid from your ear.

- Replace dead batteries with new ones of the same type. When inserting a battery, turn off the hearing aid and then match the negative (−) and positive (+) signs. If you use your hearing aid 10 to 12 hours per day, you'll probably need to replace the battery weekly.

(continued)

Using and caring for your hearing aid (*continued*)

- If you won't be using the hearing aid for several days, remove the battery to prevent it from leaking and causing corrosion. Leave the battery case open, storing your hearing aid in an airtight container with a silica-gel packet, especially in humid climates.
- To clean the battery, gently rub it with a pencil eraser to remove corrosion. If the battery gets damp, dry the contacts with a cotton swab. Store extra batteries in the freezer to lengthen shelf life.

When you have problems

- If you have pain or drainage in your ear — a sign of a skin or cartilage infection, a middle-ear infection, a tumor, or an improperly fitted earmold — call your doctor.
- If you have any questions about wearing, caring for, or maintaining your hearing aid, call your doctor or audiologist.
- If the hearing aid fails to operate, review the instructions in the operator's manual or consult the checklist below.

PROBLEM AND POSSIBLE CAUSE	POSSIBLE SOLUTIONS
No sound or weak sound	
• Incorrect battery insertion	• Reinsert battery.
• Dead battery	• Try a new battery.
• Clogged earmold opening	• Unclog the earmold opening.
• Twisted plastic tubing	• Untwist the plastic tubing.
• Switch is off or on "T" for use with telephone	• Switch to on position.
• Volume not turned high enough	• Turn volume control at least one-half rotation.
Whistling or squealing sound	
• Incorrect earmold insertion	• Reinsert earmold.
• Volume turned too high	• Turn down volume.
• Earmold not securely snapped to a receiver of a body hearing aid (a whistling sound is normal when the earmold isn't inserted and the hearing aid is turned on; such whistling indicates that the aid is working and that the battery is inserted correctly)	• Secure earmold to receiver.

Planning home care for the patient with Alzheimer's disease

Dear Caregiver:

Taking care of a person with Alzheimer's disease requires a great deal of patience and understanding. It also requires you to look at the person's typical daily routine and his environment with new eyes and make necessary changes to help him function at the highest possible level. The following tips can help you plan your daily care.

Reduce stress

Too much stress can worsen the patient's symptoms. Try to protect him from the following potential sources of stress:

- change in routine, caregiver, or environment
- fatigue
- excessive demands
- overwhelming, misleading, or competing
- stimuli
- illness and pain
- over-the-counter (nonprescription) medications.

Establish a routine

Keep the patient's daily routine stable so he can respond automatically. Adapting to change may require more thought than he can handle. Even eating a different food or going to a strange grocery store may overwhelm him.

Ask yourself: What are the patient's daily activities? Then make a schedule:

- List the activities necessary for his daily care and include ones that he especially enjoys such as weeding in the garden. Designate a time frame for each activity.
- Establish bedtime rituals — especially important to promote relaxation and a restful night's sleep for both of you.

- Stick to your schedule as closely as possible (for example, breakfast first, then dressing) so the patient won't be surprised or need to make decisions.

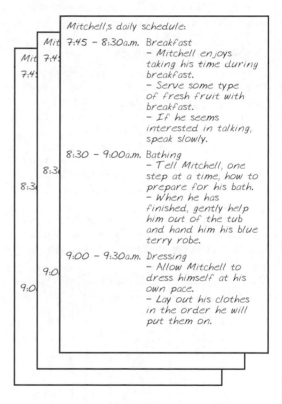

Mitchell's daily schedule:
7:45 – 8:30 a.m. Breakfast
– Mitchell enjoys taking his time during breakfast.
– Serve some type of fresh fruit with breakfast.
– If he seems interested in talking, speak slowly.

8:30 – 9:00 a.m. Bathing
– Tell Mitchell, one step at a time, how to prepare for his bath.
– When he has finished, gently help him out of the tub and hand him his blue terry robe.

9:00 – 9:30 a.m. Dressing
– Allow Mitchell to dress himself at his own pace.
– Lay out his clothes in the order he will put them on.

- Keep a copy of the patient's schedule to give to other caregivers. To help them give better care, include notes and suggestions about techniques that work for you; for instance, "Speak in a quiet voice" or "When helping Mitchell dress or take a bath, take things one step at a time and wait for him to respond."

(continued)

Planning home care for the patient with Alzheimer's disease (*continued*)

Practice validation therapy

In your conversations with the patient, use validation therapy. Don't argue with the patient — rather, acknowledge his feelings. Correcting and orienting the patient may increase agitation. For example, if the patient mistakenly says, "It's my birthday," don't correct him if he's wrong. Instead, use a statement such as, "Yes, aren't birthdays fun?"

Simplify the surroundings

The patient will eventually lose the ability to interpret correctly what he sees and hears. Protect him by trying to decrease the noise level in his environment and by avoiding busy areas, such as shopping malls and restaurants.

Does the patient mistake pictures or images in the mirror for real people? If so, remove the photos and mirrors. Also avoid rooms with busy patterns on the wallpaper and carpets because they can overstimulate his senses.

To avoid confusion and encourage the patient's independence, provide cues. For example, hang a picture of a toilet on the bathroom door.

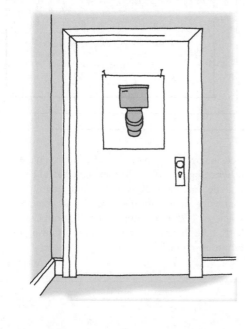

Avoid fatigue

The patient will tire easily, so plan important activities for the morning when he's functioning best. Save less demanding ones for later in the day. Remember to schedule breaks — such as one in the morning and one in the afternoon.

About 15 to 30 minutes of listening to music or just relaxing is sufficient in the early stages of Alzheimer's disease. As the disease progresses, schedule longer, more frequent breaks (perhaps 40 to 90 minutes). If the patient naps during the day, have him sleep in a reclining chair rather than in a bed to prevent him from confusing day and night.

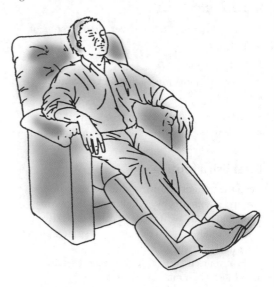

Don't expect too much

Accept the patient's limitations. Don't demand too much from him — this forces him to think about a task and causes frustration. Instead, offer help when needed, and distract him if he's trying too hard. You'll feel less stressed, too.

(continued)

Planning home care for the patient with Alzheimer's disease (*continued*)

Prepare for illness

If the patient becomes ill, expect his behavior to deteriorate and plan accordingly. He'll have a low tolerance for pain and discomfort.

Never rely on the patient to take his own medicine. He may forget to take it or miscount what he has taken. Always supervise him.

Use the sense of touch

Because the patient's visual and auditory perceptions are distorted, he has an increased need for closeness and touching. Remember to approach the patient from the front. You don't want to frighten him or provoke him into becoming belligerent or aggressive.

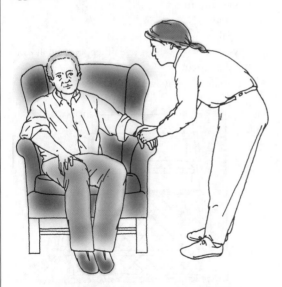

Respect the patient's need for personal space. Limit physical contact to his hands and arms at first; then move to more central parts of his body, such as his shoulders or head.

Using long or circular motions, lightly stroke the patient to help relieve muscle tension and give him a sense of his physical self. Physical contact also expresses your feelings of intimacy and caring.

Allowing the patient to touch objects in the environment can help relieve stress by providing information. Let him handle, poke, pull, or shake objects — for example, a handbag, a brush, or a comb. Make sure they're unbreakable and can't harm him.

Analyze problem behavior

Recognize that agitation may be the patient's only way of expressing himself, whether his needs are emotional or physical. Try to determine and meet the patient's needs.

Although restless and agitated behavior can be taxing for you, try to remember that the patient can't help himself. Your understanding and compassion can increase his sense of security.

Promoting patient safety

Dear Caregiver:

A person with Alzheimer's disease requires intensive physical care as well as almost constant supervision to keep him from hurting himself. This means removing potential safety hazards from his environment and installing assistive devices where needed.

You can purchase many of these devices from large pharmacies or medical supply stores. You can also use childproofing devices, such as safety caps for electrical outlets, soft plastic corners for furniture, and doorknob covers. They're available from catalogs and where baby products are sold.

Use the following guidelines to help you provide a safe environment for the person in your care.

Remove potential safety hazards

- Move knives, forks, scissors, and other sharp objects beyond the patient's reach.
- Remove the knobs from the stove and other potentially hazardous kitchen appliances. Put dangerous small appliances, such as food processors and irons, out of reach.
- Taste the patient's food before serving it so he won't burn his mouth or skin if he accidentally spills it.
- Serve the patient's food on unbreakable dishes.
- Adjust your water heater to a lower temperature (no higher than 120° F [48.8° C]) to prevent accidental burns.
- Cover unused electrical outlets, especially those above waist level, with masking tape or safety caps.
- Remove mirrors or install ones with safety glass in rooms the patient uses.

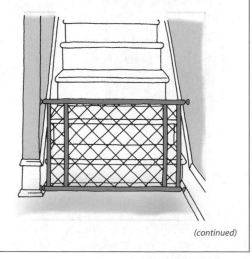

- Remove all breakable wall hangings and pictures, and attach curtains to the wall with Velcro.
- Get rid of throw rugs, and cover slippery floors with large area rugs. Place pads under the rugs, and secure them so they don't slide.
- Keep traffic patterns open by moving unsafe furniture to the walls.
- Keep floors and stairways clear of toys, shoes, and other objects that can trip the patient.
- Barricade stairways with high gates.

(continued)

Promoting patient safety (*continued*)

- Lock doors or camouflage them with murals or posters so they don't look like exits. Install locks at the bases of doors as an extra security measure, or install childproofing devices over the knobs.
- Store all medications out of the patient's reach, preferably in a locked container.
- Use child-resistant safety lids.
- Remove or lock up any guns or weapons.
- Place matches out of reach, and monitor the patient if he smokes.

Install assistive devices

- Pad sharp furniture corners with masking tape or plastic corners.
- Provide a low bed for the patient.
- Keep the house well illuminated during waking hours. Keep a night-light in the bathroom.
- If the patient uses the stairs, mark the edges with strips of yellow or orange tape to compensate for poor depth perception.
- Encourage the patient to use the bathroom by making a "path" of colored tape leading in that direction.
- Attach safety rails in the bathtub, near the toilet, and on stairways.

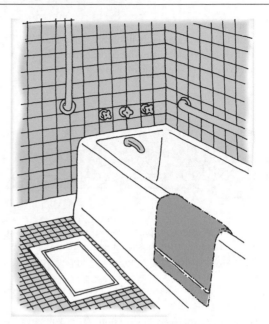

- Glue nonskid strips in the bathtub and by the toilet.
- Provide a medical identification bracelet for the patient, listing his name, address, phone number, and medical problems.

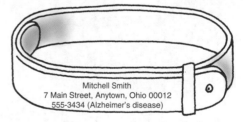

Mitchell Smith
7 Main Street, Anytown, Ohio 00012
555-3434 (Alzheimer's disease)

- Give the local police a photograph and description of the patient in case he's found wandering in the streets.

Coping with falls

Dear Patient:
If you fall, don't panic. Roll onto your stomach, turning your head in the direction of the roll. If you feel sharp pain, don't move. Call for help.

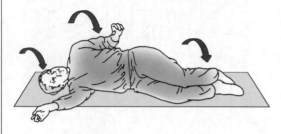

If you're free from pain, crawl to the nearest chair or sofa. Place both hands on the seat, bending slightly forward so that your hands support your weight.

Next, bend one knee and place your foot flat on the floor. Then push yourself up with your hands while swiveling to sit in the chair. After you have rested a few minutes, call a family member or your physician for help.

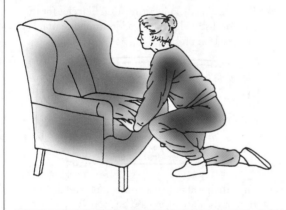

Preventing a fall

Take special care to avoid falls. Some falls result from dizziness, poor coordination, or muscle weakness. However, most result from poor safety practices at home. Follow the guidelines below to reduce your risk of falls.

Provide good lighting

- Place light switches or lamps near the entrance to each room, at the top and bottom of all stairways, and next to your bed.
- Replace low-wattage light bulbs with 75- or 100-watt bulbs.
- Use night-lights in your bedroom and bathroom.
- Outline the edges of steps with brightly colored paint or tape so they'll be easier to see.

Adapt your home

- Remove clutter, especially in hallways and on stairs. Arrange furniture to provide clear pathways, and secure electrical cords.
- Install handrails on both sides of all stairways as well as near the tub and toilet.
- Place frequently used clothing and other items where you can reach them easily. Avoid climbing on stepladders or chairs for items out of your reach.

Preventing pressure ulcers

Dear Patient:

Sitting or lying for too long in one position can damage your skin, causing pressure ulcers. These ulcers develop around areas of skin pressure such as your buttocks if you're sitting in a wheelchair. But with good skin care and frequent position changes, you can keep your skin healthy. Here are some guidelines.

Do's

- Change your position every 2 hours while awake if you're recuperating in bed. Try to follow a schedule. For example, lie on your right side, then your left side, then your back, then your stomach (if possible). Support yourself with pillows and pads.

- Shift your position every 15 minutes if you use a wheelchair. Sit on a firm seat covered by a wheelchair cushion. Avoid sling-style seats, or use a board to distribute your weight evenly.

- Check your skin for signs of pressure ulcers twice per day. Use a hand mirror, or ask your caregiver to check areas prone to these ulcers, such as your shoulders, tailbone, hips, elbows, heels, and the back of your head. Call your physician if you notice any breaks in your skin or unusual changes in your skin temperature.

- Wear cotton clothing next to your skin to absorb moisture, or wear silk to reduce friction.

- Bathe daily or as necessary in warm weather. Before you get into the tub, make sure the water is tepid, not hot. (If you can't sense the temperature, have your caregiver check it with a bath thermometer.)

- Use a footstool to keep your legs elevated, if appropriate. Also, wear antiembolism stockings to reduce swelling and prevent blood clots from forming in your legs.

- Follow your prescribed exercise program. Try to do range-of-motion exercises every 8 hours or as often as recommended.

- Keep your nails clean and short, and cut them straight across. Check your feet for ingrown toenails.

- Eat a well-balanced diet, drink lots of fluids, and try to maintain your ideal weight.

- Apply a sunblock before going outdoors.

Don'ts

- Avoid using commercial soaps or skin products that dry or irritate your skin. Instead, use oil-free lotions.

- Don't sleep on wrinkled bed sheets or tuck your covers tightly into the foot of your bed.

- Avoid exposing your skin to extreme conditions, such as hot summer sun or wintry cold.

- Avoid using heating pads, electric blankets, or other electrical devices in bed.

- Avoid wearing tight clothing or shoes or applying tight dressings or adhesive tape to your skin.

- If you smoke, don't smoke in bed. Try to stop smoking. If you can't, keep lit cigarettes away from your body.

Additional instructions:

_____

_____

_____

_____

_____

Appendix 3

How aging can affect laboratory values

This chart shows common serum and urine laboratory test values for adults, how these values change with age, and what such changes may indicate.

NORMAL VALUES (AGES 20 TO 40)	AGE-RELATED CHANGES	INDICATIONS OF CHANGES
Serum		
Albumin 3.5 to 5 g/dl	• Age 65 and older: Men and women have equal values • Values decrease at same rate after age 65 in both sexes	• Decreased values with normal liver function may indicate need for increased dietary protein intake. • Edema may signal low albumin values.
Alkaline phosphatase 30 to 85 IU/L	Values increase 8 to 10 IU/L	Increased values may reflect liver function decline or vitamin D malabsorption and bone demineralization.
Beta globulin 0.7 to 1.1 g/dl	Values increase slightly	Increased values with normal liver function (a response to decreased albumin values) indicate the need for increased dietary protein intake.
Blood urea nitrogen • Men: 10 to 25 mg/dl • Women: 8 to 20 mg/dl	Values increase, possibly to as high as 69 mg/dl (SI, 25.8 mmol/L)	In absence of such stressors as infection or surgery, slightly increased values are acceptable.
Creatine kinase 55 to 170 U/L	Values increase slightly	Increased values may reflect decreasing muscle mass and liver function.
Creatinine 0.6 to 1.3 mg/dl	Values increase, possibly to as high as 1.9 mg/L (SI, 168 μmol/L) in men	Creatinine values require close monitoring to help prevent toxicity from drugs excreted in urine.
Creatinine clearance • Men: 94 to 140 ml/min/ 1.73 m² • Women: 72 to 110 ml/min/ 1.73 m²	• Men: Rate decreases, based on the following formula: $$\frac{(140 - age) \times kg\ body\ weight}{72 \times serum\ creatine}$$ • Women: 85% of men's rate	• Decrease values reflect reduced glomerular filtration rate. • Creatinine clearance rates require close monitoring to help prevent toxicity from drugs excreted in urine.

NORMAL VALUES (AGES 20 TO 40)	AGE-RELATED CHANGES	INDICATIONS OF CHANGES
Hematocrit ● Men: 45% to 52% ● Women: 37% to 48%	Values may decrease slightly (unproven)	Decreased values reflect decreased bone marrow and hematopoiesis and increased risk for infection (because of fewer, weaker lymphocytes and immune system changes that diminish antigen-antibody response).
Hemoglobin ● Men: 14 to 18 g/dl ● Women: 12 to 16 g/dl	● Values in men decrease by 1 to 2 g/dl ● Change in values in women unknown	Decreased values reflect decreased bone marrow, hematopoiesis, and (for men) androgen levels.
Lactate dehydrogenase 71 to 207 U/L	Values increase slightly	Increased values may reflect declining muscle mass and liver function.
Leukocyte count 4,000 to 10,000/µl	Values decrease to 3,100 to 9,000/µl (SI, 3.1 to 9 × 10⁹/L)	Values decrease proportionally to lymphocyte count.
Lymphocyte count 25% to 40%	Values decrease	Values decrease proportionally to leukocyte count.
Platelet count 140,000 to 400,000/µl	Characteristics change, with decreased granular constituents and increased platelet-release factors	Changes may reflect diminished bone marrow and increased fibrinogen levels.
Potassium 3.5 to 5.5 mEq/L	Values increase slightly	Increased levels require patient to avoid salt substitutes made of potassium, carefully read food labels for potassium, and know signs and symptoms of hyperkalemia.
Thyroid-stimulating hormone 0 to 15 µIU/ml	Values increase slightly	Greatly increased values suggest primary hypothyroidism or endemic goiter.
Thyroxine 5 to 13.5 mcg/dl	Values decrease about 25%	Decreased values reflect declining thyroid function.
Triglycerides ● Men: 44 to 180 mg/dl ● Women: 10 to 190 mg/dl	Values increase slightly	More than a slight increase suggests possible abnormalities, requiring further tests such as serum cholesterol levels.
Triiodothyronine 80 to 220 ng/dl	Values decreases about 25%	Decreased values reflect declining thyroid function.
Urine		
Glucose 0 to 15 mg/dl	Values decrease slightly	● Decreased values may reflect renal disease or urinary tract infection (UTI). ● Abnormal values not a reliable check for diabetics because glucosuria may not occur until plasma glucose level exceeds 300 mg/dl.
Protein 50 to 80 mg/24 hours	Values increase slightly	Increased values may reflect renal disease or UTI.
Specific gravity 1.032	Values decrease to 1.024 (SI, 1.024) by age 80	Decreased values reflect 30% to 50% decrease in number of nephrons available to concentrate urine.

Appendix 4

Credits

Chapter 1

Katherine Hepburn, page 2, from scene in "Stage Door Canteen," 1943.

President Bill Clinton, page 3. Official White House photo by Bob McNeely taken on January 1, 1993.

Jonas Salk, page 3, at the University of Pittsburgh, where he developed the first polio vaccine. Previously published in 1957 University of Pittsburgh *The Owl* yearbook.

Chapter 2

George Herman "Babe" Ruth, Jr., page 22, played major league baseball from 1914 to 1935.

Robert Cheruiyot, page 23, as he passes through Wellesley Square during the 2006 Boston Marathon on April 17, 2006. Photo by George Roberts.

Chapter 3

Albert Einstein, page 44. Photo by Jack Turner, Princeton, NJ, originally copyrighted in 1947 and available from the Library of Congress.

Ronald Reagan, page 45, waving from limousine during the Inaugural Parade in Washington, D.C., on Inauguration Day, January 20, 1981.

Cherry angiomas, page 65, from Weber, J., and Kelley, J. *Health Assessment in Nursing,* 4th ed. Philadelphia: Lippincott Williams & Wilkins, 2009.

Seborrheic keratosis, senile or actinic purpura, solar lentigines, spider angioma, and venous lake, page 65, from Goodheart, H.P. *Goodheart's Photoguide to Common Skin Disorders,* 3rd ed. Philadelphia: Lippincott Williams & Wilkins, 2008.

Sublingual varicosities, page 67, from Neville, B., et al. *Color Atlas of Clinical Oral Pathology.* Philadelphia: Lea & Febiger, 1991.

Ectropion and entropion, page 68, from *Atlas of Pathophysiology,* 3rd ed. Philadelphia: Lippincott Williams & Wilkins, 2009.

Ptosis, page 68, from *Assessment Made Incredibly Easy,* 4th ed. Philadelphia: Lippincott Williams & Wilkins, 2008.

Arcus senilis, page 69, from Tasman, W., and Jaeger, E. *The Wills Eye Hospital Atlas of Clinical Ophthalmology,* 2nd ed. Philadelphia: Lippincott Williams & Wilkins, 2001.

Chapter 6

Neil Armstrong working on lunar module, page 141. Photo by NASA.

Chapter 7

Elvis Presley, page 311, from scene in "Jailhouse Rock," 1957.

Stonewall Inn in Greenwich Village, New York, page 311. Site of violent demonstrations in 1969 that launched gay rights movement in the United States and around the world. Photo by Diana Davies.

Chapter 8

President Jimmy Carter, page 337. Official White House photo taken on January 31, 1977.

Chapter 9

Prohibition agents destroying barrels of alcohol in 1921, page 360. From Chicago Daily News negatives collection, Chicago Historical Society.

Suffragette handing out newspapers, page 360. Circa 1919.

Supreme Court building, page 361. Photo taken June 2008.

Chapter 10

Demonstration at the Red Cross Emergency Ambulance Station in Washington, D.C., during the influenza pandemic of 1918, page 376. National Photo Company and made available from the Library of Congress.

"Tomb of the Unknowns" at Arlington National Cemetery, Washington, D.C., page 376. U.S. Navy photo by Chief Warrant Officer Seth Rossman.

Trinity Church Cemetery, New York, page 377. Photo taken April 2005.

Selected references

Boling, P. *The Past, Present, and Future of Home Health Care, an Issue of Clinics in Geriatric Medicine*. Philadelphia: W.B. Saunders, 2009.

Bradway, C., and Hirschman, K.B. "Working with Families of Hospitalized Older Adults with Dementia: Caregivers Are Useful Resources and Should Be Part of the Care Team," *AJN* 108(10):52–60, October 2008.

Brener, T., ed. *End of Life: A Nurse's Guide to Compassionate Care*. Philadelphia: Lippincott Williams & Wilkins, 2007.

Cheng, J.W., and Nayar, M. "A Review of Heart Failure Management in the Elderly Population," *American Journal of Geriatric Pharmacotherapy* 7(5):233–49, October 2009.

Dowling-Castronovo, A., and Specht, J.K. "HOW TO TRY THIS: Assessment of Transient Urinary Incontinence in Older Adults," *AJN* 109(2):62–71, February 2009.

Earl, S., et al. "Prevalence of the Metabolic Syndrome among U.S. Adults: Findings from the Third National Health and Nutrition Examination Survey," *JAMA* 287(3): 356–59, January 2002.

Eliopoulos, C. *Gerontological Nursing*, 7th ed. Philadelphia: Lippincott Williams & Wilkins, 2009.

Flory, J., et al. "Place of Death: U.S. Trends since 1980," *Health Affairs*, 23(3):194–200, 2004.

Fulmer, T. "Try This: Elder Mistreatment Assessment," *The Hartford Institute for Geriatric Nursing* 15, 2008.

Fulmer, T., et al. "Elder Neglect Assessment in the Emergency Department," *Journal of Emergency Nursing* 26 (5):436–43, October 2000.

Fulmer, T., et al., eds. *Evidence-Based Geriatric Nursing Protocols For Best Practice*, 3rd ed. New York: Springer Publishing Co., 2008.

Glauser, J. "Up to Two Million U.S. Elders May Be Abused," *Emergency Medicine News* 27(11):34–38, November 2005.

Halter, J.B., et al. *Hazzard's Geriatric Medicine & Gerontology*, 6th ed. New York: McGraw-Hill, 2009.

Kane, R.L., et al. *Essentials of Clinical Geriatrics*, 6th ed. New York: McGraw-Hill, 2008.

Katz, A. "Sexuality and Hysterectomy: Finding the Right Words: Responding to Patients' Concerns about the Potential Effects of Surgery," *AJN* 105(12):65–68, December 2005.

Killick, C., and Taylor, B.J. "Professional Decision Making on Elder Abuse: Systematic Narrative Review," *Journal of Elder Abuse & Neglect* 21(3):211–38, July 2009.

(continued)

Laumann, E., et al. "Elder Mistreatment in the United States: Prevalence Estimates from a National Representative Study," *Journals of Gerontology Series B: Psychological Sciences and Social Sciences* 63(4):S248–254, 2008.

Lewis, L. "Long-Distance Caregiving," *AJN* 108(9):49, September 2008.

Lindau, S., et al. "A Study of Sexuality and Health among Older Adults in the United States," *New England Journal of Medicine* 357(8):762–74, August 2007.

Miller, C. *Nursing for Wellness in Older Adults*, 5th ed. Philadelphia: Lippincott Williams & Wilkins, 2009.

Missotten, P., et al. "Impact of Place of Residence on Relationship Between Quality of Life and Cognitive Decline in Dementia," *Alzheimer Disease & Associated Disorders* 23(4):395–400, October/December 2009.

Morita, A. et al. "The Relationship between Slowing EEGs and the Progression of Parkinson's Disease," *Journal of Clinical Neurophysiology* 26(6):426–29, December 2009.

Murphy, E., and Williams, G.R. "The Thyroid and the Skeleton," *Clinical Endocrinology* 61:285–98, 2004.

Page, C., et al. "The Effect of Care Setting on Elder Abuse: Results from a Michigan Survey," *Journal of Elder Abuse & Neglect* 21(3):239–52, July 2009.

Reyna, C., et al. "Older Adult Stereotypes among Care Providers in Residential Care Facilities: Examining the Relationship between Contact, Education, and Agesim," *Journal of Gerontological Nursing*, 33(2):50–55, February 2007.

Rowe, M. "Wandering in Hospitalized Older Adults: Identifying Risk Is the First Step in this Approach to Preventing Wandering in Patients with Dementia," *AJN* 108(10): 62–70, October 2008.

Sawin, C.T., et al. "Low Serum Thyrotropin Concentrations as a Risk Factor for Atrial Fibrillation in Older Persons," *New England Journal of Medicine* 331:1249–52, November 1994.

Sharts-Hopko, N. and Glynn-Milley, C. "Primary Open-Angle Glaucoma," *AJN* 109(2):40–47, February 2009.

Stein, P.S., and Henry, R.G. "Poor Oral Hygiene in Long-Term Care," *AJN* 109(6):44–50, June 2009.

Teaster, P., et al. "The 2004 Survey of State Adult Protective Services: Abuse of Adults 60 Years of Age and Older," *National Center on Elder Abuse*, 2006.

Vlassara, H, et al. "Role of Oxidants/Inflammation in Declining Renal Function in Chronic Kidney Disease and Normal Aging," *Kidney International* 76(S114):S3–11, December 2009.

Wallace, M.A. "Assessment of Sexual Health in Older Adults," *AJN* 108(7):52–60, July 2008.

Yaffe, M.J. et al. "Professions Show different Enquiry Strategies for Elder Abuse Detection: Implications for Training and Interprofessional Care," *Journal of Interprofessional Care* 23(6):646–54, November 2009.

Index

---

i refers to an illustration; t refers to a table.

i refers to an illustration; t refers to a table.

i refers to an illustration; t refers to a table.

i refers to an illustration; t refers to a table.

i refers to an illustration; t refers to a table.

i refers to an illustration; t refers to a table.

---

i refers to an illustration; t refers to a table.

i refers to an illustration; t refers to a table.

i refers to an illustration; t refers to a table.